Nutrition and Central Nervous System

Nutrition and Central Nervous System

Editor

M. Hasan Mohajeri

MDPI • Basel • Beijing • Wuhan • Barcelona • Belgrade • Manchester • Tokyo • Cluj • Tianjin

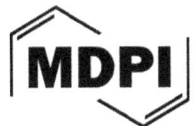

Editor
M. Hasan Mohajeri
University of Zurich
Switzerland

Editorial Office
MDPI
St. Alban-Anlage 66
4052 Basel, Switzerland

This is a reprint of articles from the Special Issue published online in the open access journal *Nutrients* (ISSN 2072-6643) (available at: https://www.mdpi.com/journal/nutrients/special_issues/Nutrition_Central_Nervous_System).

For citation purposes, cite each article independently as indicated on the article page online and as indicated below:

LastName, A.A.; LastName, B.B.; LastName, C.C. Article Title. *Journal Name* **Year**, *Article Number*, Page Range.

ISBN 978-3-03943-230-1 (Hbk)
ISBN 978-3-03943-231-8 (PDF)

© 2020 by the authors. Articles in this book are Open Access and distributed under the Creative Commons Attribution (CC BY) license, which allows users to download, copy and build upon published articles, as long as the author and publisher are properly credited, which ensures maximum dissemination and a wider impact of our publications.

The book as a whole is distributed by MDPI under the terms and conditions of the Creative Commons license CC BY-NC-ND.

Contents

About the Editor vii

Preface to "Nutrition and Central Nervous System" ix

Kristi A. Clark, Jasmin M. Alves, Sabrina Jones, Alexandra G. Yunker, Shan Luo,
Ryan P. Cabeen, Brendan Angelo, Anny H. Xiang and Kathleen A. Page
Dietary Fructose Intake and Hippocampal Structure and Connectivity during Childhood
Reprinted from: *Nutrients* **2020**, *12*, 909, doi:10.3390/nu12040909 1

Minsang Kim, Minah Song, Hee-Jin Oh, Jin Hui, Woori Bae, Jihwan Shin, Sang-Dock Ji,
Young Ho Koh, Joo Won Suh, Hyunwoo Park and Sungho Maeng
Evaluating the Memory Enhancing Effects of *Angelica gigas* in Mouse Models of Mild
Cognitive Impairments
Reprinted from: *Nutrients* **2020**, *12*, 97, doi:10.3390/nu12010097 17

Meng-Chao Tsai, Shyh-Hsiang Lin, Kiswatul Hidayah and Ching-I Lin
Equol Pretreatment Protection of SH-SY5Y Cells against Aβ (25–35)-Induced Cytotoxicity and
Cell-Cycle Reentry via Sustaining Estrogen Receptor Alpha Expression
Reprinted from: *Nutrients* **2019**, *11*, 2356, doi:10.3390/nu11102356 29

Wei Wang, Daisuke Tanokashira, Yusuke Fukui, Megumi Maruyama, Chiemi Kuroiwa,
Takashi Saito, Takaomi C. Saido and Akiko Taguchi
Serine Phosphorylation of IRS1 Correlates with Aβ-Unrelated Memory Deficits and Elevation
in Aβ Level Prior to the Onset of Memory Decline in AD
Reprinted from: *Nutrients* **2019**, *11*, 1942, doi:10.3390/nu11081942 41

Muhammad Ikram, Kamran Saeed, Amjad Khan, Tahir Muhammad,
Muhammad Sohail Khan, Min Gi Jo, Shafiq Ur Rehman and Myeong Ok Kim
Natural Dietary Supplementation of Curcumin Protects Mice Brains against
Ethanol-Induced Oxidative Stress-Mediated Neurodegeneration and Memory Impairment
via Nrf2/TLR4/RAGE Signaling
Reprinted from: *Nutrients* **2019**, *11*, 1082, doi:10.3390/nu11051082 59

Huiling Chen, Qing Huang, Shunjia Zhang, Kaiqiang Hu, Wenxiang Xiong, Lingyun Xiao,
Renhuai Cong, Qingfei Liu and Zhao Wang
The Chinese Herbal Formula PAPZ Ameliorates Behavioral Abnormalities in Depressive Mice
Reprinted from: *Nutrients* **2019**, *11*, 859, doi:10.3390/nu11040859 77

Anica Klockars, Erin L. Wood, Sarah N. Gartner, Laura K. McColl, Allen S. Levine,
Elizabeth A. Carpenter, Colin G. Prosser and Pawel K. Olszewski
Palatability of Goat's versus Cow's Milk: Insights from the Analysis of Eating Behavior and
Gene Expression in the Appetite-Relevant Brain Circuit in Laboratory Animal Models
Reprinted from: *Nutrients* **2019**, *11*, 720, doi:10.3390/nu11040720 91

Yasuhisa Ano, Tatsuhiro Ayabe, Rena Ohya, Keiji Kondo, Shiho Kitaoka
and Tomoyuki Furuyashiki
Tryptophan-Tyrosine Dipeptide, the Core Sequence of β-Lactolin, Improves Memory by
Modulating the Dopamine System
Reprinted from: *Nutrients* **2019**, *11*, 348, doi:10.3390/nu11020348 111

Stephanie Bull-Larsen and M. Hasan Mohajeri
The Potential Influence of the Bacterial Microbiome on the Development and Progression of ADHD
Reprinted from: *Nutrients* **2019**, *11*, 2805, doi:10.3390/nu11112805 . . . . **123**

Luis G. Bermúdez-Humarán, Eva Salinas, Genaro G. Ortiz, Luis J. Ramirez-Jirano, J. Alejandro Morales and Oscar K. Bitzer-Quintero
From Probiotics to Psychobiotics: Live Beneficial Bacteria Which Act on the Brain-Gut Axis
Reprinted from: *Nutrients* **2019**, *11*, 890, doi:10.3390/nu11040890 . . . . **149**

About the Editor

M. Hasan Mohajeri (Professor) is a Lecturer at the Medical Faculty of the University of Zurich, Switzerland. He has a solid publication record with more than 110 contributions in topics related to brain development and aging as well as the interaction between the nervous system and the gut microbiota (scholar_search: https://scholar.google.co.uk/citations?hl=de&user=OWHRJzEAAAAJ). He is also the co-inventor of numerous patents. He is a member of the editorial board of several journals. Dr. Mohajeri studied Biochemistry at the University of Zurich, Switzerland, and obtained his Ph.D. in Neurosciences from the Swiss Federal Institute of Technology (ETH) in Zurich, Switzerland in 1994. He has more than 20 years of scientific and managerial working experience in large international life science enterprises as well as start-up companies in Europe and the USA.

Preface to "Nutrition and Central Nervous System"

The focus of this Special Issue is "Nutrition and the Central Nervous System". The brain is, as a very specialized and one of the most metabolically active organs of the body, dependent on a steady and sufficient supply of dietary ingredients. The critical role of the diet for brain development as well as for proper CNS functioning and the possible preventative roles against neurodegenerative and neurological conditions is commonly accepted. The overarching aim of this Special Issue is pinpointing the mechanisms of action and publishing state-of-the-art contributions discussing the roles that nutritional compounds play in the development, maintenance, and aging of the CNS.

M. Hasan Mohajeri
Editor

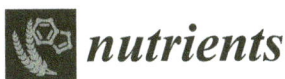

Article

Dietary Fructose Intake and Hippocampal Structure and Connectivity during Childhood

Kristi A. Clark [1], Jasmin M. Alves [2,3], Sabrina Jones [2,3], Alexandra G. Yunker [2,3], Shan Luo [2,3,4], Ryan P. Cabeen [5], Brendan Angelo [2,3], Anny H. Xiang [6] and Kathleen A. Page [2,3,*]

1. Department of Neurology, Keck School of Medicine of the University of Southern California, Los Angeles, CA 90033, USA; kristi.clark.999@gmail.com
2. Department of Internal Medicine; Division of Endocrinology, Keck School of Medicine of the University of Southern California, Los Angeles, CA 90033, USA; jalves@usc.edu (J.M.A.); sljones@usc.edu (S.J.); ayunker@usc.edu (A.G.Y.); shanluo@usc.edu (S.L.); angelob@usc.edu (B.A.)
3. Diabetes and Obesity Research Institute of the University of Southern California, Los Angeles, CA 90033, USA
4. Department of Psychology, University of Southern California, Los Angeles, CA 90089, USA
5. Laboratory of Neuro Imaging (LONI), USC Stevens Neuroimaging and Informatics Institute, Keck School of Medicine of USC, Los Angeles, CA 90033, USA; Ryan.Cabeen@loni.usc.edu
6. Department of Research and Evaluation, Kaiser Permanente Southern California, Pasadena, CA 91101, USA; Anny.H.Xiang@kp.org
* Correspondence: kpage@usc.edu

Received: 13 February 2020; Accepted: 24 March 2020; Published: 26 March 2020

Abstract: In rodent literature, there is evidence that excessive fructose consumption during development has a detrimental impact on hippocampal structure and function. In this study of 103 children ages 7–11 years old, we investigated whether dietary fructose intake was related to alterations in hippocampal volume and connectivity in humans. To examine if these associations were specific to fructose or were related to dietary sugars intake in general, we explored relationships between dietary intake of added sugars and the monosaccharide, glucose, on the same brain measures. We found that increased dietary intake of fructose, measured as a percentage of total calories, was associated with both an increase in the volume of the CA2/3 subfield of the right hippocampus and increased axial, radial, and mean diffusivity in the prefrontal connections of the right cingulum. These findings are consistent with the idea that increased fructose consumption during childhood may be associated with an inflammatory process, and/or decreases or delays in myelination and/or pruning. Increased habitual consumption of glucose or added sugar in general were associated with an increased volume of right CA2/3, but not with any changes in the connectivity of the hippocampus. These findings support animal data suggesting that higher dietary intake of added sugars, particularly fructose, are associated with alterations in hippocampal structure and connectivity during childhood.

Keywords: children; cingulum; development; dietary sugar; fructose; hippocampus

1. Introduction

Diets high in added sugars, particularly fructose, have adverse metabolic consequences and are associated with oxidative stress, insulin resistance, and cardiometabolic disorders [1–4]. Beyond its known metabolic health risks, high fructose consumption has been linked to impairments in peripheral and central appetite signaling and may promote feeding behavior [5–10]. Emerging data also indicates that high fructose diets have a profound impact on brain function [11,12], particularly within the hippocampus, a brain region involved in memory, learning, and food intake regulation that is particularly vulnerable to dietary and metabolic insults [13–15]. Experimental studies in animal models have shown that high fructose consumption leads to hippocampal insulin resistance [16,17], neuroinflammation [18,19], and reduced hippocampal neurogenesis [20], and suggests a potential mechanistic basis for fructose induced cognitive deficits [17,18,21].

The findings that hippocampal function is highly sensitive to excess fructose consumption are particularly relevant to the study of obesity and excess weight gain considering the role the hippocampus plays in energy regulation. In rodents, hippocampal lesions [14] or inactivation [15] increase food consumption and body weight. The translation of these findings to humans has been supported by experiments in patients with brain lesions. Patients with lesions to the temporal lobe have been shown to overeat in response to food presentation relative to healthy controls and patients with lesions in other brain regions, even after consuming an energy dense meal [22,23]. Considering these findings together, the hippocampus appears to be highly important in the inhibition of food consumption; therefore, in the case of hippocampal impairment by external insults, such as excessive consumption of fructose, humans and animals may overeat and consequently gain additional weight.

Human hippocampal connectivity has been found to be quite extensive [24], and evidence from animal models suggests that the ability of the hippocampus to inhibit appetitive behaviors may rely on its connections to other brain areas. Prior findings have demonstrated that disconnection lesions (the elimination of all direct and indirect connections) between the ventral hippocampus and the contralateral prefrontal cortex in rodents impairs general behavioral inhibition in a 5-choice reaction time task [25]. More specifically related to obesity, a monosynaptic glutamatergic pathway between the ventral hippocampus and the medial prefrontal cortex has been identified as important in the control of energy regulation. Chemogenic inactivation of this pathway has been shown to increase food consumption, indicating the activation of this pathway may be important in the ability to suppress overeating [26]. The hippocampus is also connected to the lateral septum, and activation of this excitatory pathway inhibits food intake [27]. Other hippocampal-dependent feeding pathways include connections with the amygdala and hypothalamus [18,28]. While diets high in fructose or other added sugars have been found to alter hippocampal physiology [18,20], and metabolic insults, such as obesity, have been shown to decrease hippocampal global brain connectivity [29], the impact of dietary fructose or added sugar intake on the microstructure of pathways that connect the hippocampus to other brain regions has not yet been studied.

Recent studies in rodents have shown that the effects of high fructose diets on hippocampal function are particularly damaging during sensitive periods of neurocognitive development, such as childhood and adolescence [18], but few studies have attempted to translate these findings to humans. To address this gap in knowledge, we used in vivo magnetic resonance imaging (MRI) methods, which provide a non-invasive way to examine the neurodevelopment of the human brain. T1-weighted acquisitions allow quantification of grey matter volume in specific regions of the brain, and diffusion tensor imaging (DTI) is a sensitive imaging method that can characterize the microstructural architecture of white matter tracts that connect distinct brain regions [30]. We used both structural MRI and diffusion MRI to examine the associations between dietary fructose and added sugar intake and hippocampal development in healthy children aged 7 to 11 years. Based on studies in animal models, we hypothesized that higher dietary intake of added sugars, particularly fructose, would be associated with alterations in hippocampal volume and in the microstructure of white matter tracts that connect the hippocampus to other brain regions.

2. Materials and Methods

2.1. Participants

Healthy, typically developing children between the ages of 7–11 years old participated in the BrainChild Study of the impact of intrauterine exposure to metabolic disorders on brain pathways during childhood. Children were born at Kaiser Permanente Southern California (KPSC), a large health care organization that uses an integrated electronic medical record (EMR) system. KPSC member demographics are broadly representative of Southern California residents [31]. Each participating Institutional Review Board approved this study (University of Southern California (USC) #HS-14-00034, KPSC #10282). Participants' parents gave written informed consent. Children provided written informed assent.

The study included two in-person visits. Visit one occurred at the Clinical Research Unit of the USC Diabetes and Obesity Research Institute. Visit two occurred at USC Dana and David Dornsife Neuroimaging Center and included a MRI scan of the brain.

2.2. Clinical Characteristics and Demographics

Child's height was measured to the nearest 0.1 cm using a stadiometer and weight to the nearest 0.1 kg using a calibrated digital scale. BMI was calculated using the standard formula, weight (kg) divided by height (m^2). BMI z-scores and BMI percentiles (age and sex-specific standard deviation scores) were determined based on Center for Disease Control (CDC) standards [32]. Participants were given the option of having Tanner stage assessed by physical exam [33,34] and/or by a validated sex-specific assessment questionnaire for children and parents, containing both illustrations and explanatory text [35]. Forty-eight participants opted for both physical exam and questionnaire, and 55 participants opted for self-reported puberty status only. The correlation between Tanner Staging assessed by physical exam and by questionnaire was 0.91.

Socioeconomic status (SES) was assessed using household income at birth, estimated based on census tract of residence and expressed as a continuous variable, and maternal education at birth, which was extracted from birth certificates in the EMR as a categorical variable with the following categories: "high-school or some high-school", "some college", and "college and post-education". Prenatal exposures to maternal gestational diabetes mellitus (GDM) and maternal pre-pregnancy BMI were assessed using the EMR.

2.3. Dietary Measures

Diet was assessed using repeated 24-h dietary recalls on non-consecutive days during two in-person visits as part of the BrainChild Study. In a subset of 35 participants, we also obtained 3-day dietary records on one of the two in-person visits, and dietary intake was estimated using a total of four days of dietary assessments for these participants. The mean interval between the two in-person visits was 34 ± 57 days. We used the multi-pass method for dietary recall, in which a trained staff member asked the participant to recall what food and beverages they had consumed over a 24-h time period with the input of both the child and the child's parent. The trained staff member then went through three other "passes" to complete quantity of food/beverages consumed as well as to include missing or forgotten food/beverages. Use of the multi-pass 24-h dietary recall method is a valid method to assess energy intake in children [36]. Once the dietary recalls were collected, the recalls were analyzed using the Nutritional Data System for Research software v.2018 developed by the Nutrition Coordinating Center (NCC), University of Minnesota, Minneapolis, MS [37]. The variables used were percent calories from fructose, percent calories from glucose, and percent calories from added sugar by available carbohydrate. Data from dietary recalls were manually checked for quality. To determine outliers, we performed linear regression analysis, using body weight to predict total energy intake. Residuals were standardized and examined for any values that were >3 or <−3 standard deviations from the mean. Records containing data that exceeded these values were not included in the analysis. Using this method, 267 dietary recalls were included in the analysis, and one dietary recall was excluded.

2.4. Magnetic Resonance Imaging (MRI) Acquisition

After a mock scanner training session, magnetic resonance imaging (MRI) was performed using a Siemens MAGNETOM Prisma^{fit} 3 Tesla MRI scanner (Siemens Medical Systems) with a 20-channel phased array coil. A high-resolution magnetic resonance imaging scan was acquired using a T1-weighted three-dimensional magnetization prepared rapid gradient echo (MP-RAGE) sequence with the parameters: 256 × 256 × 176-matrix size with 1 × 1 × 1-mm^3 resolution; inversion time = 900 ms; repetition time (TR) = 1950 ms; echo time (TE) = 2.26 ms; flip angle = 90°; Total scan duration was 4 min and 14 s. A diffusion weighted image was acquired using a dual spin echo, single shot, pulsed gradient, echo planar imaging sequence in 64 diffusion sensitized gradient directions with the following parameters: TR = 8100 ms; TE = 69 ms; flip angle = 90°; 70 axial slices; 2 mm × 2 mm × 2 mm voxel size; FOV = 256 mm; *b* value = 1000 s/mm^2; Total scan duration was 9 min and 29 s.

2.5. MRI Data Processing

The T1 MP-RAGE structural image was put into the automated segmentation software, FreeSurfer version 6.0 hippocampal module (http://surfer.nmr.mgh.harvard.edu/, RRID:SCR_001847) to examine total hippocampal grey matter volume and grey matter volume in the hippocampal subfields. The procedure uses Bayesian inference and a probabilistic atlas of the hippocampal formation based on manual delineations of subfields in ultra-high-resolution MRI scans [38]. Manual quality check of automated hippocampal segmentation was performed for each participant following an existing protocol [39]. The segmentation of the hippocampus was visually assessed by an individual trained in hippocampal neuroanatomy and then given a rating of "pass", "pass on condition", and "fail". Images that failed to have defined landmarks due to motion artifacts or segmentation error were excluded. Although twelve subfield volumes are generated by FreeSurfer 6.0, we only included subfields that have been shown to be preferentially affected by high sugar diets, including the CA1, CA2/3, CA4, DG (granule cell layer) and subiculum [40,41]. Previous studies in children have used FreeSurfer to segment the hippocampus and hippocampal subfields [42,43]. The raw volume data were included in the supplemental materials (Table S1).

Tractography models were created from the diffusion-weighted MRI (dMRI) data using FSL [44] and the Quantitative Imaging Toolkit (QIT) [45]. The dMRIs were first skull stripped using FSL BET and then corrected for motion and eddy current artifact using FSL FLIRT. For this, each diffusion scan was affinely registered to the baseline scan using the mutual information metric, and the associated gradient orientations were rotated to account for the registration. Diffusion tensor models were then estimated from the dMRI using QIT, and the following tensor parameters were extracted: fractional anisotropy (FA), mean diffusivity (MD), axial diffusivity (AD), and radial diffusivity (RD). Tensor images were upsampled to 1 mm^3 using model-based interpolation in QIT [46], and a deformation field was computed using DTI-TK [47] to register the data to the IIT brain template [48]. Tractography models of the bundles-of-interest were created using a framework for deterministic streamline integration [49]. For each bundle, seed, inclusion and exclusion masks were manually drawn in the IIT template [50] in reference to a white matter atlas [51]. The template masks were then resampled in each subject's native space image to constrain tractography. Other tractography parameters included a step size of 1.0 mm, a maximum angle of 45 degrees, a minimum FA of 0.15, and 25000 seeds per bundle. Bundle-specific metrics of fractional anisotropy (FA), mean diffusivity (MD), axial diffusivity (AD), and radial diffusivity (RD) were then computed. FA and MD were used as primary metrics of microstructure, with many studies showing that FA increases with age while MD decreases with age [52–55]. AD and RD were used as post-hoc measures in regions that showed a significant effect on MD. The MD measure is a weighted average of AD and RD, which themselves are more biologically specific than MD alone. The bundles of interest included major connections between the hippocampus and the rest of the brain, specifically: the uncinate fasciculus, fornix, and cingulum bundle (separated into prefrontal and temporal lobe sections) (See Figure 1A).

2.6. Statistical Analysis

Hierarchical regression models were implemented in R to estimate the effects of dietary consumption of fructose on the volume of the hippocampus and its connectivity with the rest of the brain. The dependent variables for the volume of the hippocampus included the following regions of interest (ROIs): (i) Whole hippocampus, (ii) CA1, (iii) CA2/3, (iv) CA4, (v) DG/GC/ML, (vi) subiculum. Left and right values were tested separately for a total of 12 tests, which led to a per-test p-value of 0.004 to reach an overall alpha of $p < 0.05$ using Bonferroni correction. The dependent variables for the connectivity between the hippocampus and the rest of the brain included the following tracts: (i) uncinate, (ii) fornix, (iii) cingulum–prefrontal section, and (iv) cingulum–temporal section. Left and right values were tested separately and MD and FA were tested separately for a total of 16 tests, which led to a per-test p-value of 0.003 to reach an overall alpha of $p < 0.05$ using Bonferroni correction. Planned post-hocs included: testing the associations of dietary added sugar and glucose intake on brain metrics that showed evidence of being affected by fructose, and testing the effects of axial and radial diffusivity for any tests that showed significant effects in FA or MD. Associations of sugar consumption with total intracranial volume were also computed as a negative control.

Model 1 was the unadjusted model for percent calories from fructose. Model 2 included age and sex (and intracranial volume for analyses of the volume of the hippocampus). Model 3 included the child's BMI z-score. Model 4 included two categorical variables aimed at measuring socioeconomic status: the highest education level attained by the mother and the family income level. Model 5 included maternal measures that impact prenatal environment, i.e., gestational diabetes (binary) and pre-pregnancy BMI. As variables were added, an F-test was used to determine whether the newly added variables showed a significant improvement in R^2. Semi-partial r values were calculated as an indication of effect size, where $r < 0.1$ is a small effect size, $0.1 < r < 0.3$ is a medium effect size, and $r > 0.3$ is a large effect size.

Effects of Tanner stage and potential interactions with sex were tested as Models 2A and 2B respectively. If either or both were found to explain significantly more variance than Model 2, then models 3–5 included a covariate for Tanner stage and/or an interaction between the dietary measure and sex.

3. Results

3.1. Participant Characteristics

A total of 103 children participated in this study. Child demographic and clinical characteristics are reported in Table 1. The mean ± SD age of the children was 8.55 ± 1.03 years old, 91% of the children were pre-pubertal (Tanner Stage <2), and 62% were girls. Children's BMI ranged from 13.62 to 34.01 kg/m^2; BMI percentiles ranged from 5.28 to 99.58; BMI z-scores ranged from −1.78 to 2.64. According to CDC standards, 61 (59%) children were healthy-weight, 16 (15%) children were overweight, and 26 (25%) children were obese. Overall, the participants consumed an average (±SD) of 1763 ± 359 kcal per day; 4.57 ± 2.19% of their total calories came from fructose, 4.32 ± 1.81% of their total calories came from glucose, and 13.91 ± 6.89% of total calories from added sugar. Total energy and added sugar intake in our cohort are in line with the general population of the children in the United States [56]. Familial demographics, including maternal education, family income, and mother's self-reported race/ethnicity, are shown in Table 2. Maternal pre-pregnancy BMI ranged from 18.97 to 50.38 kg/m^2, and 58% of mothers had GDM during pregnancy.

Table 1. Child demographic and clinical characteristics

	Mean (SD) or N (%) [1]	Range
Age, years	8.55 (1.03)	7.33–11.34
BMI, kg/m^2	19.00 (4.12)	13.62–34.01
BMI percentile	69.96 (27.33)	5.28–99.58
BMI z-score	0.77 (1.08)	−1.78–2.64
BMI category	Healthy-weight: 61 (59%) Overweight: 16 (16%) Obese: 26 (25%)	
Sex	Boys: 41 (40%) Girls: 62 (60%)	
Tanner Stage of Pubertal Development	Tanner stage 1: 94 (91%) Tanner stage 2: 5 (5%) Tanner stage 3: 3 (3%) Tanner stage 4: 1 (1%)	
Energy Intake (kcal)	1763 (359)	825–2708
Percent Calories from Added Sugar (%)	13.91 (6.89)	2.65–39.90
Percent Calories from Glucose (%)	4.32 (1.81)	1.21–8.40
Percent Calories from Fructose (%)	4.57 (2.19)	0.93–11.44

[1] Percentages were rounded to the nearest percent, therefore sum of variables do not equal 100%; BMI: body mass index.

Table 2. Familial demographics.

	Mean (SD) or N (%) [1]
Maternal education [2]	LN: 21 (20%) SC: 29 (28%) CN: 51 (50%)
Mother's race/ethnicity	Hispanic: 59 (57%) Black: 11 (11%) Non-Hispanic White: 20 (19%) Other: 13 (13%)
Family income [2]	0–$30 K: 10 (10%) $30 K–50 K: 29 (29%) $50 K–70 K: 33 (33%) $70 K–90 K: 14 (14%) ≥$90 K: 15 (15%)

[1] Percentages were rounded to the nearest percent, therefore sum of variables do not equal 100%; [2] Missing maternal education and family income data from 2 participants.

3.2. Influence of Diet on Hippocampal Volumes

A total of 101 participants were included in the hippocampal volume analyses, after excluding the two participants who were missing data for the mother's education level. The amount of fructose children consumed as a percentage of calories in their diet was significantly associated with an increase in the volume of the right CA2/3 hippocampal subfield (ß = 3.34, sr = 0.25, $p < 0.01$; Model 1)) (Table 3; Figure 1B). Results remained significant after adjusting for ICV, age, and sex (ß = 2.56, sr = 0.19, $p < 0.02$; Model 2), further adjusting for child BMI z-score (ß = 2.80, sr = 0.21, $p < 0.01$; Model 3), and additionally adjusting for SES (ß = 2.70, sr = 0.19, $p < 0.02$; Model 4), as well as in fully adjusted models (ß = 3.33, sr = 0.24, $p < 0.003$; Model 5). These findings suggest that dietary fructose has an effect on hippocampal CA 2/3 volume that is independent of child's age, sex, BMI Z-score, SES, or prenatal exposures. Of note, Model 2, which included covariates for intracranial volume, age, and sex, explained significantly more variance than the unadjusted Model 1, which only contained a covariate for percentage of calories from fructose ($F(3,96) = 16.78$, $p < 0.001$). This result is unsurprising because the volume of the hippocampus and its subfields are highly dependent upon total brain volume. Model 5, which included all covariates, explained significantly more variance than Model 4, which included all covariates except maternal GDM status and maternal pre-pregnancy BMI (F(2,90) = 6.56, $p < 0.002$). All other hippocampal subfield volumes were non-significant. None of the models tested showed significant interactions of sex with dietary intake, nor did they show significant effects of Tanner stage. Additionally, neither fructose (ß = 6893, $p < 0.30$, $R^2 = 0.0008$), glucose (ß = 7583, $p < 0.30$, $R^2 = 0.0008$), nor added sugar consumption (ß = −277, $p < 0.89$, $R^2 = -0.0097$) were significantly associated with intracranial volume.

Table 3. Associations between dietary fructose intake and the volume of right CA2/3.

Predictor Variables	Model 1 ß (sr)	Model 2 ß (sr)	Model 3 ß (sr)	Model 4 ß (sr)	Model 5 ß (sr)
Percent Calories from Fructose	3.34 (0.25) **	2.56 (0.19) *	2.80 (0.21) *	2.70 (0.19) *	3.33 (0.24) **
Age, years		−1.06 (−0.04)	−1.14 (−0.04)	−1.27 (−0.04)	−1.71 (−0.06)
Sex (1, male; 0, female)		5.17 (0.07)	5.44 (0.08)	6.18 (0.08)	2.52 (0.03)
Intracranial Volume (mm^3)		1.31 × 10^{-4} (0.49) ***	1.30 × 10^{-4} (0.48) ***	1.34 × 10^{-4} (0.47) ***	1.24 × 10^{-4} (0.43) ***
BMI z-score			3.13 (0.11)	3.05 (0.11)	5.80 (0.20) *
Family income (1: <$30 K; 5: >$90 K)				−1.67 (−0.01)	−1.90 (−0.07)
Mom's education (CN)					
LN				3.24 (0.04)	2.56 (0.03)
SC				2.01 (0.03)	1.81 (0.03)
Maternal GDM (1, yes; 0, no)					4.29 (0.07)
Maternal pre-pregnancy BMI, kg/m^2					−1.31 (−0.28) ***
R^2	0.064	0.365	0.378	0.380	0.459
ΔR^2		0.301	0.013	0.002	0.079
ΔF		16.78 ***	2.13	0.11	6.56 **

Model 1 is percent calories from fructose only; Model 2 includes age, sex and intracranial volume; Model 3 includes BMI z-score; Model 4 includes family income and mom's education; Model 5 includes prenatal exposures to maternal GDM and maternal pre-pregnancy BMI. Successive models include all covariates from earlier models. BMI: body mass index; LN: <high school; SC: some college; CN: college and post-graduate; GDM: gestational diabetes mellitus; sr = semi-partial r; * $p < 0.05$; ** $p < 0.01$; *** $p < 0.001$.

In planned post-hoc analyses, we explored whether the associations between dietary fructose intake and hippocampal CA 2/3 volume were specific to fructose, or if alternatively the associations were also observed between dietary added sugar and/or glucose intake and CA 2/3 volume. We found that associations between percent of calories from added sugar and volume of the right CA2/3 were also significant ($R^2 = 0.448$, F(10,90) = 7.29, $p < 0.001$). Likewise, planned post-hoc analyses on the effects of percent of calories from glucose on the volume of the right CA2/3 were also significant ($R^2 = 0.471$, F(10,90) = 8.00, $p < 0.001$). These findings indicated that effects of dietary fructose, added sugar, and glucose intake on right CA2/3 volume were all similar suggesting that increases in the volume of right CA2/3 were non-specific with regards to whether the increased sugar intake was from glucose, fructose, or added sugars. In fact, the effect sizes for glucose intake (sr = 0.27), fructose intake (sr = 0.25), and added sugar intake (sr = 0.23) were nearly identical, indicating each of these types of sugar explained a similar amount of variance. The percent calories from fructose and percent calories from glucose were highly correlated (r = 0.87, $p < 0.001$), and there were moderate correlations between percent calories from fructose and percent calories from added sugar (r = 0.31, $p < 0.001$) and between percent calories from glucose and percent calories from added sugar (r = 0.48, $p < 0.001$). Given that dietary intake of fructose, glucose, and added sugar were correlated, we did not include them in the same model to test independent effects. It is important to note that added sugars are classified as sugars that are added to foods or beverages when they are processed or prepared, whereas naturally occurring sugars, such as those in fruit or milk, are not classified as added sugars [57].

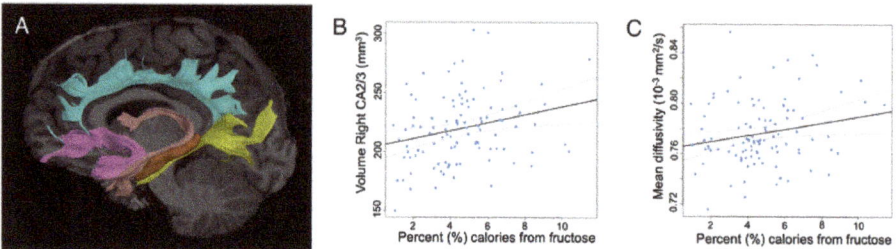

Figure 1. Associations with fructose consumption. (**A**) Using regions of interest for the hippocampus (orange) and its major connections (fornix: pink, uncinate: purple, and the cingulum, which was segmented into the temporal part: yellow and the prefrontal part: turquoise), we identified associations between fructose consumption and the volume of the right CA2/3 subfield of the hippocampus (**B**) and the mean diffusivity of the right cingulum, prefrontal connections (**C**). (**B,C**) Graphs show the unadjusted model with no covariates. Solid line indicates the best fit linear trend, with dotted lines showing the confidence interval. Notably, these graphs show the results from Model 1 (Tables 1 and 2, respectively).

3.3. Influence of Diet on Hippocampal Connectivity

A total of 98 participants were included in the diffusion imaging analyses, after excluding the 6 participants who were missing data for either the mother's education level ($n = 2$) or who failed quality control for the diffusion imaging data ($n = 4$). The amount of fructose children consumed as a percentage of calories was significantly associated with an increase in the mean diffusivity (MD) of the right cingulum, prefrontal connections ($\beta = 2.51 \times 10^{-6}$, sr = 0.21, $p < 0.04$; Model 1) (Table 4; Figure 1C). Results remained significant after adjusting for age and sex ($\beta = 2.66 \times 10^{-6}$, sr = 0.22, $p < 0.02$; Model 2), further adjusting for child BMI z-score ($\beta = 2.79 \times 10^{-6}$, sr = 0.23, $p < 0.02$; Model 3), and additionally adjusting for SES ($\beta = 3.51 \times 10^{-6}$, sr = 0.28, $p < 0.003$; Model 4), as well as in fully adjusted models ($\beta = 3.64 \times 10^{-6}$, sr = 0.29, $p < 0.002$; Model 5). The outcome of the hierarchical modeling indicated that Model 4 explained significantly more variance than Models 1–3, but Model 5 did not explain more variance than Model 4. Therefore, Model 4 was used for the planned post-hoc analyses. The MD for all other tracts and the FA for all the tracts were non-significant. None of the models tested showed significant interactions of sex with dietary intake, nor did they show significant effects of Tanner stage.

Planned post-hoc analyses on the effects of percent of calories from added sugar on the MD of the right cingulum, prefrontal connections resulted in a significant model overall ($R^2 = 0.167$, $F(7,90) = 2.58$, $p < 0.02$). Although the overall model was significant, the covariate of interest (i.e., percent calories from added sugar) was not significantly associated with MD of the right cingulum, prefrontal connections ($\beta = -2.56 \times 10^{-7}$, sr = −0.07, $p < 0.50$), indicating that the overall model for added sugar associations with MD of the right cingulum, prefrontal connections was driven by significant associations with decreased age and increased family income. Planned post-hoc analyses on the effects of percent of calories from glucose on the MD of the right cingulum, prefrontal connections also resulted in a significant model overall ($R^2 = 0.184$, $F(7,90) = 2.89$, $p < 0.009$). However, similar to findings with added sugar, there was not a significant association of percent calories from glucose on the MD of the right cingulum, prefrontal connections ($\beta = 2.25 \times 10^{-6}$, sr = 0.15, $p < 0.13$). Likewise, similar to added sugar, the overall model for glucose associations with MD of the right cingulum, prefrontal connections was driven by significant associations with decreased age and increased family income. These result are different from the effects we observed in the volume of the right CA2/3 because MD was only associated with fructose intake and not added sugar or glucose intake.

Table 4. Effects of fructose consumption on the mean diffusivity (MD) of right cingulum, prefrontal connections.

Predictor Variables	Model 1 ß (sr)	Model 2 ß (sr)	Model 3 ß (sr)	Model 4 ß (sr)	Model 5 ß (sr)
Percent Calories from Fructose	2.51×10^{-6} (0.21) *	2.66×10^{-6} (0.22) *	2.79×10^{-6} (0.23) *	3.51×10^{-6} (0.28) **	3.64×10^{-6} (0.29) **
Age, years		-7.52×10^{-6} (−0.28) **	-7.50×10^{-6} (−0.28) **	-6.78×10^{-6} (−0.25) **	-6.95×10^{-6} (−0.26) **
Sex (1, male; 0, female)		-9.79×10^{-6} (−0.19)	-9.82×10^{-6} (−0.19)	-8.65×10^{-6} (−0.17)	-8.37×10^{-6} (−0.16)
BMI z-score			1.67×10^{-6} (0.07)	1.68×10^{-6} (0.07)	2.40×10^{-6} (0.10)
Family income (1: <$30 K; 5: >$90 K)				6.71×10^{-6} (0.29) **	6.56×10^{-6} (0.28) **
Mom's education (CN)					
LN				3.64×10^{-6} (0.05)	5.09×10^{-6} (0.07)
SC				4.69×10^{-6} (0.08)	5.67×10^{-6} (0.09)
Maternal GDM (1, yes; 0, no)					-3.99×10^{-6} (−0.08)
Maternal pre-pregnancy BMI, kg/m²					-3.51×10^{-7} (−0.09)
R²	0.044	0.152	0.157	0.243	0.257
ΔR²		0.108	0.005	0.086	0.014
ΔF		6.87 **	0.57	3.42 *	0.83

Model 1 includes percent calories from fructose only; Model 2 includes age and sex; Model 3 includes BMI z-score; Model 4 includes family income and mom's education; Model 5 includes maternal GDM and maternal pre-pregnancy BMI. Successive models include all covariates from earlier models. BMI: body mass index; LN: <high school; SC: some college; CN: college and post-graduate; GDM: gestational diabetes mellitus; sr = semi-partial r; * $p < 0.05$; ** $p < 0.01$.

3.4. Post-hocs for Diffusion Imaging Measures

Because MD is defined as the average diffusivity, it is not as biologically specific as axial diffusivity (AD) or radial diffusivity (RD). Therefore, we ran post-hoc analyses using Model 4 only to determine whether the observed association of increased fructose intake on MD of the right cingulum, prefrontal connections, was driven by axial diffusivity (AD), radial diffusivity (RD), or both. The AD for the right cingulum, prefrontal connections was significantly associated with increased percentage of calories from fructose (ß = 4.62×10^{-6}, sr = 0.27, $p < 0.005$; Model 4). The RD for the right cingulum, prefrontal connections was significantly associated with increased percentage of calories from fructose (ß = 2.89×10^{-6}, sr = 0.23, $p < 0.01$; Model 4). This pattern was quite similar to the pattern observed with MD. Comparing the effect sizes of sr = 0.27 for AD and sr = 0.23 for RD, we conclude that the effects were similar, but slightly larger for AD.

4. Discussion

In this study, we examined the influence of dietary sugar intake on hippocampal neuroanatomy, both gray matter and white matter, in children. We found that increased volume in the right hippocampal CA2/3 subfield was associated with increased consumption of the monosaccharides, fructose or glucose, and/or added sugars in general, while increased MD in the right cingulate-prefrontal cortex connections were only associated with increased dietary intake of fructose. We found associations on the right but not the left hemisphere, which is broadly consistent with prior work showing lateralities on the impact of environmental insults in the hippocampus [58,59]. These associations between dietary sugar intake and hippocampal volume and fructose intake and cingulate-prefrontal cortex connections remained significant after adjusting for child's intracranial volume, age, sex, BMI, SES, and prenatal exposures suggesting an effect of dietary fructose, added sugar, and glucose intake on hippocampal volume and an effect of dietary fructose on cingulate-prefrontal cortex white matter connectivity that is independent of a number of potential confounding factors.

The observed association between dietary sugar intake and increased hippocampal volume during childhood may be driven by a few factors. A larger hippocampal CA2/3 volume during childhood could be due to a delay in synaptic pruning, a process that typically occurs during early adolescence. During adolescence, the hippocampus reaches peak volume, and begins to undergo synaptic pruning, eliminating unused connections [60,61], and prior studies have shown that the CA3 hippocampal subfield gradually begins to decrease in volume during mid childhood [61,62]. Work by Vuong et al. found that synaptic pruning is delayed in juvenile rats exposed in utero to obese mothers with GDM [63]. In their findings, inflammation and recruitment of microglial cells occurred during post-natal development in the hippocampus, along with a reduction in synaptic pruning, and the animals presented with altered hippocampal morphology. These findings suggest that prenatal environmental insults can result in hippocampal inflammation, reductions in synaptic pruning and altered hippocampal development [63]. Interestingly, Hershey et al., found that children with Type 1 diabetes had increased hippocampal volume, despite the commonly reported decreased volume in adults with Type 1 and Type 2 diabetes [64]. There is substantial research that a diet high in added sugar contributes to a pro-inflammatory environment [13,19,65]. Therefore, increased volume in the CA2/3 hippocampal subfield may be due to inflammation and/or a delay in synaptic pruning. Future studies that examine inflammation specifically, such as T2 scans for gliosis, could potentially address this possibility [66].

Notably, we found that the CA2/3 hippocampal subfield was preferentially impacted by dietary sugar intake. Coincidentally, the CA3 subfield is among the last subfields to undergo postnatal maturation, paralleling DG development [67,68]. Additionally, substantial work in animals has shown that the CA3 subfield is altered by a host of prenatal and early life environmental insults, such as prenatal exposure to GDM [69,70] or postnatal exposure to chronic stress [71–73]. Therefore, our findings are in line with prior research in animals indicating a preferential sensitivity of the CA3 subfield. It is worth noting, due to the predetermined boundaries delineated by FreeSurfer, we were unable to decipher the boundary between the CA2 and CA3 subfield. Future studies that incorporate manual tracing should be considered to confirm if excessive added sugar intake preferentially impacts the CA3 subfield of the hippocampus.

Many studies have observed that MD decreases while FA increases over the course of development [52–55]. We found that increased dietary fructose intake was associated with increased mean diffusivity (MD) in the white matter cingulum tract that connects the right hippocampus and the right prefrontal cortex. MD has been shown to increase in many different white matter diseases that lead to demyelination, dysmyelination, and/or wallerian degeneration [74–76]. For example, increases in MD have been observed prior to the appearance of lesions on a gadolinium-enhanced scan in multiple sclerosis, which is a complex disease that involves not only demyelination and wallerian degeneration, but also edema and inflammation, indicating that changes in the MD may be sensitive to pre-lesion changes in the blood brain barrier [77]. Patients with chronic epilepsy and hippocampal sclerosis show increased MD values in the hippocampus [78,79]. Together, these results are consistent with the idea that the increased MD values associated with fructose could reflect an inflammatory process, possibly associated with a loss of myelin, or delayed axonal pruning.

Because mean diffusivity is a weighted average of axial (AD) and radial diffusivity (RD), we conducted post-hoc analyses on these measures to obtain more biological specificity about what might be underlying the observed associations with MD. In general, AD is thought to reflect intracellular water mobility and is influenced by the integrity and arrangement of axonal membranes and cytoskeletal proteins, while RD is thought to reflect more of the extracellular water mobility and is primarily influenced by myelin [80]. Previous studies have shown that over the course of normal neurodevelopment, both RD and AD decrease with age [81–85]. Decreases in RD are typically attributed to myelination, while the decreases in AD are thought to correspond more to axonal pruning [86]. In our study, we found that both AD and RD were increased in the cingulum tract in children with increased dietary fructose intake, consistent with the idea that increases in fructose intake could be associated with a decrease or delay in the myelination process and the normal pruning process. Future studies could use multi-compartment diffusion imaging models, such as Neurite Orientation Dispersion and Density Imaging (NODDI), to further investigate this tract to determine whether these changes in diffusivity are more related to cellular density and/or orientation dispersion, thus adding more biological specificity [87].

Self-reported dietary assessments have known limitations, including under-reporting of dietary intake. Given that eating behavior can vary from day to day, the collection of multiple 24-hr recalls on non-consecutive days is recommended to improve the accuracy of habitual dietary intake estimates [88]. Some studies have recommended obtaining at least three 24-hr dietary recalls on non-consecutive days to provide better accuracy of energy intake [36]. Dietary assessments in our study were obtained from repeated 24-hr recalls obtained during in-person visits on non-consecutive days. We obtained two days of dietary assessments on the majority of participants, and four days of dietary assessments on a subset of 35 participants. We implemented techniques to improve the accuracy of our dietary data collection method, including the Multiple Pass 24-h recall method, which was previously shown to significantly reduce levels of under-reporting [89]. We also used a consensus recall method, in which the child and parent were interviewed together, which has been suggested to improve the accuracy of dietary assessments compared to interviews with the child or parent alone [90]. Estimates of total energy intake in our cohort are similar to national averages for children in this age range [91], while the average percent calories from added sugar in our cohort was 2.5% lower than the average of 16.4% reported in the 2009 to 2012 National Health and Nutrition Examination Survey for children age 6–11 [92]. Thus, while total energy intake estimates in our cohort are in line with those of national averages of children in the U.S., it is possible that our cohort under-reported intake of foods and beverages that contain added sugars. It is also possible that the children in our cohort consumed, on average, slightly lower amounts of added sugars than average children in the U.S. population.

In summary, our findings suggest that increases in dietary fructose are associated with alterations in hippocampal structure and connectivity in children. These findings should be interpreted cautiously given the limitations of self-reported dietary intake assessments, and it is important to note that our observations are correlational and do not confer causality. Future studies that include experimental designs that manipulate dietary intake of fructose and/or added sugars are necessary to determine the effects of fructose and added sugar on hippocampal structure and connectivity during childhood. Moreover, the potential cognitive consequences of the observed associations between dietary fructose and alterations in hippocampal structure and connectivity remains an important consideration. Our findings support the need for future studies that include cognitive testing in addition to neuroimaging to examine whether increased dietary fructose intake in childhood is associated with altered hippocampal structure and hippocampal function in childhood.

Supplementary Materials: The following are available online at http://www.mdpi.com/2072-6643/12/4/909/s1, Figure S1: Raw data plots of added sugar consumption and the mean diffusivity of the right cingulum, prefrontal connections, Figure S2: Raw data plots of added sugar consumption and the volume of the right CA2/3 subfield of the hippocampus, Figure S3: Raw data plots of glucose consumption and the mean diffusivity of the right cingulum, prefrontal connections, Figure S4: Raw data plots of glucose consumption and the volume of the right CA2/3 subfield of the hippocampus, Table S1: Table of hippocampal and total brain volumes.

Author Contributions: K.A.C., K.A.P., J.M.A., S.J. were responsible for conceptualization of the study; K.A.C., J.M.A., R.P.C., B.A. contributed to methodology and formal analysis; J.M.A., A.G.Y., B.A., S.L. were responsible for management and coordination of the study execution; K.A.P. and A.H.X. were responsible for supervision of the research activities; K.A.C., K.A.P., S.J., J.M.A. wrote the original draft; K.A.C., K.A.P., S.J., J.M.A., S.L., A.G.Y., R.C., A.H.X. provided critical review, commentary and revisions to the manuscript; K.A.P., A.H.X., S.L., J.M.A. provided funding for this study. Prior Presentation. Some of the data from the BrainChild Cohort were used to address a separate research question related to prenatal exposure to maternal obesity and hippocampal volume in children, which was accepted for publication in *Brain and Behavior* on December 8, 2019. All authors have read and agreed to the published version of the manuscript.

Funding: This work was supported by an American Diabetes Association Pathway Accelerator Award (#1-14-ACE-36; principal investigator K.A.P.) and in part by National Institute of Diabetes and Digestive and Kidney Diseases, National Institutes of Health (NIH), R01-DK-116858 (principal investigators K.A.P. and A.H.X.), K01-DK-115638 (principal investigator S.L.), and the National Institute of Mental Health, F31MH115640 (PI: J.M.A.). A Research Electronic Data Capture (REDCap) database was used for this study, which is supported by the Southern California Clinical and Translational Science Institute through NIH grant UL1-TR-001855.

Acknowledgments: The authors would like to thank the families who participate in the BrainChild Study. The authors would also like to thank Ana Romero for managing the BrainChild study, Mayra Martinez and Janet Mora-Marquez for recruiting volunteers, Alexis Defendis for helping with study execution, and the staff at Dana and David Dornsife Cognitive Neuroimaging Center at USC and at the USC Diabetes and Obesity Research Institute for their assistance with these studies.

Conflicts of Interest: The authors declare no conflict of interest.

References

1. Bray, G.A.; Nielsen, S.J.; Popkin, B.M. Consumption of high-fructose corn syrup in beverages may play a role in the epidemic of obesity. *Am. J. Clin. Nutr.* **2004**, *79*, 537–543. [CrossRef]
2. Basciano, H.; Federico, L.; Adeli, K. Fructose, insulin resistance, and metabolic dyslipidemia. *Nutr. Metab.* **2005**, *2*, 5. [CrossRef]
3. Tappy, L.; Le, K.A. Metabolic Effects of Fructose and the Worldwide Increase in Obesity. *Physiol. Rev.* **2010**, *90*, 23–46. [CrossRef]
4. Johnson, R.J.; Segal, M.S.; Sautin, Y.; Nakagawa, T.; Feig, D.I.; Kang, D.-H.; Gersch, M.S.; Benner, S.; Sánchez-Lozada, L.G. Potential role of sugar (fructose) in the epidemic of hypertension, obesity and the metabolic syndrome, diabetes, kidney disease, and cardiovascular disease. *Am. J. Clin. Nutr.* **2007**, *86*, 899–906.
5. Lindqvist, A.; Baelemans, A.; Erlanson-Albertsson, C. Effects of sucrose, glucose and fructose on peripheral and central appetite signals. *Regul. Pept.* **2008**, *150*, 26–32. [CrossRef]
6. Page, K.A.; Chan, O.; Arora, J.; Belfort-DeAguiar, R.; Dzuira, J.; Roehmholdt, B.; Cline, G.W.; Naik, S.; Sinha, R.; Constable, R.T.; et al. Effects of Fructose vs Glucose on Regional Cerebral Blood Flow in Brain Regions Involved with Appetite and Reward Pathways. *JAMA* **2013**, *309*, 63. [CrossRef]
7. Luo, S.; Monterosso, J.R.; Sarpelleh, K.; Page, K.A. Differential effects of fructose versus glucose on brain and appetitive responses to food cues and decisions for food rewards. *Proc. Natl. Acad. Sci. USA* **2015**, *112*, 6509–6514. [CrossRef]
8. Teff, K.L.; Elliott, S.S.; Tschöp, M.; Kieffer, T.J.; Rader, D.; Heiman, M.; Townsend, R.R.; Keim, N.L.; D'Alessio, D.; Havel, P.J. Dietary Fructose Reduces Circulating Insulin and Leptin, Attenuates Postprandial Suppression of Ghrelin, and Increases Triglycerides in Women. *J. Clin. Endocrinol. Metab.* **2004**, *89*, 2963–2972. [CrossRef]
9. Cha, S.H.; Wolfgang, M.; Tokutake, Y.; Chohnan, S.; Lane, M.D. Differential effects of central fructose and glucose on hypothalamic malonyl—CoA and food intake. *Proc. Natl. Acad. Sci. USA* **2008**, *105*, 16871–16875. [CrossRef]
10. Erlanson-Albertsson, C.; Lindqvist, A. Fructose affects enzymes involved in the synthesis and degradation of hypothalamic endocannabinoids. *Regul. Pept.* **2010**, *161*, 87–91. [CrossRef]

11. Lowette, K.; Roosen, L.; Tack, J.; Vanden Berghe, P. Effects of high-fructose diets on central appetite signaling and cognitive function. *Front. Nutr.* **2015**, *2*, 5. [CrossRef]
12. Lakhan, S.E.; Kirchgessner, A. The emerging role of dietary fructose in obesity and cognitive decline. *Nutr. J.* **2013**, *12*, 114. [CrossRef]
13. Hsu, T.M.; Kanoski, S.E. Blood-brain barrier disruption: Mechanistic links between Western diet consumption and dementia. *Front. Aging Neurosci.* **2014**, *6*, 88. [CrossRef]
14. Davidson, T.L.; Chan, K.; Jarrard, L.E.; Kanoski, S.E.; Clegg, D.J.; Benoit, S.C. Contributions of the Hippocampus and Medial Prefrontal Cortex to Energy and Body Weight Regulation. *Hippocampus* **2009**, *19*, 235–252. [CrossRef]
15. Hannapel, R.C.; Henderson, Y.H.; Nalloor, R.; Vazdarjanova, A.; Parent, M.B. Ventral hippocampal neurons inhibit postprandial energy intake. *Hippocampus* **2017**, *27*, 274–284. [CrossRef]
16. Agrawal, R.; Gomez-Pinilla, F. "Metabolic syndrome" in the brain: Deficiency in omega-3 fatty acid exacerbates dysfunctions in insulin receptor signalling and cognition. *J. Physiol.* **2012**, *590*, 2485–2499. [CrossRef]
17. Wu, H.-W.; Ren, L.-F.; Zhou, X.; Han, D.-W. A high-fructose diet induces hippocampal insulin resistance and exacerbates memory deficits in male Sprague-Dawley rats. *Nutr. Neurosci.* **2015**, *18*, 323–328. [CrossRef]
18. Hsu, T.M.; Konanur, V.R.; Taing, L.; Usui, R.; Kayser, B.D.; Goran, M.I.; Kanoski, S.E. Effects of sucrose and high fructose corn syrup consumption on spatial memory function and hippocampal neuroinflammation in adolescent rats. *Hippocampus* **2015**, *25*, 227–239. [CrossRef]
19. Djordjevic, A.; Bursać, B.; Veličković, N.; Vasiljević, A.; Matić, G. The impact of different fructose loads on insulin sensitivity, inflammation, and PSA-NCAM-mediated plasticity in the hippocampus of fructose-fed male rats. *Nutr. Neurosci.* **2015**, *18*, 66–75. [CrossRef]
20. Van der Borght, K.; Köhnke, R.; Göransson, N.; Deierborg, T.; Brundin, P.; Erlanson-Albertsson, C.; Lindqvist, A. Reduced neurogenesis in the rat hippocampus following high fructose consumption. *Regul. Pept.* **2011**, *167*, 26–30. [CrossRef]
21. Ross, A.P.; Bartness, T.J.; Mielke, J.G.; Parent, M.B. A high fructose diet impairs spatial memory in male rats. *Neurobiol. Learn. Mem.* **2009**, *92*, 410–416. [CrossRef]
22. Hebben, N.; Corkin, S.; Eichenbaum, H.; Shedlack, K. Diminished ability to interpret and report internal states after bilateral medial temporal resection: Case, H.M. *Behav. Neurosci.* **1985**, *99*, 1031–1039. [CrossRef]
23. Rozin, P.; Dow, S.; Moscovitch, M.; Rajaram, S. What Causes Humans to Begin and End a Meal? A Role for Memory for What Has Been Eaten, as Evidenced by a Study of Multiple Meal Eating in Amnesic Patients. *Psychol. Sci.* **1998**, *9*, 392–396. [CrossRef]
24. Maller, J.J.; Welton, T.; Middione, M.; Callaghan, F.M.; Rosenfeld, J.V.; Grieve, S.M. Revealing the Hippocampal Connectome through Super-Resolution 1150-Direction Diffusion MRI. *Sci. Rep.* **2019**, *9*, 2418. [CrossRef] [PubMed]
25. Chudasama, Y.; Doobay, V.M.; Liu, Y. Hippocampal-Prefrontal Cortical Circuit Mediates Inhibitory Response Control in the Rat. *J. Neurosci.* **2012**, *32*, 10915–10924. [CrossRef] [PubMed]
26. Hsu, T.M.; Noble, E.E.; Liu, C.M.; Cortella, A.M.; Konanur, V.R.; Suarez, A.N.; Reiner, D.J.; Hahn, J.D.; Hayes, M.R.; Kanoski, S.E. A hippocampus to prefrontal cortex neural pathway inhibits food motivation through glucagon-like peptide-1 signaling. *Mol. Psychiatry* **2018**, *23*, 1555–1565. [CrossRef] [PubMed]
27. Sweeney, P.; Yang, Y. An excitatory ventral hippocampus to lateral septum circuit that suppresses feeding. *Nat. Commun.* **2015**, *6*, 10188. [CrossRef] [PubMed]
28. Russo, C.; Russo, A.; Pellitteri, R.; Stanzani, S. Hippocampal Ghrelin-positive neurons directly project to arcuate hypothalamic and medial amygdaloid nuclei. Could they modulate food-intake? *Neurosci. Lett.* **2017**, *653*, 126–131. [CrossRef] [PubMed]
29. Geha, P.; Cecchi, G.; Constable, R.T.; Abdallah, C.; Small, D.M. Reorganization of brain connectivity in obesity. *Hum. Brain Mapp.* **2017**, *38*, 1403–1420. [CrossRef]
30. Alexander, A.L.; Lee, J.E.; Lazar, M.; Field, A.S. Diffusion Tensor Imaging of the Brain. *Neurotherapeutics* **2007**, *4*, 316–329. [CrossRef]
31. Koebnick, C.; Langer-Gould, A.M.; Gould, M.K.; Chao, C.R.; Iyer, R.L.; Smith, N.; Chen, W.; Jacobsen, S.J. Sociodemographic Characteristics of Members of a Large, Integrated Health Care System: Comparison with US Census Bureau Data. *Perm. J.* **2012**, *16*, 37–41. [CrossRef] [PubMed]

32. Defining Childhood Obesity|Overweight & Obesity|CDC. Available online: https://www.cdc.gov/obesity/childhood/defining.html (accessed on 1 November 2019).
33. Marshall, W.A.; Tanner, J.M. Variations in pattern of pubertal changes in girls. *Arch. Dis. Child.* **1969**, *44*, 291–303. [CrossRef] [PubMed]
34. Marshall, W.A.; Tanner, J.M. Variations in the pattern of pubertal changes in boys. *Arch. Dis. Child.* **1970**, *45*, 13–23. [CrossRef] [PubMed]
35. Rasmussen, A.R.; Wohlfahrt-Veje, C.; Tefre de Renzy-Martin, K.; Hagen, C.P.; Tinggaard, J.; Mouritsen, A.; Mieritz, M.G.; Main, K.M. Validity of self-assessment of pubertal maturation. *Pediatrics* **2015**, *135*, 86–93. [CrossRef]
36. Johnson, R.K.; Driscoll, P.; Goran, M.I. Comparison of Multiple-Pass 24-Hour Recall Estimates of Energy Intake with Total Energy Expenditure Determined by the Doubly Labeled Water Method in Young Children. *J. Am. Diet. Assoc.* **1996**, *96*, 1140–1144. [CrossRef]
37. Schakel, S.F.; Buzzard, I.M.; Gebhardt, S.E. Procedures for Estimating Nutrient Values for Food Composition Databases. *J. Food Compos. Anal.* **1997**, *10*, 102–114. [CrossRef]
38. Iglesias, J.E.; Augustinack, J.C.; Nguyen, K.; Player, C.M.; Player, A.; Wright, M.; Roy, N.; Frosch, M.P.; McKee, A.C.; Wald, L.L.; et al. A computational atlas of the hippocampal formation using ex vivo, ultra-high resolution MRI: Application to adaptive segmentation of in vivo MRI. *NeuroImage* **2015**, *115*, 117–137. [CrossRef]
39. Backhausen, L.L.; Herting, M.M.; Buse, J.; Roessner, V.; Smolka, M.N.; Vetter, N.C. Quality Control of Structural MRI Images Applied Using FreeSurfer—A Hands-On Workflow to Rate Motion Artifacts. *Front. Neurosci.* **2016**, *10*, 558. [CrossRef]
40. Calvo-Ochoa, E.; Hernández-Ortega, K.; Ferrera, P.; Morimoto, S.; Arias, C. Short-term high-fat-and-fructose feeding produces insulin signaling alterations accompanied by neurite and synaptic reduction and astroglial activation in the rat hippocampus. *J. Cereb. Blood Flow Metab.* **2014**, *34*, 1001–1008. [CrossRef]
41. Molteni, R.; Barnard, R.J.; Ying, Z.; Roberts, C.K.; Gómez-Pinilla, F. A high-fat, refined sugar diet reduces hippocampal brain-derived neurotrophic factor, neuronal plasticity, and learning. *Neuroscience* **2002**, *112*, 803–814. [CrossRef]
42. Al-Amin, M.; Zinchenko, A.; Geyer, T. Hippocampal subfield volume changes in subtypes of attention deficit hyperactivity disorder. *Brain Res.* **2018**, *1685*, 1–8. [CrossRef] [PubMed]
43. Tamnes, C.K.; Walhovd, K.B.; Engvig, A.; Grydeland, H.; Krogsrud, S.K.; Østby, Y.; Holland, D.; Dale, A.M.; Fjell, A.M. Regional Hippocampal Volumes and Development Predict Learning and Memory. *Dev. Neurosci.* **2014**, *36*, 161–174. [CrossRef] [PubMed]
44. Jenkinson, M.; Beckmann, C.F.; Behrens, T.E.J.; Woolrich, M.W.; Smith, S.M. FSL. *Neuroimage* **2012**, *62*, 782–790. [CrossRef] [PubMed]
45. Cabeen, R.P.; Laidlaw, D.H.; Toga, A.W. Quantitative Imaging Toolkit: Software for Interactive 3D Visualization, Processing, and Analysis of Neuroimaging Datasets. In Proceedings of the Annual Meeting of the International Society for Magnetic Resonance in Medicine (ISMRM), Paris, France, 2018.
46. Arsigny, V.; Fillard, P.; Pennec, X.; Ayache, N. Log-Euclidean metrics for fast and simple calculus on diffusion tensors. *Magn. Reson. Med.* **2006**, *56*, 411–421. [CrossRef] [PubMed]
47. Zhang, H.; Yushkevich, P.A.; Alexander, D.C.; Gee, J.C. Deformable registration of diffusion tensor MR images with explicit orientation optimization. *Med. Image Anal.* **2006**, *10*, 764–785. [CrossRef] [PubMed]
48. Zhang, S.; Peng, H.; Dawe, R.J.; Arfanakis, K. Enhanced ICBM Diffusion Tensor Template of the Human Brain. *Neuroimage* **2011**, *54*, 974–984. [CrossRef]
49. Cabeen, R.P.; Bastin, M.E.; Laidlaw, D.H. Kernel Regression Estimation of Fiber Orientation Mixtures in Diffusion MRI. *Neuroimage* **2016**, *127*, 158–172. [CrossRef]
50. Wakana, S.; Caprihan, A.; Panzenboeck, M.M.; Fallon, J.H.; Perry, M.; Gollub, R.L.; Hua, K.; Zhang, J.; Jiang, H.; Dubey, P.; et al. Reproducibility of quantitative tractography methods applied to cerebral white matter. *Neuroimage* **2007**, *36*, 630–644. [CrossRef]
51. Catani, M.; Thiebaut de Schotten, M. A diffusion tensor imaging tractography atlas for virtual in vivo dissections. *Cortex* **2008**, *44*, 1105–1132. [CrossRef]
52. Neil, J.; Miller, J.; Mukherjee, P.; Hüppi, P.S. Diffusion tensor imaging of normal and injured developing human brain—A technical review. *NMR Biomed.* **2002**, *15*, 543–552. [CrossRef]

53. Snook, L.; Paulson, L.-A.; Roy, D.; Phillips, L.; Beaulieu, C. Diffusion tensor imaging of neurodevelopment in children and young adults. *NeuroImage* **2005**, *26*, 1164–1173. [CrossRef] [PubMed]
54. Mukherjee, P.; McKinstry, R.C. Diffusion tensor imaging and tractography of human brain development. *Neuroimaging Clin. N. Am.* **2006**, *16*, 19–43. [CrossRef] [PubMed]
55. Bonekamp, D.; Nagae, L.M.; Degaonkar, M.; Matson, M.; Abdalla, W.M.; Barker, P.B.; Mori, S.; Horská, A. Diffusion tensor imaging in children and adolescents: Reproducibility, hemispheric, and age-related differences. *Neuroimage* **2007**, *34*, 733–742. [CrossRef] [PubMed]
56. Drewnowski, A.; Rehm, C.D. Energy intakes of US children and adults by food purchase location and by specific food source. *Nutr. J.* **2013**, *12*, 59. [CrossRef] [PubMed]
57. CDC Know Your Limit for Added Sugars. Available online: https://www.cdc.gov/nutrition/data-statistics/know-your-limit-for-added-sugars.html (accessed on 19 December 2019).
58. Zach, P.; Mrzílková, J.; Stuchlík, A.; Valeš, K. Delayed Effects of Elevated Corticosterone Level on Volume of Hippocampal Formation in Laboratory Rat. *Physiol. Res.* **2010**, *59*, 12.
59. Teicher, M.H.; Anderson, C.M.; Polcari, A. Childhood maltreatment is associated with reduced volume in the hippocampal subfields CA3, dentate gyrus, and subiculum. *Proc. Natl. Acad. Sci. USA* **2012**, *109*, E563–E572. [CrossRef]
60. Andersson, J.L.; Skare, S.; Ashburner, J. How to correct susceptibility distortions in spin-echo echo-planar images: Application to diffusion tensor imaging. *Neuroimage* **2003**, *20*, 870–888. [CrossRef]
61. Tamnes, C.K.; Bos, M.G.N.; van de Kamp, F.C.; Peters, S.; Crone, E.A. Longitudinal development of hippocampal subregions from childhood to adulthood. *Dev. Cogn. Neurosci.* **2018**, *30*, 212–222. [CrossRef]
62. Canada, K.L.; Ngo, C.T.; Newcombe, N.S.; Geng, F.; Riggins, T. It's All in the Details: Relations Between Young Children's Developing Pattern Separation Abilities and Hippocampal Subfield Volumes. *Cereb. Cortex* **2019**, *29*, 3427–3433. [CrossRef]
63. Vuong, B.; Odero, G.; Rozbacher, S.; Stevenson, M.; Kereliuk, S.M.; Pereira, T.J.; Dolinsky, V.W.; Kauppinen, T.M. Exposure to gestational diabetes mellitus induces neuroinflammation, derangement of hippocampal neurons, and cognitive changes in rat offspring. *J. Neuroinflamm.* **2017**, *14*, 80. [CrossRef]
64. Hershey, T.; Perantie, D.C.; Wu, J.; Weaver, P.M.; Black, K.J.; White, N.H. Hippocampal Volumes in Youth with Type 1 Diabetes. *Diabetes* **2010**, *59*, 236–241. [CrossRef]
65. Beilharz, J.E.; Maniam, J.; Morris, M.J. Short-term exposure to a diet high in fat and sugar, or liquid sugar, selectively impairs hippocampal-dependent memory, with differential impacts on inflammation. *Behav. Brain Res.* **2016**, *306*, 1–7. [CrossRef] [PubMed]
66. Lee, J.K.; Ekstrom, A.D.; Ghetti, S. Volume of hippocampal subfields and episodic memory in childhood and adolescence. *NeuroImage* **2014**, *94*, 162–171. [CrossRef] [PubMed]
67. Jabès, A.; Lavenex, P.B.; Amaral, D.G.; Lavenex, P. Postnatal Development of the Hippocampal Formation: A Stereological Study in Macaque Monkeys. *J. Comp. Neurol.* **2011**, *519*, 1051–1070. [CrossRef] [PubMed]
68. Lu, D.; He, L.; Xiang, W.; Ai, W.-M.; Cao, Y.; Wang, X.S.; Pan, A.; Luo, X.-G.; Li, Z.; Yan, X.-X. Somal and Dendritic Development of Human CA3 Pyramidal Neurons from Midgestation to Middle Childhood: A Quantitative Golgi Study. *Anat. Rec.* **2013**, *296 Pt 8*, 123–132. [CrossRef] [PubMed]
69. Golalipour, M.J.; Kafshgiri, S.K.; Ghafari, S. Gestational diabetes induced neuronal loss in CA1 and CA3 subfields of rat hippocampus in early postnatal life. *Folia Morphol.* **2012**, *71*, 71–77. [PubMed]
70. Lotfi, N.; Hami, J.; Hosseini, M.; Haghir, D.; Haghir, H. Diabetes during pregnancy enhanced neuronal death in the hippocampus of rat offspring. *Int. J. Dev. Neurosci.* **2016**, *51*, 28–35. [CrossRef]
71. Schoenfeld, T.J.; McCausland, H.C.; Morris, H.D.; Padmanaban, V.; Cameron, H.A. Stress and Loss of Adult Neurogenesis Differentially Reduce Hippocampal Volume. *Biol. Psychiatry* **2017**, *82*, 914–923. [CrossRef]
72. Kumar, R.S.; Narayanan, S.N.; Kumar, N.; Nayak, S. Exposure to Enriched Environment Restores Altered Passive Avoidance Learning and Ameliorates Hippocampal Injury in Male Albino Wistar Rats Subjected to Chronic Restraint Stress. *Int. J. Appl. Basic Med. Res.* **2018**, *8*, 231–236.
73. Baran, S.E.; Campbell, A.M.; Kleen, J.K.; Foltz, C.H.; Wright, R.L.; Diamond, D.M.; Conrad, C.D. Combination of high fat diet and chronic stress retracts hippocampal dendrites. *Neuroreport* **2005**, *16*, 39–43. [CrossRef]
74. Guo, A.C.; Jewells, V.L.; Provenzale, J.M. Analysis of normal-appearing white matter in multiple sclerosis: Comparison of diffusion tensor MR imaging and magnetization transfer imaging. *AJNR Am. J. Neuroradiol.* **2001**, *22*, 1893–1900. [PubMed]

75. Pierpaoli, C.; Barnett, A.; Pajevic, S.; Chen, R.; Penix, L.R.; Virta, A.; Basser, P. Water diffusion changes in Wallerian degeneration and their dependence on white matter architecture. *Neuroimage* **2001**, *13*, 1174–1185. [CrossRef] [PubMed]
76. Horsfield, M.A.; Jones, D.K. Applications of diffusion-weighted and diffusion tensor MRI to white matter diseases—A review. *NMR Biomed.* **2002**, *15*, 570–577. [CrossRef] [PubMed]
77. Werring, D.J.; Brassat, D.; Droogan, A.G.; Clark, C.A.; Symms, M.R.; Barker, G.J.; MacManus, D.G.; Thompson, A.J.; Miller, D.H. The pathogenesis of lesions and normal-appearing white matter changes in multiple sclerosis: A serial diffusion MRI study. *Brain* **2000**, *123*, 1667–1676. [CrossRef] [PubMed]
78. Wieshmann, U.C.; lark, C.A.C.; Symms, M.R.; Barker, G.J.; Birnie, K.D.; Shorvon, S.D. Water diffusion in the human hippocampus in epilepsy. *Magn. Reson. Imaging* **1999**, *17*, 29–36. [CrossRef]
79. Yoo, S.Y.; Chang, K.-H.; Song, I.C.; Han, M.H.; Kwon, B.J.; Lee, S.H.; Yu, I.K.; Chun, C.-K. Apparent diffusion coefficient value of the hippocampus in patients with hippocampal sclerosis and in healthy volunteers. *AJNR Am. J. Neuroradiol.* **2002**, *23*, 809–812.
80. Schwartz, E.D.; Cooper, E.T.; Fan, Y.; Jawad, A.F.; Chin, C.-L.; Nissanov, J.; Hackney, D.B. MRI diffusion coefficients in spinal cord correlate with axon morphometry. *Neuroreport* **2005**, *16*, 73–76. [CrossRef]
81. Zhang, Y.; Zhang, J.; Oishi, K.; Faria, A.V.; Jiang, H.; Li, X.; Akhter, K.; Rosa-Neto, P.; Pike, G.B.; Evans, A.; et al. Atlas-guided tract reconstruction for automated and comprehensive examination of the white matter anatomy. *Neuroimage* **2010**, *52*, 1289–1301. [CrossRef]
82. Lebel, C.; Walker, L.; Leemans, A.; Phillips, L.; Beaulieu, C. Microstructural maturation of the human brain from childhood to adulthood. *NeuroImage* **2008**, *40*, 1044–1055. [CrossRef]
83. Bava, S.; Thayer, R.; Jacobus, J.; Ward, M.; Jernigan, T.L.; Tapert, S.F. Longitudinal characterization of white matter maturation during adolescence. *Brain Res.* **2010**, *1327*, 38–46. [CrossRef]
84. Suzuki, Y.; Matsuzawa, H.; Kwee, I.L.; Nakada, T. Absolute eigenvalue diffusion tensor analysis for human brain maturation. *NMR Biomed.* **2003**, *16*, 257–260. [CrossRef]
85. Kumar, R.; Nguyen, H.D.; Macey, P.M.; Woo, M.A.; Harper, R.M. Regional brain axial and radial diffusivity changes during development. *J. Neurosci. Res.* **2012**, *90*, 346–355. [CrossRef]
86. Bockhorst, K.H.; Narayana, P.A.; Liu, R.; Ahobila-Vijjula, P.; Ramu, J.; Kamel, M.; Wosik, J.; Bockhorst, T.; Hahn, K.; Hasan, K.M.; et al. Early postnatal development of rat brain: In vivo diffusion tensor imaging. *J. Neurosci. Res.* **2008**, *86*, 1520–1528. [CrossRef]
87. Zhang, H.; Schneider, T.; Wheeler-Kingshott, C.A.; Alexander, D.C. NODDI: Practical in vivo neurite orientation dispersion and density imaging of the human brain. *NeuroImage* **2012**, *61*, 1000–1016. [CrossRef]
88. Tucker, K.L. Assessment of usual dietary intake in population studies of gene—Diet interaction. *Nutr. Metab. Cardiovasc. Dis.* **2007**, *17*, 74–81. [CrossRef]
89. Moshfegh, A.J.; Rhodes, D.G.; Baer, D.J.; Murayi, T.; Clemens, J.C.; Rumpler, W.V.; Paul, D.R.; Sebastian, R.S.; Kuczynski, K.J.; Ingwersen, L.A.; et al. The US Department of Agriculture Automated Multiple-Pass Method reduces bias in the collection of energy intakes. *Am. J. Clin. Nutr.* **2008**, *88*, 324–332. [CrossRef]
90. Foster, E.; Bradley, J. Methodological considerations and future insights for 24-hour dietary recall assessment in children. *Nutr. Res.* **2018**, *51*, 1–11. [CrossRef]
91. Herrick, K.A.; Rossen, L.; Parsons, R.; Dodd, K. Estimating usual dietary intake from National Health and Nutrition Examination Survey data using the National Cancer Institute method. *Natl. Cent. Health Stat.* **2018**, *178*, 1–63.
92. Vos, M.B.; Kaar, J.L.; Welsh, J.A.; Van Horn, L.V.; Feig, D.I.; Anderson, C.A.M.; Patel, M.J.; Munos, J.C.; Krebs, N.F.; Xanthakos, S.A.; et al. Added Sugars and Cardiovascular Disease Risk in Children. *Circulation* **2017**, *135*, e1017–e1034. [CrossRef]

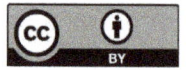

© 2020 by the authors. Licensee MDPI, Basel, Switzerland. This article is an open access article distributed under the terms and conditions of the Creative Commons Attribution (CC BY) license (http://creativecommons.org/licenses/by/4.0/).

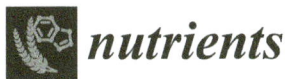

Article

Evaluating the Memory Enhancing Effects of *Angelica gigas* in Mouse Models of Mild Cognitive Impairments

Minsang Kim [1], Minah Song [2], Hee-Jin Oh [2], Jin Hui [3], Woori Bae [2], Jihwan Shin [2], Sang-Dock Ji [4], Young Ho Koh [5,6], Joo Won Suh [3], Hyunwoo Park [7,*] and Sungho Maeng [2,*]

1. Graduate School of Interdisciplinary Program of Biomodulation Collage of Natural Science, Myongji University, Yongin 17058, Korea; kms0177@naver.com
2. Graduate School of East-West Medical Science, Kyung Hee University, Yongin 17104, Korea; bungu20@naver.com (M.S.); julia110892@naver.com (H.-J.O.); wrbae0328@naver.com (W.B.); junikk0@naver.com (J.S.)
3. Center for Nutraceutical and Pharmaceutical Materials, Myongji University, Yongin 17058, Korea; kimhwi83@gmail.com (J.H.); jwsuh@mju.ac.kr (J.W.S.)
4. Department of Agricultural Biology, National Academy of Agricultural Science, Rural Development Administration, Wanju-gun, Jeollabuk-do 55365, Korea; sdji1@korea.kr
5. ILSONG Institute of Life Science, Hallym University, Anyang 14066, Korea; kohyh@hallym.ac.kr
6. Department of Bio-Medical Gerontology, Hallym University Graduate School, Chuncheon 24252, Korea
7. Health Park Co., Ltd., #2502, Gangnam-dae-Ro 305, Sucho-gu, Seoul 06628, Korea
* Correspondence: hwpark75@gmail.com (H.P.); jethrot@khu.ac.kr (S.M.); Tel.: +82-10-5440-0169 (H.P.); +82-10-5554-0155 (S.M.)

Received: 14 October 2019; Accepted: 8 November 2019; Published: 30 December 2019

Abstract: (1) Background: By 2050, it is estimated that 130 million people will be diagnosed with dementia, and currently approved medicines only slow the progression. So preventive intervention is important to treat dementia. Mild cognitive impairment is a condition characterized by some deterioration in cognitive function and increased risk of progressing to dementia. Therefore, the treatment of mild cognitive impairment (MCI) is a possible way to prevent dementia. *Angelica gigas* reduces neuroinflammation, improves circulation, and inhibits cholinesterase, which can be effective in the prevention of Alzheimer's disease and vascular dementia and the progression of mild cognitive impairment. (2) Methods: *Angelica gigas* (AG) extract 1 mg/kg was administered to mildly cognitive impaired mice, models based on mild traumatic brain injury and chronic mild stress. Then, spatial, working, and object recognition and fear memory were measured. (3) Result: *Angelica gigas* improved spatial learning, working memory, and suppressed fear memory in the mild traumatic brain injury model. It also improved spatial learning and suppressed cued fear memory in the chronic mild stress model animals. (4) Conclusions: *Angelica gigas* can improve cognitive symptoms in mild cognitive impairment model mice.

Keywords: *Angelica gigas*; mild cognitive impairment; traumatic brain injury; chronic mild stress

1. Introduction

Mild cognitive impairment (MCI) refers to a condition in which one's cognitive function is lower than that of normal peers but not considered dementia [1,2]. However, patients with MCI have an approximately 50% chance of developing Alzheimer's disease within five years [3]. Dementia is not curable. Therefore, it is important to prevent MCI from progressing into dementia. However, there is no established treatment that prevents the progression of MCI to dementia [4].

Animal models are needed to study MCI and develop therapeutics. An appropriate MCI model may have symptoms aggravating with age, but with only subtle memory impairment [5]. Animal models that meet these criteria include middle-aged rodents and transgenic mice that overexpress A β at an early stage before the dementia onset [4]. Spontaneously hypertensive rats (SHRs) appear to be appropriate as MCI models for vascular dementia, since hypertensive astrogliosis, cytoskeleton breakdown, hippocampal atrophy, and cholinergic deficit prematurely appear prematurely in this animal [6–8]. In contrast, drug-induced memory impairment models (such as those using scopolamine, NMDA blockers, and benzodiazepines) are not appropriate because they do not represent the various aspects of MCI [5].

Traumatic brain injury (TBI) is one of the most common brain injuries that causes a progressive decline of memory and cognition [9]. Unlike severe TBI, moderate to minimal TBI tends to be overlooked. However, even mild TBI can cause gradual amnesia, altered executive function, concentration disorders, depression, apathy, and anxiety [8,10,11]. In particular, repetitive head injuries, such as those caused by collision sports or motor vehicle accidents, are known to cause dementia [12]. Animal models of TBI show a decrease in cognitive function that correlates to the extent of injury, the number of impacts, and progressively worsens [13–15]. Therefore, the TBI model is a useful MCI research tool because it is simple, progressive, reproducible, and the severity of cognitive decline is relative to the number of impacts [16].

Chronic mild stress (CMS) is a behavioral model of depression that is caused by sequential exposure to variable mild stressors. CMS is characterized by anhedonia that may be reversed by chronic treatment with antidepressants [17]. However, most depression models show cognitive decline. Also, in the CMS animal model, mild cognitive deficit is accompanied, and antidepressants improve cognitive function in this model [18]. These memory deficits were related to the increased phosphorylation of Tau and APP processing, and the application of stress to wild type mice was suggested as an animal model of sporadic AD (Alzheimer's disease) [19].

Currently, there are many methods on trial to prevent the progression of MCI to dementia. In particular, nonpharmacological methods, such as cognitive leisure activities, education and exercise, and pharmacological methods, such as vitamin E, donepezil, and intranasal insulin, have been tried [20–23]. However, more research is needed to prove their efficacy.

Angelica gigas (AG) has been used in traditional medicine to improve circulation, physical weakness, headache, dizziness, joint pain, abdominal pain, constipation, irregular menstruation, and bruises, etc. [24]. Known bioactive components of AG include decursin, decursinol angelate, and nodakenin [24]. It has been shown to improve liver function in rats treated with long-term ethanol. AG also lowered LDL cholesterol and inhibited nicotine sensitization in rats [25,26]. Finally, AG attenuated acetylcholinesterase activity and was neuroprotective against beta-amyloid peptide-induced memory impairment [27]. According to these findings, the AG extract was tested in TBI and CMS models to evaluate whether it would improve memory impairment in MCI.

2. Results

2.1. AG Improved TBI- and CMS-Induced Spatial Learning Deficit

The effect of AG on spatial learning and memory was measured using the Morris water maze (Figure 1). During the five-day training, TBI impaired spatial learning. Supplementation of AG improved the TBI-induced deficit in spatial learning (Figure 1A). CMS impaired spatial learning (control vs. CMS), which improved following AG supplementation (CMS vs. CMS + AG) (Figure 1B). The sucrose preference of the CMS mice gradually decreased over six weeks. This declining preference meant that the mice developed an anhedonia-like tendency. AG did not affect this anhedonia-like behavior (Figure S1).

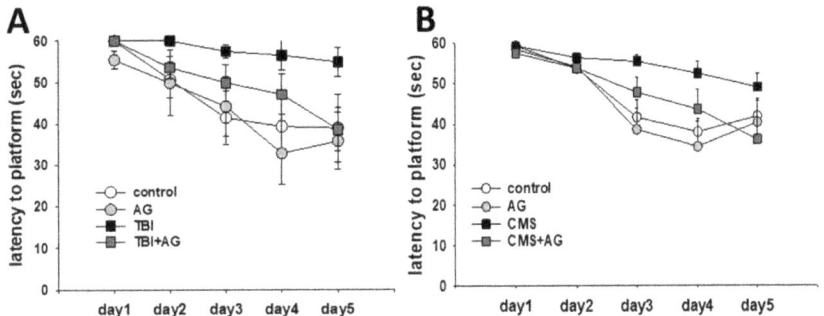

Figure 1. Spatial learning by *Angelica gigas* (AG) in traumatic brain injury (TBI) and chronic mild stress (CMS) mice as measured by the latency to the platform in the Morris water maze (MWM). (**A**) TBI model. There were repetitive training (within) effects [$F(4,104) = 13.9, p < 0.001$] and treatment group (between) effects [$F(3,26) = 2.27, p = 0.044$], but with non-significant within–between interaction differences [$F(12,104) = 1.1, p = 0.36$]. The post-hoc pairwise comparison showed a difference between control vs. TBI ($p = 0.033$), TBI vs. TBI + AG ($p = 0.041$). (**B**) CMS model. There were repetitive training effects [$F(4,196) = 31.3, p < 0.001$], treatment group effects [$F(3,49) = 3.1, p = 0.034$], and within–between interactions [$F(12,196) = 2.2, p = 0.012$]. Post-hoc pairwise comparison revealed a difference between the control and CMS groups ($p = 0.019$), AG vs. CMS ($p = 0.01$), CMS vs. CMS + AG ($p = 0.042$). All data were normally distributed and are represented as means ± S.E.M. Control: vehicle (DW) treated; AG: *Angelica gigas* 1 mg/kg; TBI: vehicle treated + traumatic brain injury; TBI + AG: *Angelica gigas* 1 mg/kg + traumatic brain injury; CMS: vehicle treated + chronic mild stress; CMS + AG: *Angelica gigas* 1 mg/kg + chronic mild stress. Repeated measure ANOVA, Tukey's HSD post-hoc test.

2.2. AG Improved Short-Term Working Memory

The effect of AG on short-term working memory was measured using the Y-maze test (Figure 2). TBI did not have a significant effect on the alternation behaviors. However, AG increased the alternation behavior in both TBI and normal mice (Figure 2A). Similarly, CMS did not affect the alternation behavior in CMS mice. In contrast, AG treatment increased the alternation behavior (Figure 2B)

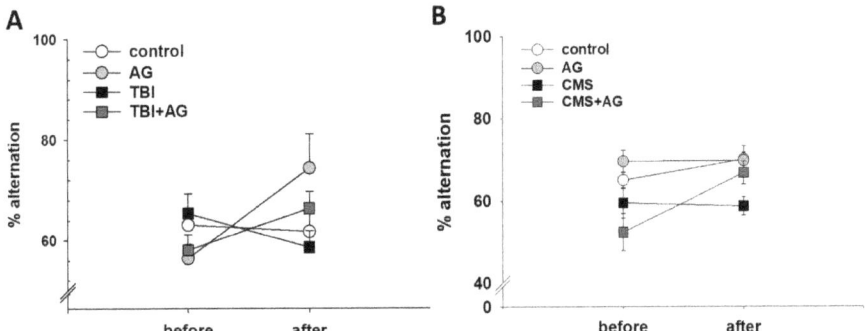

Figure 2. Short-term working memory by AG in TBI and CMS mice, measured by the percent alternation in the Y-maze. (**A**) TBI model. There were before–after (within) effects [$F(1,28) = 3.57, p = 0.012$], treatment group (between) effects [$F(3,28) = 3.23, p = 0.081$], and within–between interactions [$F(3,28) = 3.28, p = 0.036$]. There were no before–after changes in the control ($p = 0.6$) and TBI ($p = 0.38$), but improvements in the AG ($p = 0.008$) and TBI + AG ($p = 0.047$). (**B**) CMS model. There were before–after effects [$F(1,36) = 6.2, p = 0.018$] and treatment group effects [$F(3,36) = 11.8, p < 0.001$], but no significant within–between interaction differences [$F(3,36) = 1.5, p = 0.24$]. There was no before–after

change in the control group ($p = 031$), AG ($p = 0.97$) or CMS ($p = 0.33$) groups. However, there was an increase of % alternation in the CMS + AG group ($p = 0.006$). All data were normally distributed and are represented as means ± S.E.M. Control: vehicle (DW) treated; AG: *Angelica gigas* 1 mg/kg; TBI: vehicle treated + traumatic brain injury; TBI+AG: *Angelica gigas* 1 mg/kg + traumatic brain injury; CMS: vehicle treated + chronic mild stress; CMS+AG: *Angelica gigas* 1 mg/kg + chronic mild stress. Repeated measures ANOVA, Tukey's HSD post-hoc test.

2.3. AG Had No Effect on Object Recognition Memory

The effect of AG on recognition memory was measured in the novel object test (Figure 3). AG had no effect on normal mice. However, the recognition memory in TBI model mice declined with AG treatment. The absence of a before–after change in the AG treated TBI group meant that AG prevented the adverse effect of TBI (Figure 3A). There was no significant effect of CMS and AG treatment on the recognition memory (Figure 3B)

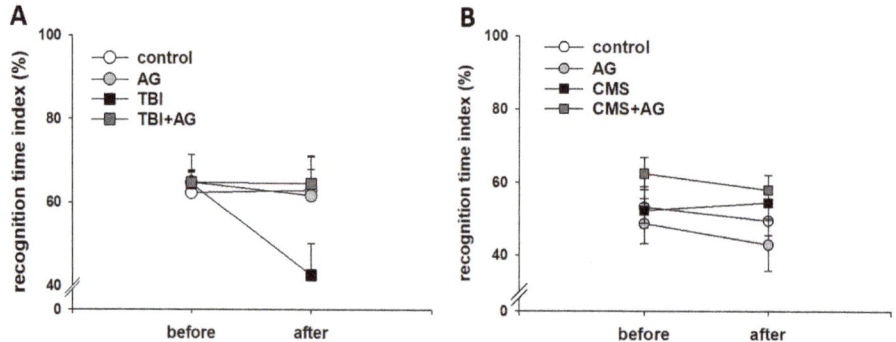

Figure 3. Object recognition memory by AG in the TBI and CMS mice as measured by the recognition time index in the novel object test. (**A**) TBI model. There were before–after (within) effects [$F(1,28) = 8.3$, $p = 0.008$], treatment group (between) effects [$F(3,28) = 0.67$, $p = 0.58$], and within–between interaction effects [$F(3,28) = 3.6$, $p = 0.026$]. There was no before–after change in the control ($p = 0.93$), AG ($p = 0.59$) and TBI + AG ($p = 0.97$) groups, but there were decreases in the TBI ($p = 0.001$) group. (**B**) CMS model. There were no before-after effects [$F(1,36) = 0.32$, $p = 0.57$], treatment group effects [$F(3,36) = 1.2$, $p = 0.31$], or within–between interactions [$F(3,36) = 0.12$, $p = 0.95$]. All data were normally distributed and are represented as means ± S.E.M. Control: vehicle (DW) treated; AG: *Angelica gigas* 1 mg/kg; TBI: vehicle treated + traumatic brain injury; TBI + AG: *Angelica gigas* 1 mg/kg + traumatic brain injury; CMS: vehicle treated + chronic mild stress; CMS+AG: *Angelica gigas* 1 mg/kg + chronic mild stress. Repeated measures ANOVA, Tukey's HSD post-hoc test.

2.4. The Effect of AG on Fear Memory

The effect of AG on fear memory was measured using the fear conditioning paradigm (Figure 4). The acquisition of fear memory in the TBI mouse model was not statistically higher than that of the control animals. AG treatment lowered the acquisition of fear memory in the TBI model mice (Figure 4A). There was no significant effect of TBI and AG on the consolidated contextual and cued fear memory (Figure 4B,C). The acquisition of fear memory in the CMS mice was lower than that of controls. There was no difference in the fear acquisition after AG treatment in CMS mice (Figure 4D). Compared to the normal mice, the CMS, AG, and CMS + AG mouse groups had lower levels of consolidated contextual fear memory. However, there were no differences among the CMS, AG, and CMS + AG groups (Figure 4E). Compared to normal mice, the AG and CMS + AG groups had lower levels of consolidated cued fear memory. In addition, AG reduced the consolidated cued fear memory in the CMS group of mice (Figure 4F).

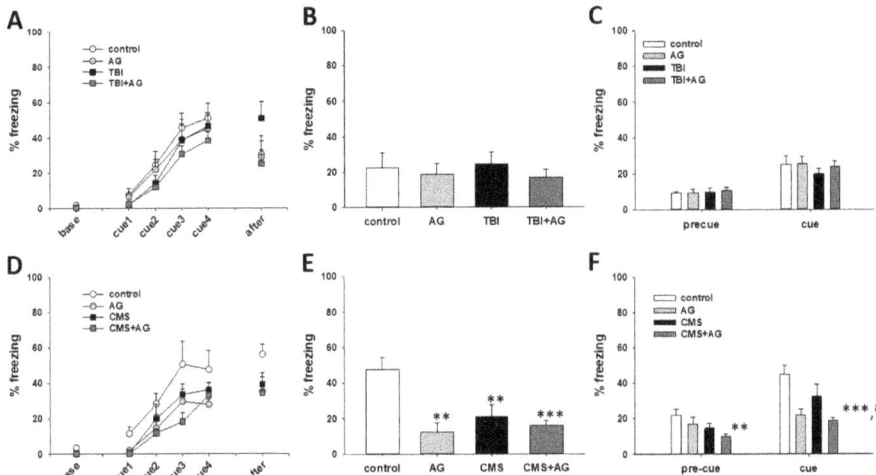

Figure 4. Fear memory by AG in TBI and CMS mice, as measured by the freezing time in the fear conditioning test. (**A**) Fear acquisition in the TBI model. There were time (within) effects [$F(5,140) = 45.7$, $p < 0.001$], treatment group (between) effects [$F(3,28) = 3.25$, $p = 0.03$], but no within–between interaction differences [$F(15,140) = 1.1$, $p = 0.36$]. There were no differences between the treatment groups at base, cue1, cue2, cue3, or cue4. However, the differences between the TBI and TBI + AG groups were significant ($p = 0.039$). In addition, the differences between the TBI and control groups ($p = 0.16$), and TBI vs. AG ($p = 0.13$) groups were not significant. (**B**) Consolidated contextual fear memory in TBI model. There were no group differences in the freezing response to the context [$F(3,28) = 0.36$, $p = 0.78$]. (**C**) Consolidated cued fear in the TBI model. There were procedure (within) effects [$F(1, 28) = 61.6$, $p < 0.001$], no treatment group (between) effects [$F(3,28) = 0.29$, $p = 0.83$], or within–between interactions [$F(3,28) = 0.64$, $p = 0.59$]. There was a significant increase in the freezing comparing cue vs. precue in the control ($p < 0.001$), AG ($p < 0.001$), TBI ($p = 0.005$), and TBI + AG groups ($p < 0.001$). (**D**) Fear acquisition in the CMS model. There were time (within) effects [$F(5,95) = 27.8$, $p < 0.001$], treatment group (between) effects [$F(3,19) = 4.9$, $p = 0.011$], but no within–between interaction effects [$F(15,95) = 0.47$, $p = 0.95$]. Fear acquisition in AG ($p = 0.021$), CMS ($p = 0.035$), and CMS + AG ($p = 0.001$) were lower than controls throughout the fear acquisition procedure. There were no statistical differences among the AG, CMS, and CMS + AG groups. (**E**) Consolidated contextual fear memory in the CMS model. There were group differences in the freezing response to the context [$F(3,19) = 9.8$, $p < 0.001$]. The contextual fear in AG ($p = 0.002$), CMS ($p = 0.008$), and CMS + AG ($p < 0.001$) was lower than those of the controls. (**F**) Consolidated cued fear in the CMS model. There were procedure (within) effects [$F(1,19) = 54.7$, $p < 0.001$], treatment group (between) effects [$F(3,19) = 9.3$, $p = 0.001$], and within–between interaction differences [$F(3,19) = 4.8$, $p = 0.012$]. There was a significant increase in freezing between cue and precue in the control ($p < 0.001$), CMS ($p < 0.001$), and CMS + AG ($p = 0.002$) groups, but not in the AG group ($p = 0.31$). At pre-cue, the control vs. CMS + AG ($p = 0.001$) groups were statistically different. At cue, the control vs. AG, ($p = 0.004$); control vs. CMS + AG, ($p < 0.001$); CMS vs. CMS + AG, ($p = 0.017$) were all statistically different. All data were normally distributed and are represented as means ± S.E.M. Control: vehicle (DW) treated; AG: *Angelica gigas* 1 mg/kg; TBI: vehicle treated + traumatic brain injury; TBI + AG: *Angelica gigas* 1 mg/kg + traumatic brain injury; CMS: vehicle treated + chronic mild stress; CMS + AG: *Angelica gigas* 1 mg/kg + chronic mild stress. ** $p < 0.01$, *** $p < 0.001$ vs. control. # $p < 0.05$ vs. CMS. ANOVA and repeated measures ANOVA, Tukey's HSD post-hoc test.

3. Discussion

We investigated whether AG extract could prevent the progression of cognitive decline or improve memory in MCI models. We found that AG improved spatial learning and working memory but suppressed fear memory in the TBI model. In the CMS model, AG improved spatial learning and suppressed the cued fear memory.

MCI is a condition that increases a patient's risk of developing dementia. Therefore, it is important that MCI is diagnosed early in order to prevent or limit dementia development [4]. Methods to improve sleep disorders, depression, one's social network, and physical exercise are considered for the treatment of MCI [28–30]. Pharmacological interventions, such as cholinesterase inhibitors, nonsteroidal anti-inflammatory drugs, estrogen replacement therapy, Gingko biloba, and vitamin E, have not shown to prevent MCI progression to dementia [4].

The roots of AG have been used in traditional medicine to improve blood flow and anemia. They have also been used for their analgesic properties [31]. AG improves spatial memory, avoidance memory, and working memory in dementia models [27]. Among the components of AG, decursinol showed the highest inhibitory activity toward acetylcholinesterase [32]. Therefore, AG is expected to improve cognitive impairment in animal models.

In order to develop a valid MCI animal model, there must be subtle memory impairment [5]. The presence of depression-like symptoms may also be an important factor in the MCI model. Dementia and depression are known to have many associations. For instance, 60% of MCI cases that progress to AD are accompanied by depression [33].

The defect in a TBI model varies depending on the hitting area and velocity [14]. In contrast with severe TBI, mild TBI has minimal histological changes but apparent cognitive and emotional problems [8]. This association suggests that mild TBI can be used as an MCI model [34]. Such spatial memory deficit occurred in our TBI model mice, but other reflexes (such as the paw withdrawal reflex, righting reflex, and corneal reflex) were maintained (data not shown). Also, TBI is commonly known to cause disturbances in working memory. TBI in the parietotemporal regions has been shown to cause working memory deficits in mice [35]. However, working memory was normal in the mild TBI model made by repeated frontal impact; therefore, working memory is not always compromised in TBI [36]. Our measurements of working memory did not differ in the TBI model. Another common problem in TBI is the inability to recognize the source of information, such as facial recognition [37]. Face recognition memory corresponds to animal object recognition memory. There was a deficit in animal object recognition memory in the TBI models [38]. The TBI mice in this study also had decreased object recognition memory. These model mice also showed heightened fear memory; however, the results are controversial. One group found that there was no difference between normal animals and a mild repeated frontal TBI model with regard to conditioned fear after a severe CCI impact to the left parietal cortex [36]. However, a single impact above the skull increased anxiety and contextual fear in rats [39]. In mice, hippocampal-dependent fear memory decreased, but cued-dependent fear memory was not affected by TBI [40]. In our results, there was an enhanced acquisition of contextual fear in the TBI mice. However, after 24 h, the consolidated level of contextual and cued memory was not different with control animals.

Stress has a variety of effects on cognitive function [41]. CMS is a depression model also characterized by a decrease in cognitive function associated with neuroimmune, neuroendocrine, and neurogenesis functions [4]. In this experiment, the CMS animals displayed anhedonia-like behaviors in the sucrose preference test and deficits in spatial memory. In other studies using CMS models, working memory was reduced in rats but was maintained in mice [42,43]. Our study similarly found that there was no working memory deficit in CMS mice. Reduction in object recognition memory in mice and increased contextual fear in rats were reported previously [42,44]. In the present study, CMS did not affect object recognition memory, but fear acquisition and contextual consolidation were reduced. These findings were inconsistent; however, rats that were exposed to social instability stress (daily 1-h isolation, change of cage partners) showed deficits in contextual and cued memory [45,46]. Taken together, in the TBI mice, spatial learning and object recognition memory were degraded. However, spatial memory, working memory, and fear memory were intact. In the CMS model, spatial memory was degraded, but working and object recognition memory were not affected, and cued fear memory was reduced.

AG has known antibacterial, immune-stimulating, antiplatelet aggregation, neuroprotective, anti-inflammatory, and antioxidant properties [31]. We found that AG did not improve spatial memory in normal mice. However, it did improve memory in TBI and CMS animals. In addition, AG treatment led to improved working memory in normal mice of the TBI cohort. AG did not increase the recognition memory of the normal mice. However, recognition memory was only abnormal in the TBI mice at baseline. In the TBI and AG co-administration group, recognition memory was maintained. This result suggests that AG can prevent TBI-induced deficit. In the CMS cohort, however, the object memory of the CMS group was not affected. Therefore, AG also did not improve object memory in either the normal or the CMS mice. With regard to fear memory, the contextual and cued consolidated fear memory of normal and CMS mice were reduced in the CMS cohort. However, consolidated fear levels were not affected in the TBI cohort. Among AG's known effects, its cholinesterase inhibition, improved blood flow, and anti-inflammatory properties may prevent cognitive decline and improve memory in these mouse models [31,32].

In conclusion, AG prevented the deterioration of spatial learning and object recognition memory in a mouse TBI model. AG also prevented the deterioration of spatial learning in the CMS model mice and improved working memory in normal mice. As TBI is a cognitive impairment gradually progresses, and chronic stress can cause AD-like pathologies, these findings suggest that AG may also prevent progressive cognitive decline in MCI animal models, which may be worth further research.

4. Materials and Methods

4.1. Preparation of AG Extract

The dried AG root was purchased from the Junbu, Bonghwa, and Jecheon area and authenticated by professor Hui Jin. A voucher specimen was deposited in the Myongji Bioefficiency Research Center, Myongji University. AG was immersed in 70% ethanol and boiled for 4 h at 90 °C, 2 times. Then, filtered extracts were concentrated up to 25 Brix at 60 °C by depressurized evaporation, and then stored at 4 °C before using. The crude extract yield was 42.1% (w/w). The extract was dissolved in distilled water for administration into animals. HPLC was used to examine whether extracts contained nodakenin and decursin (Figure S2).

4.2. Animals and Experimental Groups

Seven-week-old male C57Bl/6 mice were purchased from Central Laboratory animals Inc. (Seoul, Korea) ($n = 32$ for cohort 1, $n = 40$ for cohort 2). The mice were housed under constant temperature and humidity with 12-h cycles of light/darkness. They had *ad libitum* access to rodent chow and water. After a week of habituation, the mice were randomly assigned into experimental groups. The mice in the TBI cohort were assigned to the following assignments: (1) control ($n = 6$): DW p.o. + no TBI; (2) AG ($n = 6$): *Angelica gigas* 1 mg/kg p.o + no TBI; (3) TBI ($n = 8$): DW p.o. + TBI; (4) TBI + AG ($n = 12$): *Angelica gigas* 1 mg/kg p.o. + TBI. The mice in the CMS cohort were assigned to the following assignments: (1) control ($n = 10$): DW p.o. + no CMS; (2) AG ($n = 10$): *Angelica gigas* 1 mg/kg p.o + no CMS; 3) CMS ($n = 10$): DW p.o. + CMS; 4) CMS + AG ($n = 10$): *Angelica gigas* 1 mg/kg p.o. + CMS. The outline of the experimental procedures is schematically represented in Figure 5. Animal studies were conducted in accordance with the Guide for the Care and Use of Laboratory Animals by the NIH. The protocols were approved by the Institutional Animal Care and Use Committee of Kyung Hee University (KHUASP(GC)-17-024).

Cohort 1 : TBI

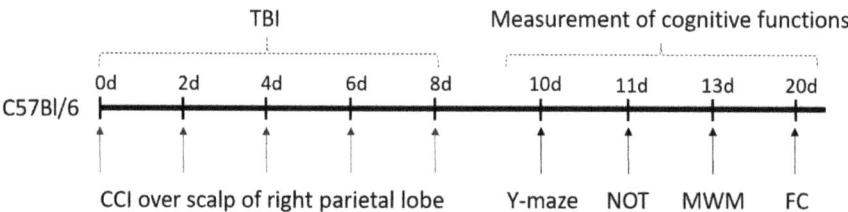

Cohort 2 : CMS

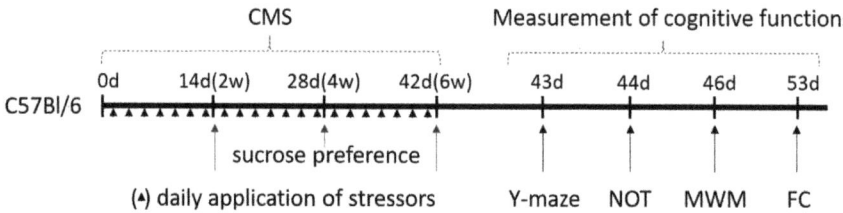

Figure 5. Experimental outline of mild cognitive impairment mice models induced by TBI (Cohort 1) and CMS (Cohort 2). TBI: Traumatic brain injury, CCI: Controlled cortical impact, Y-maze: Y shaped maze test, NOT: Novel object test, MWM: Morris water maze, FC: Fear conditioning, CMS: Chronic mild stress.

4.3. Creating Animal Models

4.3.1. TBI Model

A Cortical Contusion Injury device, which was purchased from Custom Design and Fabrication, Inc., (model eCCI-6.3), was used to simulate TBI. The mice were anesthetized with 3% isoflurane during the procedure. In order to induce TBI, a 3 mm rod impacted the scalp over the right hippocampal region at the velocity of 4 m/second and depth of 0.5 mm. This was repeated five times, with two days between each impact. Animals in the control and AG groups also underwent isoflurane anesthesia, but no impact.

4.3.2. CMS Model

The stress procedure lasted for six weeks. The mice were randomly subjected to two types of stressors each day. The potential stressors included 2 h of immobilization, strobe light exposure, white noise exposure, cat urine exposure, and overnight food deprivation, water deprivation, or light exposure. During the weekend, the mice were exposed to wet bedding or a tilted cage for 24 h. The control mice were left undisturbed in their home cage.

4.4. Behavioral Tests

4.4.1. Sucrose Preference

Anhedonia-like changes in the CMS mice were monitored using the sucrose preference test, which was performed at the 2nd, 4th, and 6th week. Consumption of water and sucrose by a single caged mouse was measured from 6 p.m. to 9 a.m. The preference index was calculated as follows: [sucrose consumption/(DW consumption + sucrose consumption)].

4.4.2. Morris Water Maze

The water tank (200 cm diameter) was filled 0.5 cm above the platform with tap water and made opaque by white paint. For 5 days, the mice were trained to locate the submerged platform within 60 s according to the symbols placed around the walls. If the mouse was unable to escape within 60 s, it was guided to the platform. Each day of training included 4 sessions, each of which started in a different quadrant.

4.4.3. Y-Maze

The maze consisted of three corridors that were joined at the center at equal angles. After placing a mouse in the maze, the movements were recorded for five minutes. An alternation was defined as a sequential visit to each arm without the repetition of either of the two previous arms. The percent alternation was calculated as the number of correct alternations per total arm visits minus 2.

4.4.4. Novel Object Test

In a plexiglas box (50 × 50 × 40 cm), two cylinder-shaped tin cans were introduced in two corners, 30 cm apart from each other. The mice were allowed to explore each object for 5 min. On the next day, the object of the right corner was replaced with a box-shaped novel object. The time that the mice spent exploring each object was recorded during the 5-min period. The animals were considered to be exploring an object when they were facing or sniffing the object. The recognition index was calculated by the ratio of time spent exploring the novel object over the total time spent exploring both objects.

4.4.5. Fear Conditioning

The fear conditioning test consisted of acquisition, contextual consolidation, and cued consolidation phases. For the acquisition, the mice were placed in the Passive/Active avoidance system chamber from Scitech Korea (model No. PAAS) and left undisturbed for two minutes. The subsequent sessions comprised a conditioned stimulus (2000 Hz tone, 30 s) that co-terminated with an unconditioned stimulus (electric foot shock, 0.45 mA, 2 s), and intertrial intervals (30 s) were repeated four times. The mice were left in the chamber for an additional two minutes. Freezing was measured during the first two minutes and last two minutes of the 4 intertrial intervals. On the following day, the animals were placed in the chamber for five minutes. Freezing was measured as a contextual fear memory. On the third day, the mice were placed in a novel chamber for three minutes, followed by three minutes of exposure to a 2000 Hz tone. Freezing was measured before and during the tone exposure.

4.5. Statistical Analysis

Analysis of variance (ANOVA) and repeated measures ANOVA, following Tukey's HSD post-hoc test, were performed using SPSS 23 (IBM). p-Values < 0.05 were considered significantly different. The normality of distribution of variables was tested by the Shapiro-Wilk test.

Supplementary Materials: The following are available online at http://www.mdpi.com/2072-6643/12/1/97/s1, Figure S1: Body weight and sucrose preference change in CMS mice; Figure S2: HPLC analysis of AG extract.

Author Contributions: Conceptualization, S.-D.J. and Y.H.K.; methodology, J.S.; formal analysis and investigation, M.K., M.S. and H.-J.O.; investigation, W.B.; data curation, J.H.; writing—original draft preparation, S.M.; writing—review and editing, H.P.; supervision, J.W.S. All authors have read and agreed to the published version of the manuscript.

Funding: This research was funded by the Cooperative Research Program for Agriculture Science and Technology Development, grant number PJ01331402.

Conflicts of Interest: The authors declare no conflict of interest. The funders had no role in the design of the study; in the collection, analyses, or interpretation of data; in the writing of the manuscript, or in the decision to publish the results.

References

1. Ebly, E.M.; Hogan, D.B.; Parhad, I.M. Cognitive impairment in the nondemented elderly. Results from the Canadian Study of Health and Aging. *Arch. Neurol.* **1995**, *52*, 612–619. [CrossRef] [PubMed]
2. Graham, J.E.; Rockwood, K.; Beattie, B.L.; Eastwood, R.; Gauthier, S.; Tuokko, H.; McDowell, I. Prevalence and severity of cognitive impairment with and without dementia in an elderly population. *Lancet* **1997**, *349*, 1793–1796. [CrossRef]
3. Tuokko, H.; Frerichs, R.; Graham, J.; Rockwood, K.; Kristjansson, B.; Fisk, J.; Bergman, H.; Kozma, A.; McDowell, I. Five-year follow-up of cognitive impairment with no dementia. *Arch. Neurol.* **2003**, *60*, 577–582. [CrossRef] [PubMed]
4. Chertkow, H.; Massoud, F.; Nasreddine, Z.; Belleville, S.; Joanette, Y.; Bocti, C.; Drolet, V.; Kirk, J.; Freedman, M.; Bergman, H. Diagnosis and treatment of dementia: 3. Mild cognitive impairment and cognitive impairment without dementia. *CMAJ Can. Med. Assoc. J. J. De L'association Med. Can.* **2008**, *178*, 1273–1285. [CrossRef]
5. Pepeu, G. Mild cognitive impairment: Animal models. *Dialogues Clin. Neurosci.* **2004**, *6*, 369–377.
6. Hernandez, C.M.; Hoifodt, H.; Terry, A.V., Jr. Spontaneously hypertensive rats: Further evaluation of age-related memory performance and cholinergic marker expression. *J. Psychiatry Neurosci. JPN* **2003**, *28*, 197–209.
7. Terry, A.V., Jr.; Hernandez, C.M.; Buccafusco, J.J.; Gattu, M. Deficits in spatial learning and nicotinic-acetylcholine receptors in older, spontaneously hypertensive rats. *Neuroscience* **2000**, *101*, 357–368. [CrossRef]
8. Kibby, M.Y.; Long, C.J. Minor head injury: Attempts at clarifying the confusion. *Brain Inj.* **1996**, *10*, 159–186. [CrossRef]
9. Stern, R.A.; Riley, D.O.; Daneshvar, D.H.; Nowinski, C.J.; Cantu, R.C.; McKee, A.C. Long-term consequences of repetitive brain trauma: Chronic traumatic encephalopathy. *PM R J. Inj. Funct. Rehabil.* **2011**, *3*, S460–S467. [CrossRef]
10. Arciniegas, D.; Adler, L.; Topkoff, J.; Cawthra, E.; Filley, C.M.; Reite, M. Attention and memory dysfunction after traumatic brain injury: Cholinergic mechanisms, sensory gating, and a hypothesis for further investigation. *Brain Inj.* **1999**, *13*, 1–13. [CrossRef]
11. Levin, H.S.; Mattis, S.; Ruff, R.M.; Eisenberg, H.M.; Marshall, L.F.; Tabaddor, K.; High, W.M., Jr.; Frankowski, R.F. Neurobehavioral outcome following minor head injury: A three-center study. *J. Neurosurg.* **1987**, *66*, 234–243. [CrossRef]
12. Guskiewicz, K.M.; Marshall, S.W.; Bailes, J.; McCrea, M.; Cantu, R.C.; Randolph, C.; Jordan, B.D. Association between recurrent concussion and late-life cognitive impairment in retired professional football players. *Neurosurgery* **2005**, *57*, 719–726. [CrossRef] [PubMed]
13. Langlois, J.A.; Rutland-Brown, W.; Wald, M.M. The epidemiology and impact of traumatic brain injury: A brief overview. *J. Head Trauma Rehabil.* **2006**, *21*, 375–378. [CrossRef] [PubMed]
14. Xiong, Y.; Mahmood, A.; Chopp, M. Animal models of traumatic brain injury. *Nat. Rev. Neurosci.* **2013**, *14*, 128–142. [CrossRef]
15. Mouzon, B.C.; Bachmeier, C.; Ferro, A.; Ojo, J.O.; Crynen, G.; Acker, C.M.; Davies, P.; Mullan, M.; Stewart, W.; Crawford, F. Chronic neuropathological and neurobehavioral changes in a repetitive mild traumatic brain injury model. *Ann. Neurol.* **2014**, *75*, 241–254. [CrossRef] [PubMed]
16. Creeley, C.E.; Wozniak, D.F.; Bayly, P.V.; Olney, J.W.; Lewis, L.M. Multiple episodes of mild traumatic brain injury result in impaired cognitive performance in mice. *Acad. Emerg. Med.* **2004**, *11*, 809–819. [CrossRef]
17. Willner, P. Validity, reliability and utility of the chronic mild stress model of depression: A 10-year review and evaluation. *Psychopharmacology* **1997**, *134*, 319–329. [CrossRef]
18. Song, L.; Che, W.; Min-Wei, W.; Murakami, Y.; Matsumoto, K. Impairment of the spatial learning and memory induced by learned helplessness and chronic mild stress. *Pharmacol. Biochem. Behav.* **2006**, *83*, 186–193. [CrossRef]

19. Cuadrado-Tejedor, M.; Ricobaraza, A.; Del Rio, J.; Frechilla, D.; Franco, R.; Perez-Mediavilla, A.; Garcia-Osta, A. Chronic mild stress in mice promotes cognitive impairment and CDK5-dependent tau hyperphosphorylation. *Behav. Brain Res.* **2011**, *220*, 338–343. [CrossRef]
20. Sattler, C.; Toro, P.; Schonknecht, P.; Schroder, J. Cognitive activity, education and socioeconomic status as preventive factors for mild cognitive impairment and Alzheimer's disease. *Psychiatry Res.* **2012**, *196*, 90–95. [CrossRef]
21. Geda, Y.E.; Roberts, R.O.; Knopman, D.S.; Christianson, T.J.; Pankratz, V.S.; Ivnik, R.J.; Boeve, B.F.; Tangalos, E.G.; Petersen, R.C.; Rocca, W.A. Physical exercise, aging, and mild cognitive impairment: A population-based study. *Arch. Neurol.* **2010**, *67*, 80–86. [CrossRef] [PubMed]
22. Craft, S.; Baker, L.D.; Montine, T.J.; Minoshima, S.; Watson, G.S.; Claxton, A.; Arbuckle, M.; Callaghan, M.; Tsai, E.; Plymate, S.R.; et al. Intranasal insulin therapy for Alzheimer disease and amnestic mild cognitive impairment: A pilot clinical trial. *Arch. Neurol.* **2012**, *69*, 29–38. [CrossRef] [PubMed]
23. Petersen, R.C.; Thomas, R.G.; Grundman, M.; Bennett, D.; Doody, R.; Ferris, S.; Galasko, D.; Jin, S.; Kaye, J.; Levey, A.; et al. Alzheimer's Disease Cooperative Study Group. Vitamin E and donepezil for the treatment of mild cognitive impairment. *N. Engl. J. Med.* **2005**, *352*, 2379–2388. [CrossRef] [PubMed]
24. Sarker, S.D.; Nahar, L. Natural medicine: The genus Angelica. *Curr. Med. Chem.* **2004**, *11*, 1479–1500. [CrossRef]
25. Cha, Y.S.; Choi, D.S.; Oh, S.H. Effects of *Angelica gigas* Nakai diet on lipid metabolism, alcohol metabolism and liver function of rats administered with chronic ethanol. *Appl. Biol. Chem.* **1999**, *42*, 29–33.
26. Zhao, R.J.; Koo, B.S.; Kim, G.W.; Jang, E.Y.; Lee, J.R.; Kim, M.R.; Kim, S.C.; Kwon, Y.K.; Kim, K.J.; Huh, T.L.; et al. The essential oil from *Angelica gigas* NAKAI suppresses nicotine sensitization. *Biol. Pharm. Bull.* **2005**, *28*, 2323–2326. [CrossRef]
27. Yan, J.J.; Kim, D.H.; Moon, Y.S.; Jung, J.S.; Ahn, E.M.; Baek, N.I.; Song, D.K. Protection against beta-amyloid peptide-induced memory impairment with long-term administration of extract of *Angelica gigas* or decursinol in mice. *Prog. Neuro-Psychopharmacol. Biol. Psychiatry* **2004**, *28*, 25–30. [CrossRef]
28. Reischies, F.M.; Neu, P. Comorbidity of mild cognitive disorder and depression–a neuropsychological analysis. *Eur. Arch. Psychiatry Clin. Neurosci.* **2000**, *250*, 186–193. [CrossRef]
29. Fratiglioni, L.; Wang, H.X.; Ericsson, K.; Maytan, M.; Winblad, B. Influence of social network on occurrence of dementia: A community-based longitudinal study. *Lancet* **2000**, *355*, 1315–1319. [CrossRef]
30. Laurin, D.; Verreault, R.; Lindsay, J.; MacPherson, K.; Rockwood, K. Physical activity and risk of cognitive impairment and dementia in elderly persons. *Arch. Neurol.* **2001**, *58*, 498–504. [CrossRef]
31. Sowndhararajan, K.; Kim, S. Neuroprotective and Cognitive Enhancement Potentials of *Angelica gigas* Nakai Root: A Review. *Sci. Pharm.* **2017**, *85*, 21. [CrossRef] [PubMed]
32. Kang, S.Y.; Lee, K.Y.; Sung, S.H.; Park, M.J.; Kim, Y.C. Coumarins isolated from *Angelica gigas* inhibit acetylcholinesterase: Structure-activity relationships. *J. Nat. Prod.* **2001**, *64*, 683–685. [CrossRef] [PubMed]
33. Visser, P.J.; Verhey, F.R.; Ponds, R.W.; Kester, A.; Jolles, J. Distinction between preclinical Alzheimer's disease and depression. *J. Am. Geriatr. Soc.* **2000**, *48*, 479–484. [CrossRef] [PubMed]
34. Milman, A.; Rosenberg, A.; Weizman, R.; Pick, C.G. Mild traumatic brain injury induces persistent cognitive deficits and behavioral disturbances in mice. *J. Neurotrauma* **2005**, *22*, 1003–1010. [CrossRef]
35. Eakin, K.; Baratz-Goldstein, R.; Pick, C.G.; Zindel, O.; Balaban, C.D.; Hoffer, M.E.; Lockwood, M.; Miller, J.; Hoffer, B.J. Efficacy of N-acetyl cysteine in traumatic brain injury. *PLoS ONE* **2014**, *9*, e90617. [CrossRef]
36. Cheng, J.S.; Craft, R.; Yu, G.Q.; Ho, K.; Wang, X.; Mohan, G.; Mangnitsky, S.; Ponnusamy, R.; Mucke, L. Tau reduction diminishes spatial learning and memory deficits after mild repetitive traumatic brain injury in mice. *PLoS ONE* **2014**, *9*, e115369. [CrossRef]
37. Dywan, J.; Segalowitz, S.J.; Henderson, D.; Jacoby, L. Memory for source after traumatic brain injury. *Brain Cogn.* **1993**, *21*, 20–43. [CrossRef]
38. Gauthier, I.; Tarr, M.J.; Anderson, A.W.; Skudlarski, P.; Gore, J.C. Activation of the middle fusiform 'face area' increases with expertise in recognizing novel objects. *Nat. Neurosci.* **1999**, *2*, 568–573. [CrossRef]
39. Meyer, D.L.; Davies, D.R.; Barr, J.L.; Manzerra, P.; Forster, G.L. Mild traumatic brain injury in the rat alters neuronal number in the limbic system and increases conditioned fear and anxiety-like behaviors. *Exp. Neurol.* **2012**, *235*, 574–587. [CrossRef]

40. Lifshitz, J.; Witgen, B.M.; Grady, M.S. Acute cognitive impairment after lateral fluid percussion brain injury recovers by 1 month: Evaluation by conditioned fear response. *Behav. Brain Res.* **2007**, *177*, 347–357. [CrossRef]
41. McEwen, B.S.; Sapolsky, R.M. Stress and cognitive function. *Curr. Opin. Neurobiol.* **1995**, *5*, 205–216. [CrossRef]
42. Henningsen, K.; Andreasen, J.T.; Bouzinova, E.V.; Jayatissa, M.N.; Jensen, M.S.; Redrobe, J.P.; Wiborg, O. Cognitive deficits in the rat chronic mild stress model for depression: Relation to anhedonic-like responses. *Behav. Brain Res.* **2009**, *198*, 136–141. [CrossRef] [PubMed]
43. Pothion, S.; Bizot, J.C.; Trovero, F.; Belzung, C. Strain differences in sucrose preference and in the consequences of unpredictable chronic mild stress. *Behav. Brain Res.* **2004**, *155*, 135–146. [CrossRef] [PubMed]
44. Haridas, S.; Kumar, M.; Manda, K. Melatonin ameliorates chronic mild stress induced behavioral dysfunctions in mice. *Physiol. Behav.* **2013**, *119*, 201–207. [CrossRef]
45. Wright, R.L.; Conrad, C.D. Chronic stress leaves novelty-seeking behavior intact while impairing spatial recognition memory in the Y-maze. *Stress* **2005**, *8*, 151–154. [CrossRef]
46. Morrissey, M.D.; Mathews, I.Z.; McCormick, C.M. Enduring deficits in contextual and auditory fear conditioning after adolescent, not adult, social instability stress in male rats. *Neurobiol. Learn. Mem.* **2011**, *95*, 46–56. [CrossRef]

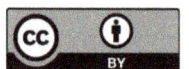

© 2019 by the authors. Licensee MDPI, Basel, Switzerland. This article is an open access article distributed under the terms and conditions of the Creative Commons Attribution (CC BY) license (http://creativecommons.org/licenses/by/4.0/).

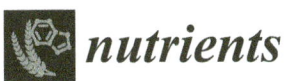

Article

Equol Pretreatment Protection of SH-SY5Y Cells against Aβ (25–35)-Induced Cytotoxicity and Cell-Cycle Reentry via Sustaining Estrogen Receptor Alpha Expression

Meng-Chao Tsai [1,†], Shyh-Hsiang Lin [2,3,4,†], Kiswatul Hidayah [2] and Ching-I Lin [5,*]

1. Department of Psychiatry, Taoyuan General Hospital, Taoyuan 33004, Taiwan; mctsai1981@gmail.com
2. School of Nutrition and Health Sciences, Taipei Medical University, Taipei 11042, Taiwan; lin5611@tmu.edu.tw (S.-H.L.); kiswatul.hidayah@gmail.com (K.H.)
3. Master Program in Food Safety, Taipei Medical University, Taipei 11042, Taiwan
4. Research Center of Geriatric Nutrition, Taipei Medical University, Taipei 11042, Taiwan
5. Department of Nutrition and Health Sciences, Kainan University, Taoyuan 33857, Taiwan
* Correspondence: drcilin@gmail.com or cilin@mail.knu.edu.tw; Tel.: +886-3-341-2500 (ext.6193); Fax: +886-3-270-5904
† Meng-Chao Tsai and Shyh-Hsiang Lin equally contributed to this work.

Received: 2 August 2019; Accepted: 23 September 2019; Published: 3 October 2019

Abstract: β-amyloid formation in the brain is one of the characteristics of Alzheimer's disease. Exposure to this peptide may result in reentry into the cell cycle leading to cell death. The phytoestrogen equol has similar biological effects as estrogen without the side effects. This study investigated the possible mechanism of the neuron cell-protecting effect of equol during treatment with Aβ. SH-SY5Y neuroblastoma cells were treated with either 1 μM S-equol or 10 nM 17β-estradiol for 24 h prior to 1 μM Aβ (25–35) exposure. After 24 h exposure to Aβ (25–35), a significant reduction in cell survival and a reentry into the cell cycle process accompanied by increased levels of cyclin D1 were observed. The expressions of estrogen receptor alpha (ERα) and its coactivator, steroid receptor coactivator-1 (SRC-1), were also significantly downregulated by Aβ (25–35) in parallel with activated extracellular signal-regulated kinase (ERK)1/2. However, pretreatment of cells with S-equol or 17β-estradiol reversed these effects. Treatment with the ER antagonist, ICI-182,780 (1 μM), completely blocked the effects of S-equol and 17β-estradiol on cell viability, ERα, and ERK1/2 after Aβ (25–35) exposure. These data suggest that S-equol possesses a neuroprotective potential as it effectively antagonizes Aβ (25–35)-induced cell cytotoxicity and prevents cell cycle reentry in SH-SY5Y cells. The mechanism underlying S-equol neuroprotection might involve ERα-mediated pathways.

Keywords: S-equol; 17β-estradiol; estrogen receptor alpha; cell cycle; β-Amyloid; Alzheimer's disease

1. Introduction

Neuronal cell death is an important feature of human neurodegenerative diseases such as Alzheimer's disease (AD). This cell death is considered to occur as a consequence of aberrant activation of the cell cycle in neurodegeneration [1]. Under normal conduction, the cell cycle is tightly controlled by specific regulatory proteins. For instance, cyclins and cyclin-dependent kinases (CDKs) are two key classes of regulatory molecules that determine a cell's progress in the cell cycle [2]. As a key regulator of the G1-S transition, cyclin D1 interacts with CDK4 to form the cyclin D1-CDK4 complex and moves to the nuclei, thereby promoting cell cycle progression. Normal adult neuron cells never reenter the cell cycle (but stay in the G_0 stage) and are thus recognized as permanently postmitotic cells [3]. Conversely, neurons reenter the cycle, undergo DNA replication, and die after they are exposed to DNA-damaging agents, oxidative stress, or certain neurotoxins such as beta-amyloid (Aβ) aggregates [3]. The Aβ peptide is the major component of senile plaque derived from the Aβ precursor protein (APP); this peptide is a neuropathological hallmark of AD [4]. There are numerous different Aβ species including Aβ (1–40), Aβ (1–42), and Aβ (25–35). The Aβ (25–35) fragment is universally used in research as it has been found to elicit profound toxic manifestations in elderly people and to physiologically play a role in AD [5]. It has been previously shown that cell cycle activation accompanied by the upregulation of cyclin D1 in primary cultured rat cortical neurons was observed in response to exposure to Aβ (25–35) and that such activation was followed by apoptotic neuronal death [6]. To elucidate the possible intracellular signaling pathway involved in the activation of the cell cycle by Aβ, extracellular signal-regulated kinase (ERK) 1/2-related pathways are the major focus of the present study because there is evidence of the involvement of ERK1/2 activation in Aβ-induced neuronal cell death [7]. It has been documented that activation of ERK 1/2 appears to be critical for G1 to S phase progression in cell cycle regulation [8]. A previous study showed that the overexpression of ERK 1/2 in cells exposed to Aβ was followed by an elevation in cyclin D1 expression, which resulted in changes in the cell-cycle distribution, particularly in the G1-S phase [9].

ERK1/2 is also the target of the regulatory action of estrogen and its regulation requires interaction with the known estrogen receptors (ERs), ERα and ERβ [10]. In addition to the reproductive system, both ERα and ERβ are broadly expressed in nonreproductive systems including the central nervous system [11]. Particularly, brain regions such as the hypothalamus, amygdala, and hippocampus appear to have distinct expression patterns of both ER subtypes [12]. Although it is recognized that ERβ is the predominant receptor in the hippocampus, where its absence has an impact on memory and cognitive function [13], ERα co-exists, and its coregulation may be important for ERβ to fulfill its cellular roles [14]. In other words, ERβ collaborating with ERα in its molecular actions is crucial for estrogen-mediated beneficial effects on hippocampus-dependent memory and cognition. The ERα subtype is of particular interest in the present study as it exhibits stronger transcription activity than ERβ and thus appears to be functionally superior to ERβ in the modulation of age-related memory decline [13–15]. It is noteworthy that ERα diminishing in the hippocampus with age leads to a decrease in the relative expression of ERα and ERβ, and nuclear ERα-mediated effects, all of which are putative molecular mechanisms for age-related memory decline in the presence of low estrogen levels [13]. In this regard, the molecular actions of both ER subtypes have been reported to be involved in the neuroprotection of estrogen against the pathogenic processes of AD [16]. Evidence suggests that estrogen is capable of protecting against Aβ-induced toxicity through ERα-mediated signaling pathways [17]. Moreover, the other major neuropathological hallmark of AD is intracellular aggregates of hyperphosphorylated Tau protein, which has recently been found to interact with ERα potentiating the reduction of ERα's transcriptional activity [18]. SRC-1 is one of the nuclear receptor coactivators which enhance the transcriptional activity of ERs to manipulate the relevant molecular events [19]. Studies performed in a human astrocytoma cell line demonstrated that estradiol treatment increased the cell number through the mediation of ERα, whereas the coactivator silencing by RNA interference of SRC-1 was able to block this effect [19].

Equol is a metabolite of daidzein, one of the major isoflavones in soybean food products, and is known as an ERs agonist [20]. Equol is capable of inducing transcriptional responses, especially through the binding of ERα [21]. The oral bioavailability of equol in humans seems to be high, resulting in a plasma concentration of 0.4~2 μM after taking a single bolus of 2 mg of equol [22]. Consumption of phytoestrogens has been found to avoid many side effects from estrogens [23]. Intriguingly, equol has been shown to be a promising neuroprotectant in in vitro models, and its neuroprotective effects are exerted through anti-neuroinflammatory mechanisms with the regulation of relevant signaling pathways at molecular levels [24]. However, whether the cell cycle regulatory event and ER-dependent signaling pathways involve the neuroprotective properties of equol remains an enigma. Thus, in this study, we investigated the effects of equol on protecting SH-SY5Y cells against

Aβ-induced perturbations and the cellular mechanisms underlying equol's neuroprotective action in cell cycle events and ER pathways.

2. Materials and Methods

2.1. Cell Culture

Human SH-SY5Y neuroblastoma cells were cultured at 37 °C and 5% CO_2 in Dulbecco's modified Eagle medium (DMEM) (Invitrogen™, Life Technologies, Grand Island, NY, USA) mixed with F12 (Invitrogen™, Life Technologies, Grand Island, NY, USA), 10% fetal bovine serum (FBS) (Biowest LLC, Miami, FL, USA), and glutamine (Biological Industries, Kibbutz Beit Haemek, Israel). The medium was changed twice per week. Cells were grown to 80% confluence before treatment.

2.2. Treatments

Aβ (25–35) (Sigma Aldrich, St. Louis, MO, USA) was dissolved in sterile distilled water at a concentration of 1 mM, then incubated in a capped vial at 37 °C for 5 days to allow formation of the aggregated form. It was then stored frozen at −20 °C until use. 17β-Estradiol, S-equol, and ICI-182,780 (all from Cayman Chemical, Ann Arbor, MI, USA) were dissolved in 99.5% ethanol to make stock solutions, which were used for experiments at a final concentration of 10 nM for estradiol and 1 μM for equol and ICI-182,780 in culture medium. It should be noted that no cytotoxic effect of the vehicle (99.5% ethanol) *per se* on cells was observed via the analysis of cell viability in our preliminary experiments that were conducted to determine the appropriate concentrations of the aforementioned treatments for the present study.

To induce cell death, cells were incubated with (Aβ) or without (C) 1 μM Aβ (25–35) for 24 h. To study the effects of estradiol (E2) and equol (Eq), cells were preincubated with estradiol (E2 + Aβ) or equol (Eq + Aβ) for 24 h prior to Aβ (25–35) exposure. Estradiol was used as a positive control and ICI-182,780 was used as an ER antagonist. It was added 1 h before the estradiol or equol treatment.

2.3. Cell Viability Analysis

Cell viability was assessed using a modified 3-[4,5-dimethylthiazol-2]-2,5 diphenyltetrazolium bromide (MTT) assay (Sigma, St. Louis, MO, USA). Cells were seeded in 24-well dishes at a seeding density of 2×10^5 cells/well. After treatment, 300 μL of the MTT solution (5 mg/mL) was added to each well and incubated at 37 °C for 3 h. After removing the culture medium, 250 μL of dimethyl sulfoxide (DMSO) was added to each well to dissolve the formazan, and then 200 μL of the solution was moved to a 96-well dish. The optical density was measured at 570 nm using a microplate reader. The absorbance of the control group was considered to have 100% cell viability.

2.4. Protein Extraction and Quantification

After treatment, cells were harvested, washed three times with PBS, and lysed using a cold RIPA lysis buffer supplemented with a protease inhibitor and an EDTA solution (Thermo, Hudson, NH, USA) at a ratio of 100:1:1, then centrifuged at 13,000 rpm and 4 °C for 30 min. The supernatant was collected, and the protein concentration was estimated with a BCA Protein Assay Kit (Sigma, St. Louis, MO, USA) using BSA as the standard.

2.5. Cell-Cycle Analysis

Cells (8×10^5) were seeded in 6-well dishes. After treatment, cells were trypsinized, washed in PBS, and centrifuged at 2000× *g* at 25 °C for 5 min, and then they were washed with PBS at least twice. Cells were fixed in 70% ethanol overnight. Before removing the ethanol, samples were centrifuged at 11 °C and 2200× *g* for 10 min. The pellet was then resuspended in 200 μL of DNA extraction buffer (containing 192 mL 0.2 M Na_2HPO_4 and 8 mL 0.1 M citric acid at pH 7.8) and incubated for 30 min at 37 °C. PI dye (200 μL, containing 0.1% Triton-X100, 100 μg/mL RNase-A, and 80 μg/mL PI in PBS) was added, gently mixed, and incubated for 30 min at room temperature in the dark. After removing the PI dye, samples were resuspended with 1 mL of cold PBS prior to analysis by flow cytometry.

2.6. Western Blot Analysis

A western blot analysis was performed to examine the expression levels of the proteins. Equal quantities (30 μg) of protein were separated by 10% sodium dodecyl sulfate polyacrylamide gel electrophoresis (SDS-PAGE) and then transferred onto nitrocellulose membranes. After transfer, membranes were blocked with Tris-buffered saline (TBS) containing 0.1% Tween-20 (TBST) and 5% non-fat-milk for 1 h. The membranes were then incubated with specific primary antibodies (Cell Signaling Technology, Danvers, MA, USA): Anti-cyclin D1 (1:1000), anti-p-ERK 1/2 (1:1000), anti-ERK 1/2 (1:1000), anti-ERα (1:1000), anti-SRC-1 (1:1000), and anti-β-actin (1:5000) overnight at 4 °C. After washing three times with TBST for 30 min, membranes were incubated with an anti-rabbit (1:80000) or anti-mouse (1:5000) immunoglobulin G (IgG) secondary antibody (Sigma) for 1 h, and then washed with TBST three times for 30 min. Immunoreactive proteins were detected by enhanced chemiluminescence (ECL) (Bionovas, Toronto, Canada) Western blot detection system.

2.7. Statistical Analysis

Data are shown as the mean and standard deviation (SD). Statistical comparisons were performed using SAS 9.3 (Cary, NC, USA). One-way analysis of variance (ANOVA) and least squared difference (LSD) post-hoc analysis of multiple comparisons were used. The statistical significance was accepted at $p < 0.05$.

3. Results

3.1. Cell Viability

As shown in Figure 1, the cell viability of the Aβ group decreased to 62.6% compared to the C group ($p < 0.05$), suggesting that Aβ (25–35) is cytotoxic to SH-SY5Y cells in the present study. After pretreatment with equol (Eq + Aβ), the cell viability was significantly increased by 9.6% compared to the Aβ group, and the same effect was observed in the E2 group which exhibited increased cell viability of up to 12.9% compared to the Aβ group ($p < 0.05$). No cytotoxic effect on cells was found from the treatments of 17β-estradiol (E2) and S-equol (Eq). These findings indicate that Eq, like E2, had the potential to provide the neuroprotective effects against Aβ cytotoxicity *in vitro*. Moreover, in order to confirm that the neuroprotective effects of S-equol and 17β-estradiol against Aβ (25–35) cytotoxicity are mediated by the estrogen receptors, cells were pretreated with 1 μM ER antagonist ICI-182,780 for 1 h prior to Eq or E2 treatment. In the presence of Aβ (25–35), pretreatment with ER antagonism of ICI-182,780 prior to Eq or E2 treatments significantly abolished their effects on SH-SY5Y cell viability ($p < 0.05$). These results suggest that Eq and E2 antagonized the reduced cell viability-induced by Aβ (25–35), at least in part, by mediating the ERs.

3.2. Estrogen Receptor Alpha (ERα) Protein Expression

Figure 2 shows that Aβ (25–35) alone markedly reduced the protein expression of ERα ($p < 0.05$), whereas pretreatments of Eq and E2 significantly attenuated the decreased protein expressions of ERα induced by Aβ (25–35) ($p < 0.05$). However, in the presence of ICI-182,780, the effects of the Eq and E2 pretreatments on ERα expression were significantly blocked ($p < 0.05$).

3.3. SRC-1 Protein Expression

Figure 3 shows the effects of the Eq and E2 pretreatments on the expression of the estrogen receptor coactivator SRC-1. Treatment of 1 μM Aβ (25–35) (Aβ) for 24 h significantly decreased the SRC-1 protein expression ($p < 0.05$). Pretreatment with either Eq or E2 significantly prevented Aβ (25–35)-induced reduction in SRC-1 protein expression ($p < 0.05$).

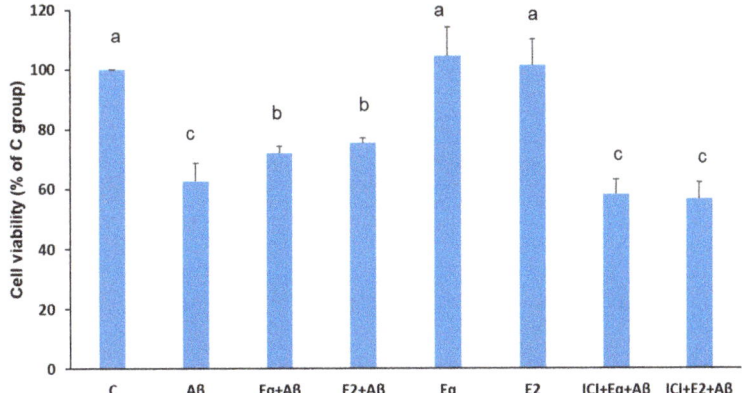

Figure 1. Cell viability of SH-SY5Y cells assessed with a modified 3-[4,5-dimethylthiazol-2]-2,5 diphenyltetrazolium bromide (MTT) assay. Data were analyzed by one-way ANOVA followed by the LSD post-hoc test and are representative of three independent experiments ($n = 3$). Values are presented as the mean + SD. Bars with different letters significantly differ at a level of $p < 0.05$. Eq, S-equol; E2, 17β-estradiol; ICI, ICI-182,780.

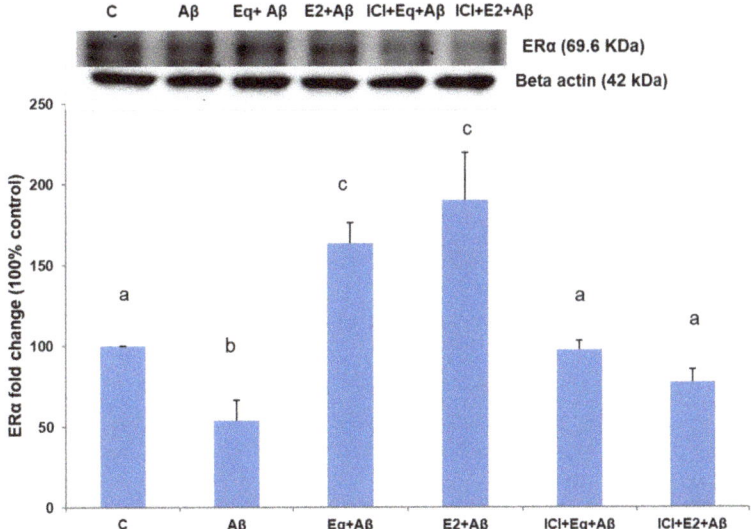

Figure 2. The estrogen receptor alpha (ERα) expressions of SH-SH5Y cells from different treatments. Data were analyzed by a one-way ANOVA followed by the LSD post-hoc test and are representative of three independent experiments ($n = 3$). Values are presented as the mean + SD. Bars with different letters are significantly different at $p < 0.05$.

3.4. Cell Cycle

Figure 4 shows the distribution of different phases of cell cycle. A significant increase of cells in the S phase in the Aβ group is observed compared to the C group as well as a concomitant reduction of cells in the G$_2$/M phases of the cycle (Figure 4). This result indicates that SH-SY5Y cells exposed to Aβ (25–35) escaped from the G$_2$/M phase. Pretreatment with either Eq (Eq + Aβ) or E2 (E2 + Aβ) showed a decreasing number of cells in the S phase and a significantly increasing number in the G$_2$/M phase compared to that in the Aβ group ($p < 0.05$). Cell cycle analysis showed that the cell cycle profiles were markedly altered by the treatment of Aβ (25–35), and pretreatment with Eq or E2 significantly blocked Aβ (25–35)-induced changes in the cell cycle profiles of the SH-SY5Y cells.

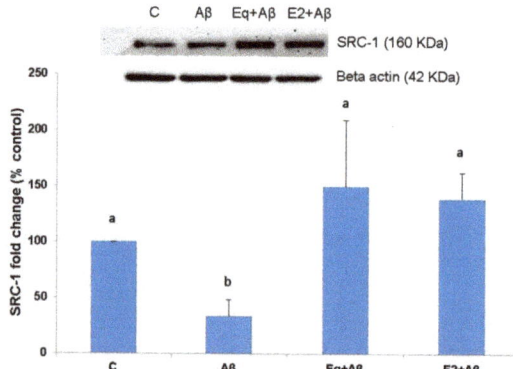

Figure 3. The SRC-1 expressions of SH-SH5Y cells from different treatments. Protein expressions were assessed by Western blotting. Data were analyzed by a one-way ANOVA followed by the LSD post-hoc test and are representative of three independent experiments ($n = 3$). Values are presented as the mean + SD. Bars with different letters are significantly different at $p < 0.05$.

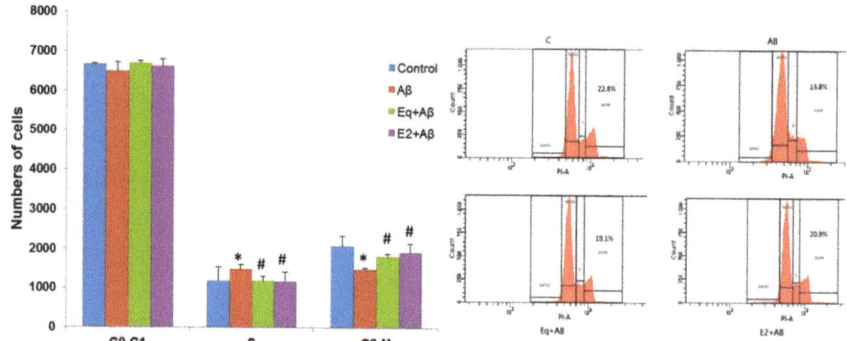

Figure 4. Cell cycle events of SH-SH5Y cells from different treatments. The cell cycle was assessed by PI staining with flow cytometry. Data were analyzed by one-way ANOVA followed by the LSD post-hoc test and are representative of three independent experiments ($n = 3$). Values are presented as the mean + SD. * $p < 0.05$ vs. the control; # $p < 0.05$ vs. the Aβ group.

3.5. Cyclin D1 Protein Expression

Figure 5 shows the relative expressions of cyclin D1, a protein marker for the G_0/G_1 phase, in different treatments. The relative expression increased markedly after cells were treated with Aβ (25–35) (Aβ group) in comparison to the untreated cells (C group). A decreased level of expression was observed in cells which underwent 24-h Eq or E2 pretreatment (Eq + Aβ group and E2 + Aβ group, respectively), compared to the Aβ group ($p < 0.05$).

3.6. Activation of ERK 1/2

Figure 6 shows that Aβ (25–35) treatment significantly increased the expression of phosphorylated (p)-ERK 1/2 ($p < 0.05$). The pretreatments of Eq and E2 significantly prevented the Aβ (25–35)-induced activation of ERK 1/2 ($p < 0.05$). On the other hand, when the ER activity was inhibited by ICI-182,780, the effect of Eq and E2 on deactivation of ERK 1/2 was significantly reduced ($p < 0.05$).

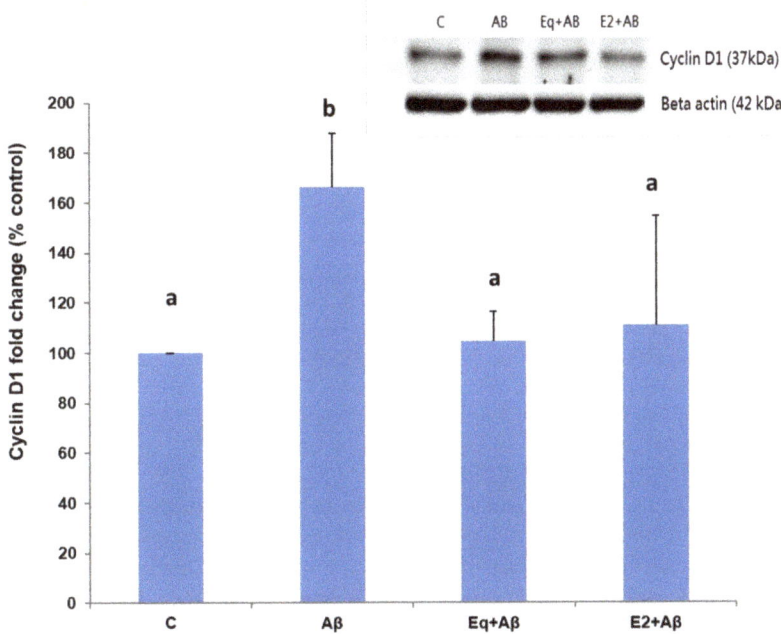

Figure 5. The cyclin D1 expressions of the SH-SH5Y cells from different treatments. Protein expressions were assessed by Western blotting. Data were analyzed by a one-way ANOVA followed by the LSD post-hoc test and are representative of three independent experiments ($n = 3$). Values are presented as the mean + SD. Bars with different letters are significantly different at $p < 0.05$.

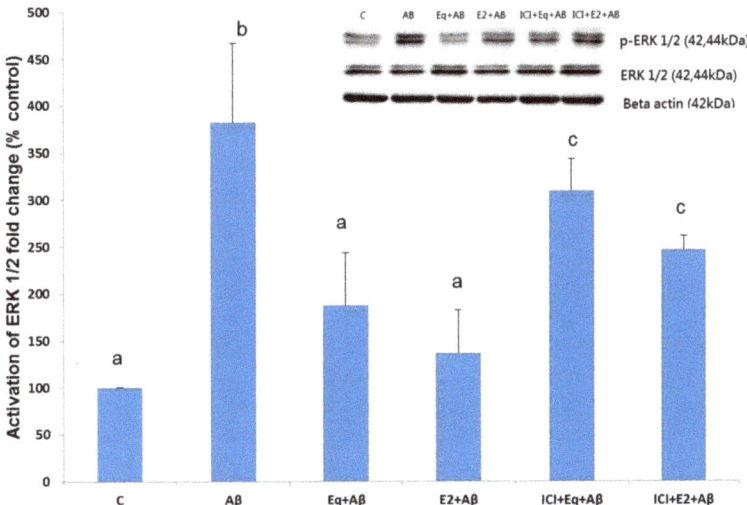

Figure 6. The phosphorylated (activated) ERK 1/2 expressions of SH-SH5Y cells from different treatments. Data were analyzed by a one-way ANOVA followed by the LSD post-hoc test and are representative of three independent experiments ($n = 3$). Values are presented as the mean + SD. Bars with different letters are significantly different at $p < 0.05$.

4. Discussion

Evidence from previous clinical and experimental studies showed that estrogen replacement therapy may have beneficial effects on AD in postmenopausal women [25,26]. However, the use of estrogen as treatment is known to have side effects, such as the development of breast and endometrial cancers in women [23]. Phytoestrogens may be an alternative treatment for AD with fewer side effects. A previous study showed that the phytoestrogen, α-zearanol, elevated the cell survival of Aβ (25–35)-induced PC-12 cells by attenuating oxidative stress and apoptotic cell death in a manner similar to 17β-estradiol [27]. In the present study, both S-equol and 17β-estradiol were also found to increase cell survival followed by Aβ (25–35) treatment. These results would predict that phytoestrogen, S-equol, possessed putative neuroprotective effects against Aβ (25–35)-induced cytotoxicity on SH-SH5Y cells analogous to those of 17β-estradiol [28,29]. In addition, the result of the inhibition of ER with antagonist ICI-182,780 prior to the Eq and E2 treatments suggested that ER may have a role in the neuroprotection of S-equol and 17β-estradiol against Aβ (25–35) cytotoxicity. The critical roles of ERs have been implicated in the cognitive function [14]. The loss of ERα expression has been noted to more likely contribute to AD-related memory impairment and amyloidogenesis [30,31]. Our observations showed the downregulation of ERα protein expression in SH-SH5Y cells exposed to Aβ (25–35) alone, emphasizing the importance of the ERα functional role in response to Aβ (25–35)-induced cytotoxicity. Under normal conditions, the ERα function can be enhanced by its coactivators, such as SRC-1, for efficient transcriptional regulation [32]. The decreased SRC-1 protein expression in the Aβ (25–35)-treated group was seen in the present study showing the Aβ (25–35)-induced disruption of the SRC-1 coactivator. These results support the notion that Aβ (25–35)-induced perturbation of ERα was further evident from the corresponding decrease in the expression of SRC-1. Furthermore, S-equol or 17β-estradiol pretreatments efficiently attenuated the effects of Aβ (25–35) in the current study, demonstrating that to provide a neuroprotective effect, equol binds with ERα and recruits SRC-1 to enhance its effect. On the other hand, the actions of both compounds were blocked by anti-estrogen ICI-182,780 in the present study, observing that ERα is required for the neuroprotective response of S-equol or 17β-estradiol to Aβ (25–35) cytotoxicity.

17β-estradiol binding to ERα is able to trigger transcriptional regulation of target genes, such as cyclin D1 [33]. In this regard, a recent study has reported that 17β-estradiol bound ERα has a role in controlling cell cycles [34]. In the present data, we presume that downregulated ERα expression in the presence of Aβ (25–35) might partially contribute to aberrant cell cycles. In normal conditions, neuron cells are postmitotic and stay in the G_0 phase, as indicated by the downregulation of proteins related to the cell cycle [35]. For instance, cyclin D1, a protein marker of the G_0/G_1 phase, is expressed at the beginning of the G1 phase and continually accumulates in the nucleus during the G1 phase in the presence of the cell cycle reactivation [36]. When the cells progress into the S phase, cyclin D1 can secrete into the cytoplasm and its overexpression can reduce cell sizes and shorten the G1 phase resulting in the accelerated entry into the S phase [37]. Likewise, our results showed that Aβ (25–35) caused cells to leave the postmitotic phase and reenter the cell cycle in parallel with the increasing level of cyclin D1. This finding is in line with previous studies which found that Aβ (25–35) toxicity induces cell-cycle reentry [9,38]. However, only a tendency toward a decrease in cell number of the G1 phase in the Aβ-treated group was observed in this study. Such observation might be ascribed to a more rapid cell cycle progression in response to a higher level of cyclin D1 followed by Aβ treatment as mentioned above. Alternatively, it is plausible that there is a high degree of variability in the G1-phase progression due to the differences in nature between cells, which indicates that the cell itself may enter into G1 or exit from G1 at different time points from its neighboring cells [39]. In presenilin (PS)-1 familial AD brains, the presence of cyclin D1 accumulation was observed to be linked to cell-cycle activation and subsequently led to cell death [40]. Our results are in accordance with previous findings showing that when exposed to 25 μM Aβ (25–35), SH-SY5Y cells accumulated in the S phase, indicating that they did not progress beyond the S phase accompanied by apoptosis [9,41]. Taken together, we speculate that changes in ERα and cyclin D1 expressions concomitantly occurring with aberrant cell cycle reentry appear likely to underlie the cytotoxic mechanisms of Aβ (25–35). Thus, apoptotic neuronal death is presumably the consequence of Aβ (25–35)-induced cytotoxicity [42]. However, it is noteworthy that more recent evidence indicates neuronal cell death triggered by a cell cycle reentry event could be independent of an apoptotic mechanism in AD [43]. More in-depth investigation is warranted to resolve this discrepancy. Nevertheless, S-equol prevented Aβ (25–35)-induced changes in the cell-cycle behavior, ERα, and cyclin D1 expressions, indicative of the neuroprotective potential of S-equol.

A common target for estrogen signaling and Aβ neurotoxicity is ERK 1/2 [9,10,44]. It was shown that ERK 1 and 2 are expressed in the pooled cerebrospinal fluid (CSF) of patients with AD, and elevated levels of ERK 1/2 in CSF are accompanied by increased levels of tau protein and the Aβ42 peptide [45]. Rapid activation of ERK 1/2 was reported in SH-SY5Y neuroblastoma cells exposed to Aβ (25–35) [9] and in mature hippocampal neurons [46]. Aberrant activation of ERK 1/2 was correlated with an elevated level of cyclin D1 that has been shown to be responsible for cell cycle reentry in neurons under Aβ-induced toxicity conditions, thereby potentiating the neuronal apoptosis responses [38]. The present data showed that Aβ (25–35) triggered ERK 1/2 activation, and pretreatments of S-equol and 17β-estradiol were able to prevent this response. In contrast, treatment with ICI-182,780 appeared to diminish the protective effects of S-equol and 17β-estradiol. These observations led us to propose that the neuroprotective mechanisms of the actions of S-equol and 17β-estradiol against Aβ (25–35) cytotoxicity might be mediated by the ERK1/2 pathways via ERα. Previous studies have shown that estrogen prevents cytotoxic effects of Aβ by activating MAPK which regulates ERK 1/2 expression and cyclin D1 to control cell cycle reentry [9,29]. Herein, we have shown that S-equol exhibited neuroprotective effects that mimicked the action of 17β-estradiol on Aβ (25–35)-treated SH-SY5Y cells through preventing cell cycle reentry downregulating cyclin D1 and ERα-mediated ERK 1/2 expressions, all of which might have involved suppression of Aβ (25–35)-induced cell cycle reentry by S-equol or 17β-estradiol pretreatments in the current study.

5. Conclusions

This study concludes that Aβ (25–35) caused diminished ERα levels, which mediated estrogen actions to disrupt normal cell cycle regulation and thus potentiates cell death. S-equol might act as a putative neuroprotective agent against Aβ (25–35) cytotoxicity, and its neuroprotective role might be, at least in part, attributed to its estrogenic potency. The observed putative neuroprotective effects of equol were associated with sustaining ERα levels and cell survival in our cell models. Furthermore, the molecular mechanism underlying this putative neuroprotection of S-equol is shown to involve the suppression of cell cycle reentry which might be synergized with ERα-involved activation of ERK 1/2 along with the prevented activation of cyclin D1.

Author Contributions: Conceptualization, M.-C.T., S.-H.L., K.H., and C.-I.L.; methodology, S-H.L., K.H., and C.-I.L.; software, S.-H.L. and K.H.; validation, M.-C.T, S-H.L., K.H., and C.-I.L.; formal analysis, S.-H.L. and K.H.; resources, M.-C.T. and S-H.L.; data curation, S.-H.L., K.H., and C.-I.L.; writing—original draft preparation, review, and editing, C.-I.L.; supervision, M.-C.T. and S.-H.L.; project administration, M.-C.T. and C.-I.L.; funding acquisition, M.-C.T.

Funding: This study was funded by the Research Program of Taoyuan General Hospital, Taiwan; grant number PTH10542.

Conflicts of Interest: The authors declare that there is no conflict of interest regarding the publication of this paper.

References

1. Nagy, Z. Cell cycle regulatory failure in neurones: Causes and consequences. *Neurobiol. Aging* **2000**, *21*, 761–769. [CrossRef]
2. Frade, J.M.; Ovejero-Benito, M.C. Neuronal cell cycle: The neuron itself and its circumstances. *Cell Cycle* **2015**, *14*, 712–720. [CrossRef] [PubMed]
3. Herrup, K. The involvement of cell cycle events in the pathogenesis of Alzheimer's disease. *Alzheimer's Res. Ther.* **2010**, *2*, 13. [CrossRef] [PubMed]

4. Querfurth, H.W.; LaFerla, F.M. Alzheimer's disease. *N. Engl. J. Med.* **2010**, *362*, 329–344. [CrossRef] [PubMed]
5. Clementi, M.E.; Marini, S.; Coletta, M.; Orsini, F.; Giardina, B.; Misiti, F. Abeta(31–35) and Abeta(25–35) fragments of amyloid beta-protein induce cellular death through apoptotic signals: Role of the redox state of methionine-35. *FEBS Lett.* **2005**, *579*, 2913–2918. [CrossRef] [PubMed]
6. Wang, J.; Zhang, Y.J.; Du, S. The protective effect of curcumin on Abeta induced aberrant cell cycle reentry on primary cultured rat cortical neurons. *Eur. Rev. Med. Pharmacol. Sci.* **2012**, *16*, 445–454. [PubMed]
7. Frasca, G.; Carbonaro, V.; Merlo, S.; Copani, A.; Sortino, M.A. Integrins mediate beta-amyloid-induced cell-cycle activation and neuronal death. *J. Neurosci. Res.* **2008**, *86*, 350–355. [CrossRef] [PubMed]
8. Mebratu, Y.; Tesfaigzi, Y. How ERK1/2 activation controls cell proliferation and cell death: Is subcellular localization the answer? *Cell Cycle* **2009**, *8*, 1168–1175. [CrossRef]
9. Frasca, G.; Chiechio, S.; Vancheri, C.; Nicoletti, F.; Copani, A.; Angela Sortino, M. Beta-amyloid-activated cell cycle in SH-SY5Y neuroblastoma cells: Correlation with the MAP kinase pathway. *J. Mol. Neurosci.* **2004**, *22*, 231–236. [CrossRef]
10. Mannella, P.; Brinton, R.D. Estrogen receptor protein interaction with phosphatidylinositol 3-kinase leads to activation of phosphorylated Akt and extracellular signal-regulated kinase 1/2 in the same population of cortical neurons: A unified mechanism of estrogen action. *J. Neurosci.* **2006**, *26*, 9439–9447. [CrossRef]
11. Paterni, I.; Granchi, C.; Katzenellenbogen, J.A.; Minutolo, F. Estrogen receptors alpha (ERalpha) and beta (ERbeta): Subtype-selective ligands and clinical potential. *Steroids* **2014**, *90*, 13–29. [CrossRef] [PubMed]
12. Jung, M.E.; Gatch, M.B.; Simpkins, J.W. Estrogen neuroprotection against the neurotoxic effects of ethanol withdrawal: Potential mechanisms. *Exp. Biol. Med.* **2005**, *230*, 8–22. [CrossRef] [PubMed]
13. Foster, T.C. Role of estrogen receptor alpha and beta expression and signaling on cognitive function during aging. *Hippocampus* **2012**, *22*, 656–669. [CrossRef] [PubMed]
14. Bean, L.A.; Ianov, L.; Foster, T.C. Estrogen receptors, the hippocampus, and memory. *Neuroscientist* **2014**, *20*, 534–545. [CrossRef] [PubMed]
15. Carroll, J.C.; Pike, C.J. Selective estrogen receptor modulators differentially regulate Alzheimer-like changes in female 3xTg-AD mice. *Endocrinology* **2008**, *149*, 2607–2611. [CrossRef]
16. Zhao, L.; Wu, T.W.; Brinton, R.D. Estrogen receptor subtypes alpha and beta contribute to neuroprotection and increased Bcl-2 expression in primary hippocampal neurons. *Brain Res.* **2004**, *1010*, 22–34. [CrossRef]
17. Kim, H.; Bang, O.Y.; Jung, M.W.; Ha, S.D.; Hong, H.S.; Huh, K.; Kim, S.U.; Mook-Jung, I. Neuroprotective effects of estrogen against beta-amyloid toxicity are mediated by estrogen receptors in cultured neuronal cells. *Neurosci. Lett.* **2001**, *302*, 58–62. [CrossRef]
18. Wang, C.; Zhang, F.; Jiang, S.; Siedlak, S.L.; Shen, L.; Perry, G.; Wang, X.; Tang, B.; Zhu, X. Estrogen receptor-alpha is localized to neurofibrillary tangles in Alzheimer's disease. *Sci. Rep.* **2016**, *6*, 20352. [CrossRef]
19. Gonzalez-Arenas, A.; Hansberg-Pastor, V.; Hernandez-Hernandez, O.T.; Gonzalez-Garcia, T.K.; Henderson-Villalpando, J.; Lemus-Hernandez, D.; Cruz-Barrios, A.; Rivas-Suarez, M.; Camacho-Arroyo, I. Estradiol increases cell growth in human astrocytoma cell lines through ERalpha activation and its interaction with SRC-1 and SRC-3 coactivators. *Biochim. Biophys. Acta* **2012**, *1823*, 379–386. [CrossRef]
20. Mueller, S.O.; Simon, S.; Chae, K.; Metzler, M.; Korach, K.S. Phytoestrogens and their human metabolites show distinct agonistic and antagonistic properties on estrogen receptor alpha (ERalpha) and ERbeta in human cells. *Toxicol. Sci.* **2004**, *80*, 14–25. [CrossRef]
21. Setchell, K.D.; Clerici, C. Equol: Pharmacokinetics and biological actions. *J. Nutr.* **2010**, *140*, 1363s–1368s. [CrossRef] [PubMed]
22. Setchell, K.D.; Zhao, X.; Shoaf, S.E.; Ragland, K. The pharmacokinetics of S-(-)equol administered as SE5-OH tablets to healthy postmenopausal women. *J. Nutr.* **2009**, *139*, 2037–2043. [CrossRef] [PubMed]
23. Morabito, N.; Crisafulli, A.; Vergara, C.; Gaudio, A.; Lasco, A.; Frisina, N.; D'Anna, R.; Corrado, F.; Pizzoleo, M.A.; Cincotta, M.; et al. Effects of genistein and hormone-replacement therapy on bone loss in early postmenopausal women: A randomized double-blind placebo-controlled study. *J. Bone Miner. Res.* **2002**, *17*, 1904–1912. [CrossRef] [PubMed]
24. Subedi, L.; Ji, E.; Shin, D.; Jin, J.; Yeo, J.H.; Kim, S.Y. Equol, a Dietary Daidzein Gut Metabolite Attenuates Microglial Activation and Potentiates Neuroprotection In Vitro. *Nutrients* **2017**, *9*, 207. [CrossRef]
25. Merlo, S.; Spampinato, S.F.; Sortino, M.A. Estrogen and Alzheimer's disease: Still an attractive topic despite disappointment from early clinical results. *Eur. J. Pharmacol.* **2017**, *817*, 51–58. [CrossRef]

26. Christensen, A.; Pike, C.J. Age-dependent regulation of obesity and Alzheimer-related outcomes by hormone therapy in female 3xTg-AD mice. *PLoS ONE* **2017**, *12*, e0178490. [CrossRef]
27. Dong, Y.; Yang, N.; Liu, Y.; Li, Q.; Zuo, P. The neuroprotective effects of phytoestrogen alpha-zearalanol on beta-amyloid-induced toxicity in differentiated PC-12 cells. *Eur. J. Pharmacol.* **2011**, *670*, 392–398. [CrossRef]
28. Zhao, L.; Mao, Z.; Brinton, R.D. A select combination of clinically relevant phytoestrogens enhances estrogen receptor beta-binding selectivity and neuroprotective activities in vitro and in vivo. *Endocrinology* **2009**, *150*, 770–783. [CrossRef]
29. Valles, S.L.; Borras, C.; Gambini, J.; Furriol, J.; Ortega, A.; Sastre, J.; Pallardo, F.V.; Vina, J. Oestradiol or genistein rescues neurons from amyloid beta-induced cell death by inhibiting activation of p38. *Aging Cell* **2008**, *7*, 112–118. [CrossRef]
30. Hwang, C.J.; Yun, H.M.; Park, K.R.; Song, J.K.; Seo, H.O.; Hyun, B.K.; Choi, D.Y.; Yoo, H.S.; Oh, K.W.; Hwang, D.Y.; et al. Memory Impairment in Estrogen Receptor alpha Knockout Mice Through Accumulation of Amyloid-beta Peptides. *Mol. Neurobiol.* **2015**, *52*, 176–186. [CrossRef]
31. Tang, Y.; Min, Z.; Xiang, X.J.; Liu, L.; Ma, Y.L.; Zhu, B.L.; Song, L.; Tang, J.; Deng, X.J.; Yan, Z.; et al. Estrogen-related receptor alpha is involved in Alzheimer's disease-like pathology. *Exp. Neurol.* **2018**, *305*, 89–96. [CrossRef] [PubMed]
32. Tetel, M.J.; Acharya, K.D. Nuclear receptor coactivators: Regulators of steroid action in brain and behaviour. *J. Neuroendocrinol.* **2013**, *25*, 1209–1218. [CrossRef]
33. Cicatiello, L.; Addeo, R.; Sasso, A.; Altucci, L.; Petrizzi, V.B.; Borgo, R.; Cancemi, M.; Caporali, S.; Caristi, S.; Scafoglio, C.; et al. Estrogens and progesterone promote persistent CCND1 gene activation during G1 by inducing transcriptional derepression via c-Jun/c-Fos/estrogen receptor (progesterone receptor) complex assembly to a distal regulatory element and recruitment of cyclin D1 to its own gene promoter. *Mol. Cell. Biol.* **2004**, *24*, 7260–7274. [CrossRef] [PubMed]
34. JavanMoghadam, S.; Weihua, Z.; Hunt, K.K.; Keyomarsi, K. Estrogen receptor alpha is cell cycle-regulated and regulates the cell cycle in a ligand-dependent fashion. *Cell Cycle* **2016**, *15*, 1579–1590. [CrossRef] [PubMed]
35. Negis, Y.; Unal, A.Y.; Korulu, S.; Karabay, A. Cell cycle markers have different expression and localization patterns in neuron-like PC12 cells and primary hippocampal neurons. *Neurosci. Lett.* **2011**, *496*, 135–140. [CrossRef]
36. Sumrejkanchanakij, P.; Tamamori-Adachi, M.; Matsunaga, Y.; Eto, K.; Ikeda, M.A. Role of cyclin D1 cytoplasmic sequestration in the survival of postmitotic neurons. *Oncogene* **2003**, *22*, 8723–8730. [CrossRef]
37. Quelle, D.E.; Ashmun, R.A.; Shurtleff, S.A.; Kato, J.Y.; Bar-Sagi, D.; Roussel, M.F.; Sherr, C.J. Overexpression of mouse D-type cyclins accelerates G1 phase in rodent fibroblasts. *Genes Dev.* **1993**, *7*, 1559–1571. [CrossRef]
38. Modi, P.K.; Komaravelli, N.; Singh, N.; Sharma, P. Interplay between MEK-ERK signaling, cyclin D1, and cyclin-dependent kinase 5 regulates cell cycle reentry and apoptosis of neurons. *Mol. Biol. Cell* **2012**, *23*, 3722–3730. [CrossRef]
39. Jackman, J.; O'Connor, P.M. Methods for synchronizing cells at specific stages of the cell cycle. *Curr. Protoc. Cell Biol.* **2001**. [CrossRef]
40. Malik, B.; Currais, A.; Andres, A.; Towlson, C.; Pitsi, D.; Nunes, A.; Niblock, M.; Cooper, J.; Hortobagyi, T.; Soriano, S. Loss of neuronal cell cycle control as a mechanism of neurodegeneration in the presenilin-1 Alzheimer's disease brain. *Cell Cycle* **2008**, *7*, 637–646. [CrossRef]
41. Copani, A.; Condorelli, F.; Caruso, A.; Vancheri, C.; Sala, A.; Giuffrida Stella, A.M.; Canonico, P.L.; Nicoletti, F.; Sortino, M.A. Mitotic signaling by beta-amyloid causes neuronal death. *FASEB J.* **1999**, *13*, 2225–2234. [CrossRef] [PubMed]
42. Millucci, L.; Ghezzi, L.; Bernardini, G.; Santucci, A. Conformations and biological activities of amyloid beta peptide 25–35. *Curr. Protein Pept. Sci.* **2010**, *11*, 54–67. [CrossRef] [PubMed]
43. Barrio-Alonso, E.; Hernandez-Vivanco, A.; Walton, C.C. Cell cycle reentry triggers hyperploidization and synaptic dysfunction followed by delayed cell death in differentiated cortical neurons. *Sci. Rep.* **2018**, *8*, 14316. [CrossRef] [PubMed]
44. Fitzpatrick, J.L.; Mize, A.L.; Wade, C.B.; Harris, J.A.; Shapiro, R.A.; Dorsa, D.M. Estrogen-mediated neuroprotection against beta-amyloid toxicity requires expression of estrogen receptor alpha or beta and activation of the MAPK pathway. *J. Neurochem.* **2002**, *82*, 674–682. [CrossRef] [PubMed]

45. Spitzer, P.; Schieb, H.; Kamrowski-Kruck, H.; Otto, M.; Chiasserini, D.; Parnetti, L.; Herukka, S.K.; Schuchhardt, J.; Wiltfang, J.; Klafki, H.W. Evidence for Elevated Cerebrospinal Fluid ERK1/2 Levels in Alzheimer Dementia. *Int. J. Alzheimer's Dis.* **2011**, *2011*, 739847. [CrossRef] [PubMed]
46. Rapoport, M.; Ferreira, A. PD98059 prevents neurite degeneration induced by fibrillar beta-amyloid in mature hippocampal neurons. *J. Neurochem.* **2000**, *74*, 125–133. [CrossRef]

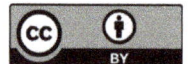

© 2019 by the authors. Licensee MDPI, Basel, Switzerland. This article is an open access article distributed under the terms and conditions of the Creative Commons Attribution (CC BY) license (http://creativecommons.org/licenses/by/4.0/).

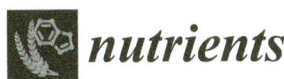

Article

Serine Phosphorylation of IRS1 Correlates with Aβ-Unrelated Memory Deficits and Elevation in Aβ Level Prior to the Onset of Memory Decline in AD

Wei Wang [1,†], Daisuke Tanokashira [1,†], Yusuke Fukui [1], Megumi Maruyama [1], Chiemi Kuroiwa [1], Takashi Saito [2,3], Takaomi C. Saido [2] and Akiko Taguchi [1,*]

1. Department of Integrative Aging Neuroscience, National Center for Geriatrics and Gerontology, Obu, Aichi 474-8511, Japan
2. Laboratory for Proteolytic Neuroscience, RIKEN Center for Brain Science, Wako, Saitama 351-0106, Japan
3. Department of Neurocognitive Science, Nagoya City University Graduate School of Medical Science, Nagoya, Aichi 467-8601, Japan
* Correspondence: taguchia@ncgg.go.jp; Tel.: +81-562-46-2311
† These authors contributed equally.

Received: 23 July 2019; Accepted: 14 August 2019; Published: 17 August 2019

Abstract: The biological effects of insulin signaling are regulated by the phosphorylation of insulin receptor substrate 1 (IRS1) at serine (Ser) residues. In the brain, phosphorylation of IRS1 at specific Ser sites increases in patients with Alzheimer's disease (AD) and its animal models. However, whether the activation of Ser sites on neural IRS1 is related to any type of memory decline remains unclear. Here, we show the modifications of IRS1 through its phosphorylation at etiology-specific Ser sites in various animal models of memory decline, such as diabetic, aged, and amyloid precursor protein (APP) knock-in $^{\text{NL-G-F}}$ (APPKI$^{\text{NL-G-F}}$) mice. Substantial phosphorylation of IRS1 at specific Ser sites occurs in type 2 diabetes- or age-related memory deficits independently of amyloid-β (Aβ). Furthermore, we present the first evidence that, in APPKI$^{\text{NL-G-F}}$ mice showing Aβ42 elevation, the increased phosphorylation of IRS1 at multiple Ser sites occurs without memory impairment. Our findings suggest that the phosphorylation of IRS1 at specific Ser sites is a potential marker of Aβ-unrelated memory deficits caused by type 2 diabetes and aging; however, in Aβ-related memory decline, the modifications of IRS1 may be a marker of early detection of Aβ42 elevation prior to the onset of memory decline in AD.

Keywords: IRS1; serine phosphorylation; hippocampus; diabetes; aging; Alzheimer's disease; memory decline; Aβ; AMPK; energy depletion

1. Introduction

Insulin signaling mediated by insulin receptor substrates 1 and 2 (IRS1 and IRS2) is involved in the regulation of growth, glucose homeostasis, energy metabolism, and lifespan [1–4]. The biological effects of insulin signaling are regulated by the modulation of IRS proteins through serine (Ser) and threonine (Thr) phosphorylation [5,6]. Notably, IRS1 is known to be abundantly phosphorylated at Ser and Thr residues regardless of insulin or IGF1 stimulation [5,7]. In vitro studies have demonstrated the relationship between IRS1 Ser/Thr phosphorylation and canonical downstream signaling components, including Akt/protein kinase B, glycogen synthase kinase 3 beta (GSK3β), and ribosomal protein S6 kinase (S6K) [5]. Under physiological and pathological conditions, Ser/Thr phosphorylation of IRS1 is potentially mediated by multiple kinases, including AMP-activated protein kinase (AMPK), conventional and novel protein kinase C (PKC), and c-Jun N-terminal kinases (JNKs), in response to intracellular energy status, nutritional conditions, and inflammatory stimulation [5,6,8].

Among the numerous Ser residues on IRS1, a few sites, including human(h)Ser312/mouse(m)Ser307, hSer616/mSer612, hSer636/mSer632, hSer639/mSer635, and hSer1101/mSer1097, have been studied because a limited number of phosphospecific antibodies were previously commercially available.

Nonetheless, hSer312/mSer307 has been widely investigated and implicated in insulin resistance under metabolic stress conditions and in inflammatory conditions such as obesity, hyperinsulinemia, and dyslipidemia [5,9,10]. However, IRS1 mSer307 knock-in mice display insulin resistance rather than increased insulin sensitivity, suggesting that IRS1 mSer307 is a positive regulatory site and is essential for normal insulin signaling [11]. IRS1 mSer612 and mSer632/635 have been cited as negative regulatory sites for IRS1 signaling through tyrosine phosphorylation [5], and mSer1097, regarded as a potential mammalian target of rapamycin (mTOR) /S6K signaling pathway, is activated in the liver of model animals of obesity [12]. However, the roles of these sites remain largely unknown because they have been examined in different context.

In the central nervous system, studies on postmortem brain tissues of patients with Alzheimer's disease (AD) have revealed increased phosphorylation of IRS1 at hSer312/mSer307, hSer616/mSer612, hSer636/mSer632, and hSer639/mSer635 compared with that in non-AD control subjects [13–16]. The phosphorylation levels of IRS1 at hSer312/mSer307 and hSer616/mSer612 are considerably elevated in the brains of patients with AD [15]. In animal studies, multiple AD mouse models display increased phosphorylation of IRS1 at mSer307 and/or mSer632 or mSer612 [16–18]. However, whether the modifications of IRS1 via Ser phosphorylation are involved in memory decline in amyloid precursor protein (APP) knock-in (KI)$^{NL-G-F}$ (APPKI^{NL-G-F}) mice, a novel AD mouse model, remains unclear [19]. Meanwhile, animals with diet-induced obesity (DIO), a model of type 2 diabetes mellitus (T2DM), that were fed a 40% or 60% high-fat diet (HFD) during different periods displayed cognitive impairment accompanied by increased phosphorylation of neural IRS1 at different Ser residues (mSer1097, mSer307, or mSer612) at different ages [20–22]. Few studies have reported the relationship between streptozotocin (STZ)-induced type 1 diabetes-related cognitive impairment and phosphorylation of neural IRS1 at Ser sites. Similarly, in aged animals, the phosphorylation of IRS1 at mSer307 has been shown to increase in the cortex; however, whether this alteration is correlated with age-related decline in cognitive function has not been explored [23].

In the present study, we investigated whether the modification of hippocampal IRS1 by Ser phosphorylation is commonly associated with different types of memory decline in DIO, STZ, aged, and APPKI^{NL-G-F} mice and whether it occurs before or after the onset of memory decline in APPKI^{NL-G-F} mice. We demonstrate that the concomitant activation of specific Ser sites on hippocampal IRS1 with amyloid-β (Aβ)-unrelated memory decline occurs in DIO and aged mice, whereas STZ mice exhibit memory deficits independent of IRS1 activity. We further show that increased phosphorylation of hippocampal IRS1 at Ser sites is already observed in young APPKI^{NL-G-F} mice showing normal memory function despite increased Aβ42 level. These data suggest that the activation of Ser residues on hippocampal IRS1 is associated with non-AD-related memory impairment in T2DM and aging and with Aβ42 level, which is related to the onset of cognitive decline in AD.

2. Materials and Methods

2.1. Animals

C57BL/6J male mice (4 weeks of age) supplied by Japan SLC, Inc. (Shizuoka, Japan) were used to establish type 1 and 2 diabetes mellitus (T1DM, T2DM) mice and their respective control mice. Generation of high-fat-diet (HFD)-induced type 2 diabetes mice (DIO mice) was carried out as previously described [20]. Briefly, C57BL/6J mice were assigned to control wild-type (WT) mice] and HFD (DIO mice) groups, and were fed a normal diet (CE-2; CLEA Japan Inc., Tokyo, Japan) or a HFD (D12492, 60% kcal from fat; Research Diets, Inc., New Brunswick, NJ, USA) for 32 weeks, respectively. To generate Streptozotocin (STZ)-induced type 1 diabetes mice (STZ mice), eight-week-old C57BL/6J mice were intraperitoneally administered with 150 mg/kg STZ (Wako Pure Chemical Industries, Ltd.,

Osaka, Japan) dissolved in sodium citrate (pH 4.5) after overnight fasting, and control mice were injected with the sodium citrate buffer alone. Young and aged WT male mice, which were all pure C57BL/6J strains, were purchased from Charles River Inc., Kanagawa, Japan, or/and bred within our animal facility. APPKI$^{NL\text{-}G\text{-}F}$ (Swedish (NL), Arctic (G), and Beyreuther/Iberian (F) mutations) homozygous mice were obtained from Dr. Saido at the Laboratory for Proteolytic Neuroscience, RIKEN Brain Science Institute, Saitama, Japan [19]. Age-matched WT mice of a similar strain (C57BL/6J) were used in the control experiments. All experiments were performed using DIO, STZ, and young and middle-aged APPKI$^{NL\text{-}G\text{-}F}$ mice, and their respective age-matched control mice (DIO mice: 34–36 weeks, WT mice: 34–36 weeks; STZ mice: 10 weeks, WT mice: 10 weeks; young APPKI$^{NL\text{-}G\text{-}F}$ mice: 12 weeks, WT mice: 12 weeks; middle-aged APPKI$^{NL\text{-}G\text{-}F}$ mice: 34–36 weeks, WT mice: 34–36 weeks; young WT mice: 8–13 weeks, aged WT mice: 84 weeks). All mice were housed in a standard 12 h light–dark cycle with free access to water and food (room temperature: 25 ± 2 °C). Animal experiments were performed in compliance with the guidelines and with the approval of the ethics committee in Animal Care and Use of the National Center for Geriatrics and Gerontology in Obu, Aichi, Japan (Approval ID: 31-5).

2.2. Western Blotting

The protocol of western blotting used has been previously described [20]. In brief, hippocampal tissue was isolated on ice and homogenized in lysis buffer with a pellet mixer. The aliquot of hippocampal lysates was boiled for 5 min in Laemmli sodium dodecyl sulfate (SDS) sample buffer [60 mm Tris-Cl (pH 6.8), 2% sodium dodecyl sulfate, 10% glycerol, 4% β-mercaptoethanol, and 0.01% bromophenol blue]. A total of 10 μg of each SDS protein sample was loaded per lane, separated by 7.5% sodium dodecyl sulfate polyacrylamide gel electrophoresis (SDS-PAGE), and transferred to polyvinylidene difluoride membranes. Membranes were blocked using 4% Block Ace (Yukijirushi Ltd., Sapporo, Japan), incubated with the indicated primary antibodies, followed by incubation with horseradish peroxidase-conjugated secondary antibodies. Primary antibodies were rabbit anti-phospho-IRS1 [mouse Ser307/human Ser312 (mSer307/hSer312), mouse Ser612/human Ser616 (mSer612/hSer616), mouse Ser632/Ser635/human Ser636/Ser639 (mSer632/Ser635/hSer636/hSer639), mouse Ser1097/human Ser1101 (mSer1097/hSer1101)] (1:500; Cell Signaling Technology(CST)), rabbit anti-IRS1 (1:1000; CST), rabbit anti-phospho-Akt (Ser473) (1:1000; CST), rabbit anti-Akt (1:1000; CST), rabbit anti-phospho-p70S6K (Thr389) (1:1000; CST), rabbit anti-p70S6K (1:1000; CST), rabbit anti-phospho-AMPK (Thr172) (1:1000; CST), rabbit anti-AMPK (1:1000; CST), rabbit anti-phospho-GSK3β (Ser9)(1:1000; CST), rabbit anti-GSK3β (Ser9) (1:1000; CST), rabbit anti-phospho-JNK (Thr183/Tyr185) (1:1000; CST), rabbit anti-JNK (1:1000; CST), rabbit anti-phospho-aPKCζ/λ(Thr410/Thr403) (1:1000; CST), rabbit anti-aPKCζ/λ(1:1000; CST), and rabbit anti-β-tubulin (1:1000; CST). Immunodetection was performed with horseradish peroxidase-conjugated secondary antibodies (1:2000; CST) and chemiluminescence detection reagent Chemi-Lumi one L (Nacalai tesque, Kyoto, Japan) or the ImmunoStar LD (Fujifilm Wako Pure Chemical Corporation Japan, Osaka, Japan). The images were scanned using the Amersham Imager 680 (GE Healthcare UK Ltd., Little Chalfont, Buckinghamshire HP7 9NA, England).

2.3. Water T Maze Test

Hippocampal-dependent spatial memory was tested using a water T maze [24,25] according to our previous report [20]. The maze consisted of a start box, a left arm, and a right arm, which was filled with water at 23 ± 1 °C up to 1 cm above the surface of the platform. Mice were allowed to swim to the right or left arm. This screening step was repeated three times at 15 s intervals. The platform was placed on the side that the mice reached less often. After the screening step, mice were allowed to explore the maze freely. If mice reached the platform, they were allowed to rest there for 5 s (correct choice). If not, the arm entry was closed with a board and they were forced to swim for 15 s as a deterrent (incorrect choice). This trial step was repeated five times at 4-min intervals. Mice were subjected to this trial step for five days. To evaluate the results of the trial, the percentage of correct responses per day was determined. After two days of rest, to test hippocampal and prefrontal cortex (PFC)-dependent working memory, the platform was moved to the opposite arm. Similarly, mice were allowed to explore the maze freely. The trial step was repeated 15 times at 4-min intervals in a day. To evaluate the results of the trial, the percentage of the correct responses were calculated after every three responses.

2.4. Measurement of Metabolic Parameters

Body weight and the blood glucose levels were recorded after 6 h of fasting. Blood glucose levels were measured using a portable glucose meter (ACCU-CHEK® Aviva; Roche DC Japan K.K.). The level of plasma insulin at 6 h fasting was determined using an insulin enzyme-linked immunosorbent assay kit (Morinaga, Yokohama, Japan).

2.5. Enzyme-Linked Immunosorbent Assay (ELISA) Quantitation of Aβ

In order to measure the Aβ levels in the hippocampus, hippocampal tissue was isolated on ice and homogenized in a lysis buffer (T-PER® Tissue Protein Extraction Reagent; Thermo Fisher Scientific, Waltham, MA, USA) containing a protease inhibitor cocktail (Nacalai Tesque, Kyoto, Japan) and a phosphatase inhibitor cocktail (Nacalai Tesque) with a pellet mixer. After incubation on ice for 15 min, the lysates were centrifuged at $14,200 \times g$ for 5 min at 4 °C and the supernatants were placed in a fresh tube. Protein concentration was determined using a Bicinchoninic acid (BCA) protein assay kit (Thermo Fisher Scientific, Waltham, MA, USA). The levels of T-PER-extractable Aβ were measured with the Human β Amyloid (1–40) enzyme-linked immunosorbent assay (ELISA) Kit Wako II (#298-64601; Fujifilm Wako Pure Chemical Corp., Osaka, Japan), the Human β Amyloid (1–42) ELISA Kit Wako, High Sensitivity (#296-64401, Fujifilm Wako Pure Chemical Corp.), the Human/Rat/Mouse β Amyloid (1–40) ELISA Kit Wako II (#294-64701; Fujifilm Wako Pure Chemical Corp., Osaka, Japan), and the Human/Rat/Mouse β Amyloid (1–42) ELISA Kit Wako, High Sensitivity (#292-64501, Fujifilm Wako Pure Chemical Corp.) in accordance with the manufacturers' instructions.

2.6. Statistics

All results are presented as mean ± standard error of the mean (SEM) in the text. Statistical analyses were performed using Prism7 for Mac OS X v.7.0d (GrapPad Software Inc., La Jolla, CA, USA). Data were statistically analyzed using Student's *t*-test and two-way analysis of variance (ANOVA). Significance is indicated as * $p < 0.05$ and ** $p < 0.01$.

3. Results

3.1. Activation of Specific Ser Residues on Hippocampal Insulin Receptor Substrate 1 (IRS1) Is Associated with T2DM-Induced Memory Impairment

We recently reported that T2DM-related cognitive declines in 45-week-old DIO mice fed a 60% HFD for 42 weeks were accompanied by an increased phosphorylation of hippocampal IRS1 at mSer1097 [20]. While mice fed a 60% HFD for 17 days and mice or rats fed a 40% HFD for 6–8 weeks exhibited memory impairment accompanied by increased phosphorylation at hSer616/mSer612 or hSer312/mSer307 [21,22], 12-week-old DIO mice fed a 60% HFD for 9 weeks exhibited normal memory function under our experimental conditions (Figure S1), suggesting that changes in neural IRS1 Ser residues are variable on a temporal scale in DIO mice. Therefore, we investigated the phosphorylation levels of hippocampal IRS1 at Ser sites and the activities of downstream factors involved in memory impairment in 35-week-old (middle-aged) DIO mice fed a 60% HFD for 32 weeks (Figure 1A,C). At 35 weeks of age, DIO mice displayed significant weight gain, hyperglycemia, and hyperinsulinemia (Figure 1B, Figure S2A), as observed at other time points [20–22,26].

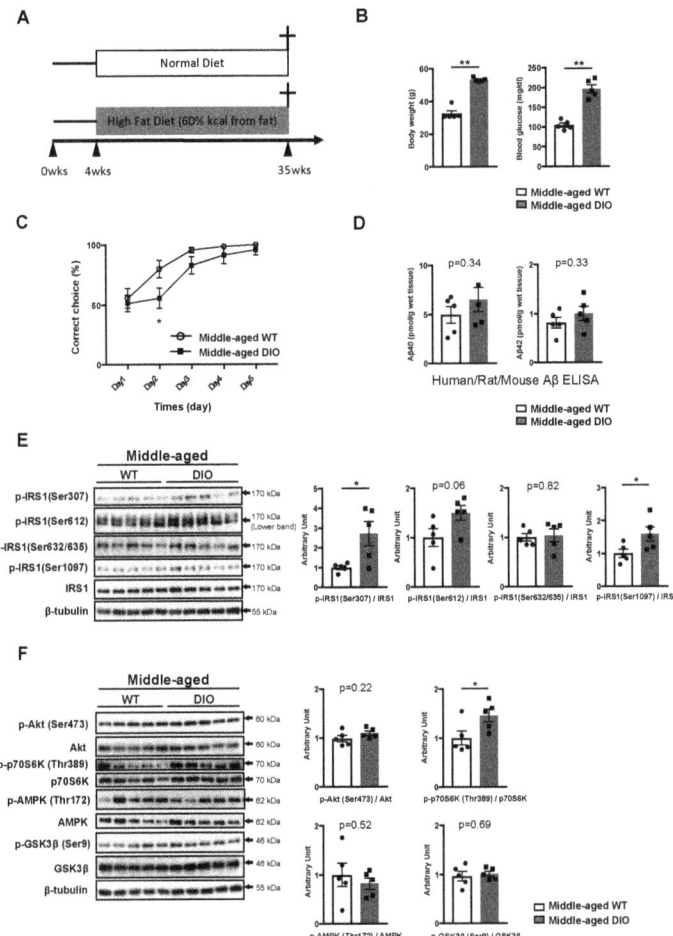

Figure 1. Changes in specific Ser sites on hippocampal insulin receptor substrate 1 (IRS1) in type 2 diabetes (T2DM)-induced memory impairment. (**A**) Schematic diagram of the experimental procedure. (**B**) Graphs of body weight and blood glucose level in wild-type (WT) and diet-induced obesity (DIO) mice (35 weeks of age, n = 5 mice per group). (**C**) Evaluation of learning memory function in middle-aged WT and DIO mice (n = 14 mice per group) using the water T-maze test. (**D**) Quantitative analysis of T-PER (Tissue Protein Extraction Reagent)-extractable Aβ40 and Aβ42 levels in the hippocampi of middle-aged WT and DIO mice using the human/rat/mouse β amyloid (1–40 and 1–42) enzyme-linked immunosorbent assay (ELISA) (35 weeks of age, n = 5 biologically independent samples per group). (**E**) Western blot analysis of phosphorylated insulin receptor substrates 1 mouse Ser307 [p-IRS1 (mSer307)], p-IRS1 (mSer612), p-IRS1 (mSer632/635), p-IRS1 (mSer1097), IRS1, and β-tubulin in the hippocampi of middle-aged WT and DIO mice (35 weeks of age, n = 5 biologically independent samples per group). Arrow indicates the p-IRS1 mSer612-corresponding band (lower band) in (**E**). Quantitative analysis of the phosphorylation of IRS1 at mSer307, mSer612, mSer632/635, and mSer1097 normalized to total protein. (**F**) Western blot analysis of phosphorylation levels of Akt Ser473, p70S6K Thr389, AMP-activated protein kinase (AMPK) Thr172, and glycogen synthase kinase 3 beta (GSK3β) Ser9 as well as total protein levels of Akt, p70 S6K, AMPK, GSK3β, and ß-tubulin in the hippocampi of middle-aged WT and DIO mice (35 weeks of age, n = 5 biologically independent samples per group). Quantitative analysis of the phosphorylation of Akt Ser473, p70S6K Thr389, AMPK Thr172, and GSK3β Ser9 normalized to the respective total protein contents. Results are presented as mean ± standard error of the mean (SEM), * $p < 0.05$; ** $p < 0.01$.

Furthermore, we examined whether memory impairment in middle-aged DIO mice is linked to increased levels of Aβ42, a pathological feature of AD. Biochemical analysis with specific kits (see Materials and Methods) demonstrated that, compared with age-matched wild-type (WT) mice, there was no change in Aβ40 and Aβ42 levels in the T-PER fractions obtained from the hippocampi of 35-week-old DIO mice (Figure 1D).

In contrast to DIO mice at 45 weeks of age, the phosphorylation of IRS1 at mSer307, which increases in insulin resistance, diabetes, and obesity [5], with phosphorylation at mSer1097 significantly increased in the hippocampus of DIO mice at 35 weeks of age, although there were no significant differences in phosphorylation at mSer612 and mSer632/635 between DIO and age-matched WT mice (Figure 1E, Figure S4A). Consistent with previous studies [27,28], the basal phosphorylation level of p70S6K slightly but significantly increased in the hippocampus of middle-aged DIO mice compared with that in the hippocampus of age-matched WT mice, whereas the basal phosphorylation of Akt and GSK3β and activation of AMPK and atypical protein kinase C ζ/λ (aPKC ζ/λ), downstream factors of insulin signaling, in the hippocampus were comparable between middle-aged WT and DIO mice (Figure 1F, Figures S3A, S4B and S5A). Additionally, the basal phosphorylation of JNK, an inflammation- and stress-related factor, remained unchanged in the hippocampus between the two groups (Figures S3A and S5A), although a relationship between the phosphorylation of IRS1 at mSer307 and activation of these factors in yeast cells, culture cells, and muscles has been reported [5]. These results indicate that T2DM-induced memory decline is provoked by an Aβ-independent mechanism and that the concomitant activation of IRS1 mSer307 and mSer1097 with p70S6K activation in the hippocampus is associated with memory deficits in 35-week-old DIO mice.

3.2. Type 1 Diabetes Mellitus (T1DM)-Induced Memory Deficits Occur Independently of IRS1 Activity

To investigate whether the alteration of IRS1 through Ser phosphorylation is associated with type 1 diabetes mellitus (T1DM)-induced memory deficits, we generated STZ-induced insulin-deficient T1DM mice. Two weeks after STZ injection, STZ mice exhibited weight loss, elevated blood glucose levels (>400 mg/dL), and low insulin levels (Figure 2A, Figure S2B). While there were no significant differences in hippocampus-dependent spatial memory between WT and STZ mice, STZ mice displayed hippocampus- and prefrontal cortex-related memory decline (Figure 2B), consistent with the findings reported in previous studies [29–32]. However, STZ-induced T1DM had no effect on Aβ40 and Aβ42 levels in the T-PER fractions of the hippocampus (Figure 2C).

Subsequently, we examined the impact of STZ-induced T1DM on the phosphorylation of IRS1 at Ser residues and downstream components in the hippocampus. In STZ mice that had already developed memory impairment, the phosphorylation levels of hippocampal IRS1 at Ser residues in STZ mice were comparable to those in WT mice (Figure 2D, Figure S4C). Although the activation of p70S6K and the monotonous activities of Akt, AMPK, aPKC ζ/λ, and JNK were observed in STZ mice as well as in middle-aged DIO mice regardless of the presence or absence of Ser phosphorylation on hippocampal IRS1, the phosphorylation of GSK3β at Ser9 significantly increased in the hippocampus of STZ mice (Figure 2E, Figure S3B, S4D and S5B). These data indicate that T1DM-induced memory deficits accompanied by increased phosphorylation of GSK3β arises independently of the modification of IRS1 signaling via Ser phosphorylation and independently of Aβ elevation.

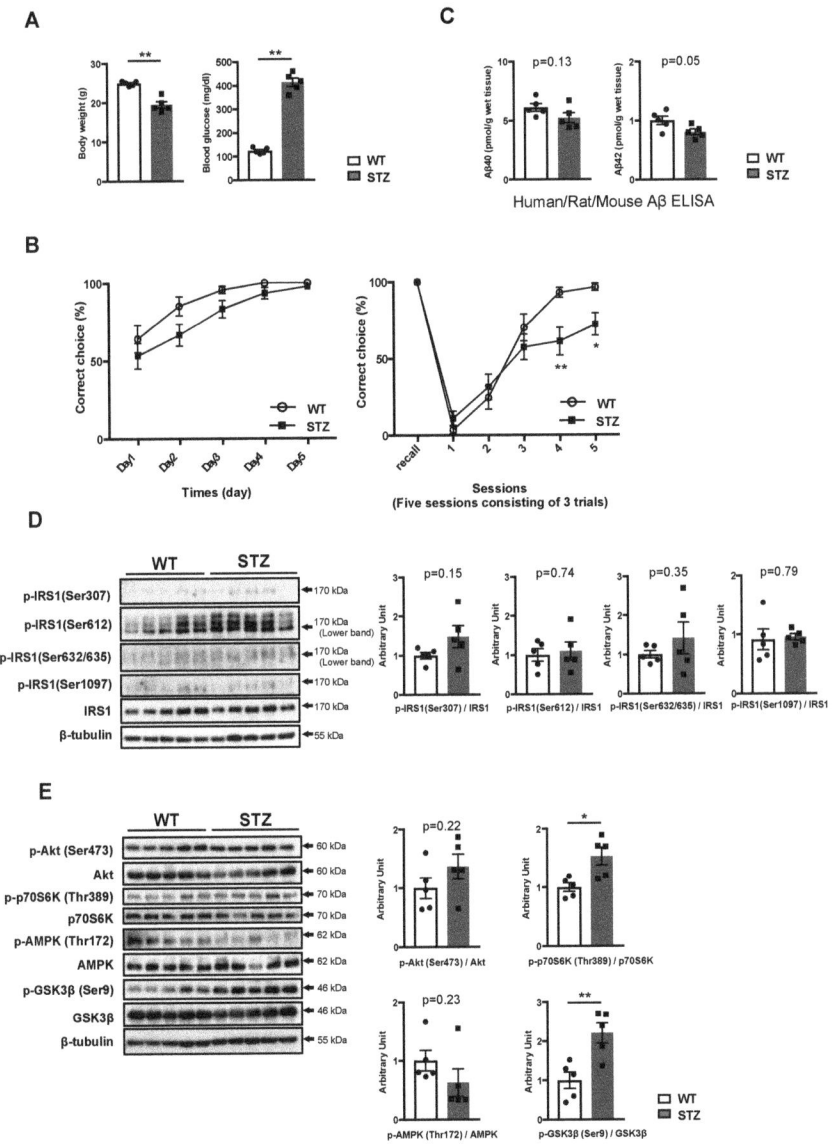

Figure 2. No alteration of IRS1 Ser phosphorylation in the hippocampus of T1DM mouse models. (**A**) Graphs of body weight and blood glucose level in wild-type (WT) and streptozotocin (STZ)-induced insulin-deficient type 1 diabetes (T1DM) model mice (10 weeks of age, n = 5 mice per group). (**B**) Evaluation of hippocampus-dependent learning and memory function and hippocampus/prefrontal cortex associated working memory function in WT (10 weeks of age, n = 19 mice per group) and STZ mice (10 weeks of age, n = 18 mice per group) using the water T-maze test and reverse water T-maze test. (**C**) Quantitative analysis of T-PER-extractable Aβ40 and Aβ42 levels in the hippocampi of WT and STZ mice using the human/rat/mouse β amyloid (1–40 and 1–42) ELISA (10 weeks of age, n = 5 biologically independent samples per group). (**D**) In WT and STZ-induced type 1 diabetes mice (10 weeks of age, n = 5 biologically independent samples per group), western blot analysis of phosphorylated insulin receptor substrates 1 mouse Ser307 [p-IRS1 (mSer307)], p-IRS1 (mSer612), p-IRS1 (mSer632/635), p-IRS1 (mSer1097), IRS1, and ß-tubulin was performed. Quantitative analysis of the phosphorylation of IRS1 at mSer307, mSer612, mSer632/635, and mSer1097 normalized to total protein. (**E**) Western blot analysis of phosphorylation levels of Akt Ser473, p70S6K Thr389, AMPK Thr172, and GSK3β Ser9 as well as total protein levels of Akt, p70S6K, AMPK, GSK3β, ß-tubulin in WT and STZ mice (10 weeks of age, n = 5 biologically independent samples per group). Arrows indicate the p-IRS1 mSer612-corresponding band (lower band) and the p-IRS1 mSer632/635-corresponding band (lower band) in (**D**). Quantitative analysis of the phosphorylation of Akt Ser473, p70 S6K Thr389, AMPK Thr172, and GSK3β Ser9 normalized to the respective total protein contents. Results are presented as mean ± SEM, * $p < 0.05$; ** $p < 0.01$.

3.3. Phosphorylation of IRS1 at Age-Specific Ser Residues with the Activation of Downstream Kinases Is Linked to Age-Related Memory Deficits

Although memory decline associated with physiological aging can occur naturally, in contrast to pathogenic memory deficits, whether the onset processes of age-related memory impairment are related to the mechanisms underlying pathogenic memory deficits in T2DM and AD remains unclear. We examined the modification of IRS1 at Ser residues and the activity of downstream factors in the hippocampi of 21-month-old mice (aged mice). Aged mice displayed memory impairments without an increase in blood glucose and plasma insulin levels, despite an increase in body weight (Figure 3A,B, Figure S2C). Meanwhile, the Aβ40 and Aβ42 levels in the T-PER fractions of the hippocampus were comparable between young and aged WT mice (Figure 3C).

In common with DIO mice, the activation of mSer307, but not of mSer1097, on IRS1 accompanied by p70S6K activation and unchanged AMPK was observed with increased phosphorylation of IRS1 at mSer612 and mSer632/635 in the hippocampi of aged mice (Figure 3D, Figure S4E). Nonetheless, unlike in DIO mice, the basal phosphorylation levels of Akt and GSK3β prominently increased in the hippocampus of aged mice (Figure 3E, Figure S4F); however, the basal activities of aPKC ζ/λ, and JNKs remained unchanged, similar to those in DIO mice (Figure S3C and S5C). These results suggest that aging causes the concomitant phosphorylation of hippocampal IRS1 at mSer307, mSer612, and mSer632/635 with the activation of canonical downstream kinases, which may be associated with Aβ-unrelated physiological decline in memory function.

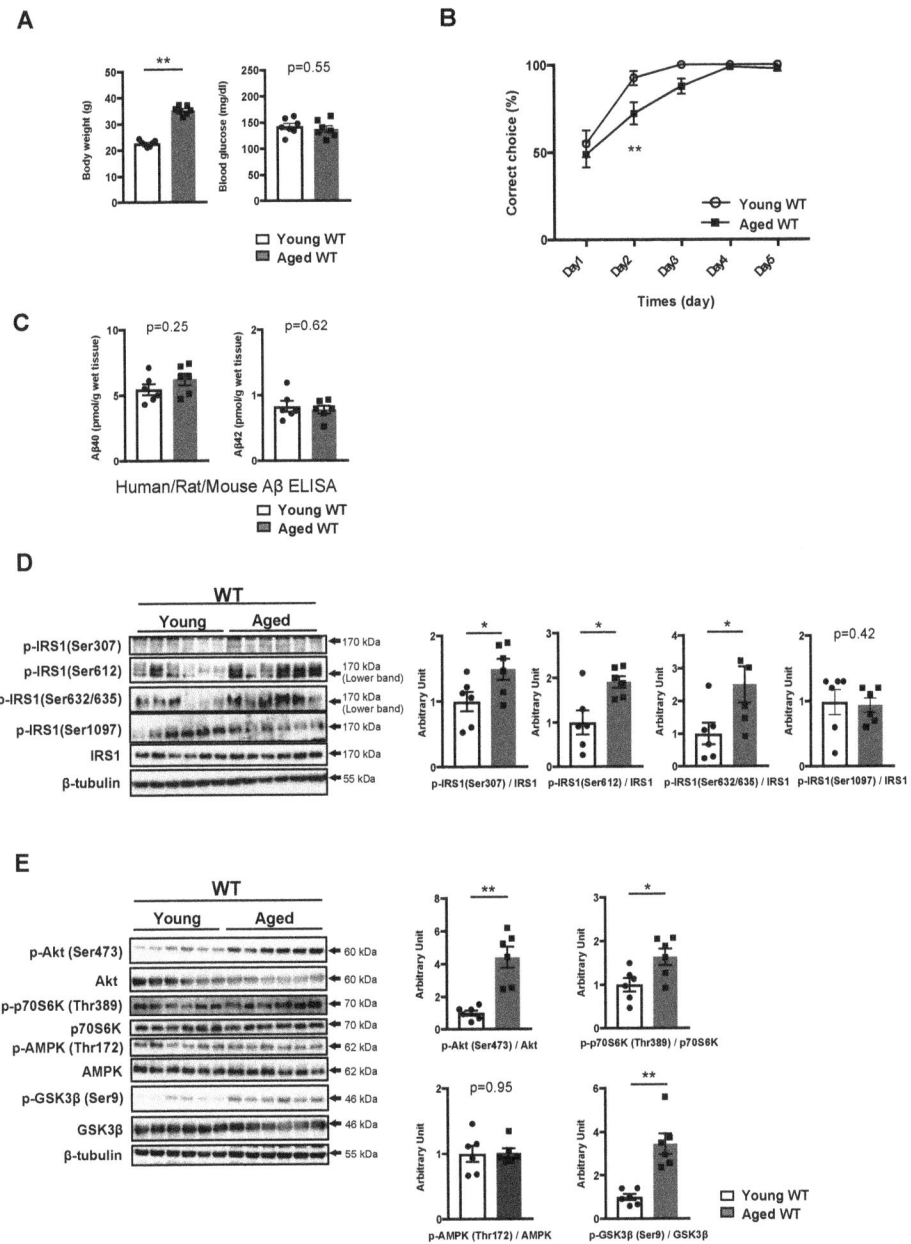

Figure 3. Age-related memory deficits accompanied by increased phosphorylation of IRS1 Ser sites in the hippocampus. (**A**) The graphs of body weight and blood glucose levels in young (12 weeks of age, n = 7 mice per group) and aged (84 weeks of age, n = 7 mice per group) wild-type (WT) mice. (**B**) Evaluation of learning memory functions in young WT mice (n = 16 mice per group) and aged WT mice (n = 18 mice per group) using the water T-maze test. (**C**) Quantitative analysis of T-PER-extractable Aβ40 and Aβ42 levels in the hippocampi of young (12 weeks of age, n = 6 biologically independent samples) and aged (84 weeks of age, n = 6 biologically independent samples) WT mice using the human/rat/mouse β amyloid (1–40 and 1–42) ELISA. (**D**) Western blot analysis of phosphorylated insulin receptor substrates 1 mouse Ser307 [p-IRS1 (mSer307)], p-IRS1 (mSer612), p-IRS1 (mSer632/635), p-IRS1 (mSer1097), IRS1, and ß-tubulin in the hippocampi of young WT mice (12 weeks of age, n = 6 biologically independent samples) and aged WT mice (84 weeks of age, n = 6 biologically independent samples). Quantitative analysis of the phosphorylation of IRS1 at mSer307, mSer612, mSer632/635, and mSer1097 normalized to total protein. (**E**) Western blot analysis of phosphorylation levels of Akt Ser473, p70S6K Thr389, AMPK Thr172, and GSK3β Ser9 as well as total protein levels of Akt, p70S6K, AMPK, GSK3β, and ß-tubulin in the hippocampi of young WT mice (12 weeks of age, n = 6 biologically independent samples) and aged WT mice (84 weeks of age, n = 6 biologically independent samples). Arrows indicate the p-IRS1 mSer612-corresponding band (lower band) and the p-IRS1 mSer632/635-corresponding band (lower band) in (**D**). Quantitative analysis of the phosphorylation of Akt Ser473, p70S6K Thr389, AMPK Thr172, and GSK3β Ser9 normalized to the respective total protein contents. Results are presented as mean ± SEM, * $p < 0.05$; ** $p < 0.01$.

3.4. Increased Phosphorylation of Hippocampal IRS1 at Ser Residues in Young Amyloid Precursor Protein (APP) Knock-In (APP KI^{NL-G-F}) Mice Occurs Prior to the Onset of Memory Decline

To investigate whether AD-related activation of Ser residues on neural IRS1 emerges before or after the onset of memory decline, we employed a novel AD mouse model, APPKI^{NL-G-F} mice carrying a humanized Aβ sequence and three AD mutations, i.e., Swedish, Beyreuther/Iberian, and Arctic mutations, in the endogenous *App* gene [19]. First, we measured body weight and glucose metabolism in 12-week-old (young) APPKI^{NL-G-F} mice. There were no differences in terms of body weight, blood glucose level, and plasma insulin concentration between WT and APPKI^{NL-G-F} mice at 12 weeks of age (Figure 4A, Figure S2B). Next, we confirmed memory function as well as Aβ40 and Aβ42 levels in the hippocampi of young APPKI^{NL-G-F} mice. At 12 weeks of age, APPKI^{NL-G-F} mice exhibited normal memory function (Figure 4B).

Using monoclonal antibody (BNT77/BC05)-based sandwich ELISA for human/rat/mouse Aβ42, we successfully confirmed that T-PER-extractable Aβ42 level had already increased in young APP KI^{NL-G-F} mice (Figure 4C, right). A conspicuous increase in T-PER-extractable Aβ42 level in these mice was detected by human Aβ42 sandwich ELISA using monoclonal antibodies (BAN50/BC05) (Figure 4D, right). However, T-PER-extractable Aβ42 levels in both ELISA were comparable to the range of Tris-buffered saline (TBS)-extractable Aβ42 level in the brain and cortex of APPKI^{NL-G-F} mice reported by Saito et al. (2019) and Saito et al. (2014). Similarly, human/rat/mouse Aβ40 and human Aβ40 sandwich ELISA revealed the same range for Aβ40 level in the T-PER fractions of the hippocampi of young APPKI^{NL-G-F} mice (black bar on the left in Figure 4C,D and Figure 5C,D). Meanwhile, regardless of age, human/rat/mouse Aβ40 or human Aβ40 sandwich ELISA showed almost the same levels (white bar on the left in Figures 1D, 2C, 3C, 4C and 5C) or range (white bar on the left in Figures 4D and 5D) of T-PER-extractable Aβ40 in WT mice, respectively.

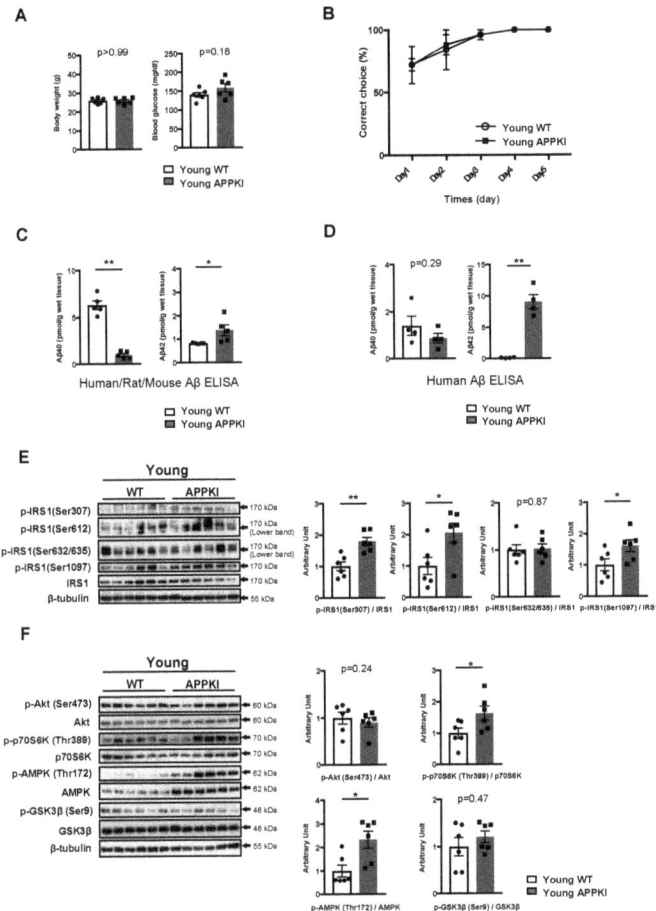

Figure 4. Activation of multiple Ser residues on hippocampal IRS1 unrelated to memory decline in young amyloid precursor protein (APP) knock-in (APPKI^{NL-G-F}) mice. (**A**) The graphs of body weight and blood glucose levels in young wild-type (WT) and APPKI^{NL-G-F} mice (12 weeks of age, n = 6 mice per group). (**B**) Evaluation of learning memory function in young WT (n = 5 mice per group) and APP KI^{NL-G-F} mice (n = 5 mice per group) using the water T-maze test. (**C**) Quantitative analysis of T-PER-extractable Aβ40 and Aβ42 levels in the hippocampi of young WT and APPKI^{NL-G-F} mice using the human/rat/mouse β amyloid (1–40 and 1–42) ELISA (12 weeks of age, n = 5 biologically independent samples per group). (**D**) Quantitative analysis of T-PER-extractable Aβ40 and Aβ42 levels in the hippocampi of young WT and APPKI^{NL-G-F} mice using the human β amyloid (1–40 and 1–42) ELISA (12 weeks of age, n = 5 biologically independent samples per group). (**E**) Western blot analysis of phosphorylated insulin receptor substrates 1 mouse Ser307 [p-IRS1 (mSer307)], p-IRS1 (mSer612), p-IRS1 (mSer632/635), p-IRS1 (mSer1097), IRS1, and ß-tubulin in the hippocampi of young WT and APP KI^{NL-G-F} mice (12 weeks of age, n = 6 biologically independent samples per group). Arrows indicate the p-IRS1 mSer612-corresponding band (lower band) and p-IRS1 mSer632/635-corresponding band (lower band) in (**E**). Quantitative analysis of the phosphorylation of IRS1 at mSer307, mSer612, mSer632/635, and mSer1097 normalized to the respective total protein contents. (**F**) Western blot analysis of phosphorylation levels of Akt Ser473, p70S6K Thr389, AMPK Thr172, and GSK3β Ser9 as well as total protein levels of Akt, p70S6K, AMPK, GSK3β, and ß-tubulin in the hippocampi of young WT and APPKI^{NL-G-F} mice (12 weeks of age, n = 6 biologically independent samples per group). Quantitative analysis of phosphorylation of Akt Ser473, p70S6K Thr389, AMPK Thr172, and GSK3β Ser9 normalized to the respective total protein contents. Results are presented as mean ± SEM, * $p < 0.05$; ** $p < 0.01$.

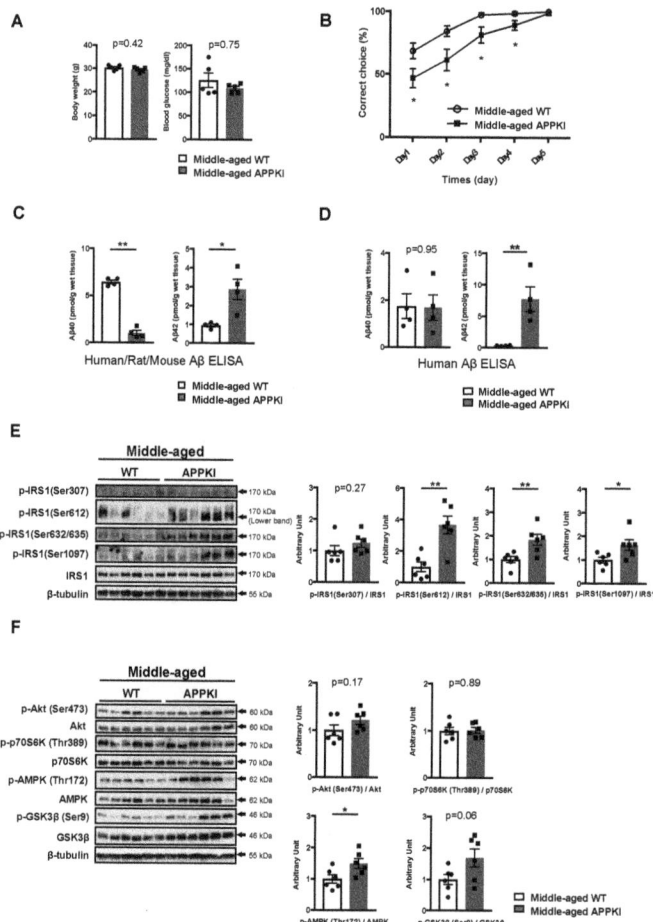

Figure 5. Memory decline accompanied by sustained phosphorylation of IRS1 Ser residues in the hippocampus of middle-aged APPKI^{NL-G-F} mice. (**A**) The graphs of body weight and blood glucose levels in middle-aged wild-type (WT) and APPKI^{NL-G-F} mice (34–36 weeks of age, n = 5 mice per group). (**B**) Evaluation of learning memory function in middle-aged WT (n = 14) and APPKI^{NL-G-F} mice (n = 15 mice per group) using the water T-maze test. (**C**) Quantitative analysis of T-PER-extractable Aβ40 and Aβ42 levels in the hippocampi of middle-aged WT and APPKI^{NL-G-F} mice using the human/rat/mouse β amyloid (1–40 and 1–42) ELISA (34–36 weeks of age, n = 4 biologically independent samples per group). (**D**) Quantitative analysis of T-PER-extractable Aβ40 and Aβ42 levels in the hippocampi of middle-aged WT and APPKI^{NL-G-F} mice using the human β amyloid (1–40 and 1–42) ELISA (34–36 weeks of age, n = 4 biologically independent samples per group). (**E**) Western blot analysis of phosphorylated insulin receptor substrates 1 mouse Ser307 [p-IRS1 (mSer307)], p-IRS1 (mSer612), p-IRS1 (mSer632/635), p-IRS1 (mSer1097), IRS1, and ß-tubulin in the hippocampi of middle-aged WT and APPKI^{NL-G-F} mice (34–36 weeks of age, n = 6 biologically independent samples per group). Arrow indicates the p-IRS1 mSer612 -corresponding band (lower band) in (**E**). Quantitative analysis of the phosphorylation of IRS1 at mSer307, mSer612, mSer632/635, and mSer1097 normalized to total protein. (**F**) Western blot analysis of phosphorylation levels of Akt Ser473, p70S6K Thr389, AMPK Thr172, and GSK3β Ser9 as well as total protein levels of Akt, p70S6K, AMPK, GSK3β, and ß-tubulin in the hippocampi of middle-aged WT and APPKI^{NL-G-F} mice (34–36 weeks of age, n = 6 biologically independent samples per group). Quantitative analysis of the phosphorylation of Akt Ser473, p70S6K Thr389, AMPK Thr172, and GSK3β Ser9 normalized to the respective total protein contents. Results are presented as mean ± SEM, * $p < 0.05$; ** $p < 0.01$.

Subsequently, we investigated the phosphorylation levels of hippocampal IRS1 at Ser residues in young APPKI[NL-G-F] mice. Importantly, the phosphorylation of hippocampal IRS1 at mSer307, mSer612, and mSer1097, but not at mSer632/635, significantly increased in 12-week-old APPKI[NL-G-F] mice (Figure 4E, Figure S4G) displaying normal memory function (Figure 4B). In parallel to these increases, a concomitant elevation in the basal phosphorylation of AMPK, a metabolic energy sensor, with p70S6K activation and a slight decrease in basal JNK phosphorylation were observed in these mice, along with monotonous Akt, GSK3β, and aPKC ζ/λ activity (Figure 4F, Figure S3D, S4H and S5D). Thus, in young APPKI[NL-G-F] mice exhibiting normal memory function, the increased phosphorylation of hippocampal IRS1 at multiple Ser sites accompanied by AMPK-related low energy conditions had already occurred in the presence of increased Aβ42 level, suggesting that the elevation of Aβ42 level and/or AMPK activation provokes the activation of Ser sites on IRS1 in brains of patients with AD prior to the onset of memory decline.

3.5. Memory Decline in Middle-Aged APPKI[NL-G-F] Mice Is Accompanied by the Activation of Specific Ser Sites on IRS1 and Energy Depletion

Next, we examined age-related alterations in the patterns of phosphorylation of IRS1 at Ser sites and its downstream components in the hippocampi of middle-aged APPKI[NL-G-F] mice at 34–36 weeks of age. Consistently, body weight, blood glucose level, and plasma insulin concentration were comparable between middle-aged WT and APPKI[NL-G-F] mice (Figure 5A, Figure S2A).

Although the onset of memory deficits was reported by 6 months in APPKI[NL-G-F] mice [19], 6-month-old APPKI[NL-G-F] mice did not display memory decline under our experimental conditions (data not shown). However, the water T-maze test demonstrated that middle-aged APPKI[NL-G-F] mice exhibited memory decline after 34 weeks under our experimental conditions (Figure 5B). Meanwhile, both human/rat/mouse Aβ42 and human Aβ42 sandwich ELISA demonstrated increased levels of T-PER-extractable Aβ42 in the hippocampi of middle-aged APPKI[NL-G-F] mice (right in Figure 5C, D) and young APPKI[NL-G-F] mice, which were comparable to TBS-extractable Aβ42 levels in the brain and cortex of APPKI[NL-G-F] mice [33].

While an age-related increase in the phosphorylation of IRS1 at mSer612 and mSer632/635 accompanied by sustained phosphorylation of IRS1 at T2DM-related mSer1097 site and of AMPK was observed in the hippocampi of middle-aged APPKI[NL-G-F] mice showing memory decline (Figure 5E, Figure S4I, Table S1), there were no significant differences in phosphorylation levels at mSer307 site and of p70S6K between middle-aged WT and APPKI[NL-G-F] mice (Figure 5E,F) owing to the age-related elevation of these factors (Figure 3D,E). Regardless of age, the activity of downstream components, such as Akt, GSK3β, aPKC ζ/λ, and JNKs, remained almost unchanged in the hippocampi of APPKI[NL-G-F] mice (Figure 5F, Figure S3E, S4J and S5E). Our data suggest that the increased phosphorylation of hippocampal IRS1 at multiple Ser residues and persistent AMPK activation that corresponds to energy depletion accompanied by age-related elevation of Aβ42 levels are associated with the onset of memory decline in these mice.

4. Discussion

The present study demonstrates that memory decline in T1DM and T2DM in middle age occurs in an Aβ-independent manner, which is consistent with the findings of previous studies [34–36]. Similarly, age-related memory impairments arise with no alteration in Aβ levels.

In middle-aged DIO and aged mice, Aβ-unrelated memory deficits are accompanied by increased basal phosphorylation of hippocampal IRS1 at specific Ser residues, whereas Aβ-unrelated memory impairments develop in STZ mice without the modification of IRS1. Although p70S6K activation accompanied by unchanged AMPK activity in the hippocampus is mutually observed with Aβ-unrelated memory deficits in middle-aged DIO, STZ, and aged mice regardless of the presence or absence of the phosphorylation of IRS1 at Ser residues, different alterations in other downstream components were observed in these mouse models. Furthermore, we found that, in APPKI[NL-G-F] mice, a concomitant increase in the basal phosphorylation of hippocampal IRS1 at multiple Ser sites with the activation of AMPK and elevation of Aβ42 level had already arisen at a young age, before the onset of memory decline, and that memory decline in middle age was accompanied by the persistence of these changes with age-related increase in the phosphorylation of IRS1 at specific Ser sites and in Aβ42 level.

HFD and genetically obese animals exhibit increased phosphorylation at mSer307 and p70S6K-induced phosphorylation at mSer1097 in peripheral tissues [37,38]. In the central nervous system, the involvement of non-activated AMPK with/without phosphorylation of IRS1 at mSer307 accompanied by p70S6K activation or different combinations of alterations in Akt and GSK3β activity (i.e., increased or decreased phosphorylation) in cognitive impairment in 40–45% HFD-fed and STZ mice has been reported [21,22,27,28,32,34,39,40], whereas the monotonous levels of phosphorylation of IRS1 at Ser sites and of downstream kinases including Akt, AMPK, GSK3β, and p70S6K are observed in 45% HFD-induced cognitive deficits [41]. Consistent with these results, memory decline in middle-aged DIO mice is accompanied by a concomitant increase in the basal phosphorylation of IRS1 at mSer307 and mSer1097 with p70S6K activation and monotonous activity of Akt, GSK3β, and AMPK in the hippocampus. On the other hand, in aged mice, the concomitant activation of Akt and GSK3β with an increase in the basal phosphorylation of hippocampal IRS1 at mSer307, mSer612, and mSer632/635 with p70S6K activation is observed, which is consistent with previous studies showing that the increased phosphorylation of mSer632/635 or mSer1097 on IRS1 is associated with p70S6K [5,37,38]. Given that the activation of mSer612 on IRS1 may negatively correlate with intracellular signaling and that the activation of Ser632/635 on IRS1 may occur independently of Akt [5], it is likely that, in aged mice, the increased phosphorylation of IRS1 at mSer307, mSer612, and mSer632/635 with the activation of multiple downstream factors other than AMPK may arise through reciprocal feedback regulation.

Additionally, HFD- and STZ-induced diabetes increases the phosphorylation of JNK accompanied by the activation of mSer307 on IRS1 in the brain [21,32]. The activity of JNK is elevated in aged mice and transgenic mouse models of AD, although the involvement of phosphorylation of IRS1 at Ser sites in the altered activation of JNK has not been reported [16,42]. Furthermore, the activation of aPKC ζ/λ is associated with the phosphorylation of IRS1 at Ser sites, including mSer1097 [5,20]. However, in all types of mouse models of memory impairment in the present study, the basal phosphorylation levels of JNK and aPKC ζ/λ consistently remained unchanged under our experimental conditions. These discrepancies may be due to the differences in observation time, animal species, and HFD or STZ protocols, such as age, duration of exposure, diet fat content, and drug dosages. Taken together, these results suggest that the reciprocal effects of the phosphorylation of IRS1 at T2DM- or age-related Ser sites and downstream components via feedback loops that may lead to the common alterations in the activity of p70S6K and AMPK are involved in Aβ-unrelated memory decline; however, the modification of IRS1 through Ser sites is not required for the onset of memory deficits in STZ-induced T1DM mice.

Although a link between the phosphorylation of neural IRS1 at mSer307, mSer612, and mSer632/635 and brain insulin resistance has been proposed [14,16,43], brain insulin resistance is not yet defined, and the phosphorylation of IRS1 at Ser sites emerges in insulin-dependent and insulin-independent manners [5,6]. Given that diabetes- and obesity-induced memory impairments were accompanied by the phosphorylation of IRS1 at mSer307 [5], we found that young APPKI^{NL-G-F} mice showing normal metabolism and memory function displayed increased phosphorylation of hippocampal IRS1 at three Ser residues including mSer307, mSer612, and mSer1097, in which the Aβ42 level had already increased before the onset of memory decline. Consistent with previous studies [13–16], the increased phosphorylation at mSer612 and mSer 632/635 and persistent activation of mSer1097 are observed in the hippocampus of middle-aged APPKI^{NL-G-F} mice exhibiting memory decline with age-associated increase in the Aβ42 level.

Interestingly, in both young and middle-aged APPKI^{NL-G-F} mice, the concomitant phosphorylation of hippocampal IRS1 at mSer612 and mSer1097 with the activation of AMPK is constantly observed regardless of the presence or absence of the activation of mSer307 or mSer 632/635, suggesting that persistent phosphorylation of mSer612 and mSer1097 accompanied by AMPK activation may contribute to memory dysfunction in AD.

Reportedly, the Arctic mutation in APPKI^{NL-G-F} mice reduces immunoreactivity in ELISA because the location of this mutation on the Aβ sequences is overlapped with the binding region of monoclonal antibody to Aβ used in human/rat/mouse Aβ sandwich ELISA [19]; however, T-PER-extractable Aβ40 and Aβ42 levels were successfully determined by human/rat/mouse Aβ sandwich ELISA using BNT77 (binds to the location of the Arctic mutation) and human Aβ sandwich ELISA using BAN50 (does not bind to the location of the Arctic mutation). We confirmed that the elevation of Aβ42 level is evident in young APPKI^{NL-G-F} mice and that the Aβ42 level increased in middle-aged APPKI^{NL-G-F} mice. Owing to the elevation of Aβ42 level in the hippocampi of APPKI^{NL-G-F} mice from a young age, it is likely that the increased phosphorylation of IRS1 at Ser sites is associated with Aβ42 level but not with memory decline. Consistent with this finding, a previous study showed that the phosphorylation of IRS1 at mSer307/hSer312 and mSer612/hSer616 increased in cultured hippocampal neurons exposed to Aβ oligomers prepared from synthetic Aβ1–42 peptide and in the AβO-injected hippocampi of non-human primates [16]. Interestingly, the increased basal phosphorylation of hippocampal IRS1 at multiple Ser sites in APPKI^{NL-G-F} mice is accompanied by AMPK activation regardless of the presence or absence of memory decline. Consistent with our findings, recent studies suggest that AMPK activation is implicated in brain aging and development of neurodegenerative diseases, including AD [44,45]. These results suggest that the elevation of Aβ42 accompanied by AMPK activation induced by energy depletion that occurs from a young age before the onset of memory decline is associated with increased phosphorylation of hippocampal IRS1 at multiple Ser sites and that sustained activation of these factors contributes to the onset of memory decline in middle-aged APPKI^{NL-G-F} mice.

In summary, whether the modification of IRS1 through its phosphorylation at Ser sites in the hippocampus has a pathogenic or an adaptive function remains unknown because the phosphorylation of hippocampal IRS1 at mSer307, mSer612, and mSer1097 increased when metformin improves memory deficits in middle-aged DIO mice [20,46]. Studies using mutant mice with IRS1 Ser residues in the brain will help us to understand the roles of Ser sites in memory function and to identify unrecognized downstream pathways.

5. Conclusions

Our findings indicate that the phosphorylation of IRS1 at disease-specific Ser residues in the hippocampus may be a potential marker of Aβ-unrelated memory impairments induced by T2DM and aging. Alternatively, in Aβ-related memory decline in AD, the modification of IRS1 via its phosphorylation at multiple Ser sites accompanied by the activation of AMPK, a sensor of energy metabolism, may be a marker of the response to an early detection of elevated Aβ42 level before the onset of memory decline in AD.

Supplementary Materials: The following are available online at http://www.mdpi.com/2072-6643/11/8/1942/s1: Figure S1: No difference in memory function between wild-type (WT) and DIO mice at a young age.; Figure S2: Levels of blood insulin in the respective mouse models.; Figure S3: Evaluation of the other signaling factors associated with IRS1 signaling in the hippocampus.; Figures S4 and S5: Full images of Western blots; Table S1: Summary of phosphorylated Ser residues on hippocampal IRS1 in all models.

Author Contributions: W.W., D.T., Y.F., M.M., and C.K. researched data. W.W. and D.T. analyzed data. W.W., D.T., and Y.F. wrote the manuscript. T.S. and T.C.S. provided the APPKI mice and interpreted the data. A.T. designed experiments, analyzed data, and wrote and edited the manuscript. All authors read and approved the final manuscript.

Funding: This work was supported by JSPS KAKENHI (JP26282026, JP17K19951, JP17H02188) (A.T.), the Research Funding for Longevity Science from National Center for Geriatrics and Gerontology, Japan (A.T.), and grants from the Mitsubishi Foundation (A.T.)

Acknowledgments: We thank Kohei Tomita (Laboratory of Experimental Animal, National Center for Geriatrics and Gerontology) for animal care and M. Sawaura and K. Tabata for providing aged wild-type mice (Charles river, Japan).

Conflicts of Interest: The authors declare no conflict of interest.

References

1. Lin, X.; Taguchi, A.; Park, S.; Kushner, J.A.; Li, F.; Li, Y.; White, M.F. Dysregulation of insulin receptor substrate 2 in beta cells and brain causes obesity and diabetes. *J. Clin. Invest.* **2004**, *114*, 908–916. [CrossRef] [PubMed]
2. Dong, X.; Park, S.; Lin, X.; Copps, K.; Yi, X.; White, M.F. Irs1 and Irs2 signaling is essential for hepatic glucose homeostasis and systemic growth. *J. Clin. Invest.* **2006**, *116*, 101–114. [CrossRef] [PubMed]
3. Taguchi, A.; Wartschow, L.M.; White, M.F. Brain IRS2 signaling coordinates life span and nutrient homeostasis. *Science* **2007**, *317*, 369–372. [CrossRef] [PubMed]
4. Long, Y.C.; Cheng, Z.; Copps, K.D.; White, M.F. Insulin receptor substrates Irs1 and Irs2 coordinate skeletal muscle growth and metabolism via the Akt and AMPK pathways. *Mol. Cell. Biol.* **2011**, *31*, 430–441. [CrossRef] [PubMed]
5. Copps, K.D.; White, M.F. Regulation of insulin sensitivity by serine/threonine phosphorylation of insulin receptor substrate proteins IRS1 and IRS2. *Diabetologia* **2012**, *55*, 2565–2582. [CrossRef] [PubMed]
6. Hancer, N.J.; Qiu, W.; Cherella, C.; Li, Y.; Copps, K.D.; White, M.F. Insulin and metabolic stress stimulate multisite serine/threonine phosphorylation of insulin receptor substrate 1 and inhibit tyrosine phosphorylation. *J. Biol. Chem.* **2014**, *289*, 12467–12484. [CrossRef]
7. White, M.F.; Maron, R.; Kahn, C.R. Insulin rapidly stimulates tyrosine phosphorylation of a Mr-185,000 protein in intact cells. *Nature* **1985**, *318*, 183–186. [CrossRef]
8. Samuel, V.T.; Shulman, G.I. Mechanisms for insulin resistance: Common threads and missing links. *Cell* **2012**, *148*, 852–871. [CrossRef]
9. Jiang, G.; Dallas-Yang, Q.; Biswas, S.; Li, Z.; Zhang, B.B. Rosiglitazone, an agonist of peroxisome-proliferator-activated receptor gamma (PPARgamma), decreases inhibitory serine phosphorylation of IRS1 in vitro and in vivo. *Biochem. J.* **2004**, *377 Pt 2*, 339–346. [CrossRef]
10. Morino, K.; Petersen, K.F.; Dufour, S.; Befroy, D.; Frattini, J.; Shatzkes, N.; Neschen, S.; White, M.F.; Bilz, S.; Sono, S.; et al. Reduced mitochondrial density and increased IRS-1 serine phosphorylation in muscle of insulin-resistant offspring of type 2 diabetic parents. *J. Clin. Invest.* **2005**, *115*, 3587–3593. [CrossRef]
11. Copps, K.D.; Hancer, N.J.; Opare-Ado, L.; Qiu, W.; Walsh, C.; White, M.F. Irs1 serine 307 promotes insulin sensitivity in mice. *Cell Metab.* **2010**, *11*, 84–92. [CrossRef] [PubMed]
12. Tremblay, F.; Brule, S.; Hee Um, S.; Li, Y.; Masuda, K.; Roden, M.; Sun, X.J.; Krebs, M.; Polakiewicz, R.D.; Thomas, G.; et al. Identification of IRS-1 Ser-1101 as a target of S6K1 in nutrient- and obesity-induced insulin resistance. *Proc. Nat. Acad. Sci. USA* **2007**, *104*, 14056–14061. [CrossRef] [PubMed]
13. Moloney, A.M.; Griffin, R.J.; Timmons, S.; O'Connor, R.; Ravid, R.; O'Neill, C. Defects in IGF-1 receptor, insulin receptor and IRS-1/2 in Alzheimer's disease indicate possible resistance to IGF-1 and insulin signalling. *Neurobiol. Aging* **2010**, *31*, 224–243. [CrossRef] [PubMed]
14. Talbot, K.; Wang, H.Y.; Kazi, H.; Han, L.Y.; Bakshi, K.P.; Stucky, A.; Fuino, R.L.; Kawaguchi, K.R.; Samoyedny, A.J.; Wilson, R.S.; et al. Demonstrated brain insulin resistance in Alzheimer's disease patients is associated with IGF-1 resistance, IRS-1 dysregulation, and cognitive decline. *J. Clin. Invest.* **2012**, *122*, 1316–1338. [CrossRef] [PubMed]
15. Yarchoan, M.; Toledo, J.B.; Lee, E.B.; Arvanitakis, Z.; Kazi, H.; Han, L.Y.; Louneva, N.; Lee, V.M.; Kim, S.F.; Trojanowski, J.Q.; et al. Abnormal serine phosphorylation of insulin receptor substrate 1 is associated with tau pathology in Alzheimer's disease and tauopathies. *Acta Neuropathol.* **2014**, *128*, 679–689. [CrossRef] [PubMed]
16. Bomfim, T.R.; Forny-Germano, L.; Sathler, L.B.; Brito-Moreira, J.; Houzel, J.C.; Decker, H.; Silverman, M.A.; Kazi, H.; Melo, H.M.; McClean, P.L.; et al. An anti-diabetes agent protects the mouse brain from defective insulin signaling caused by Alzheimer's disease- associated Abeta oligomers. *J. Clin. Invest.* **2012**, *122*, 1339–1353. [CrossRef] [PubMed]
17. Lourenco, M.V.; Clarke, J.R.; Frozza, R.L.; Bomfim, T.R.; Forny-Germano, L.; Batista, A.F.; Sathler, L.B.; Brito-Moreira, J.; Amaral, O.B.; Silva, C.A.; et al. TNF-alpha mediates PKR-dependent memory impairment and brain IRS-1 inhibition induced by Alzheimer's beta-amyloid oligomers in mice and monkeys. *Cell Metab.* **2013**, *18*, 831–843. [CrossRef]

18. Ma, Q.L.; Yang, F.; Rosario, E.R.; Ubeda, O.J.; Beech, W.; Gant, D.J.; Chen, P.P.; Hudspeth, B.; Chen, C.; Zhao, Y.; et al. Beta-amyloid oligomers induce phosphorylation of tau and inactivation of insulin receptor substrate via c-Jun N-terminal kinase signaling: Suppression by omega-3 fatty acids and curcumin. *J. Neurosci. Off. J. Soc. Neurosci.* **2009**, *29*, 9078–9089. [CrossRef]
19. Saito, T.; Matsuba, Y.; Mihira, N.; Takano, J.; Nilsson, P.; Itohara, S.; Iwata, N.; Saido, T.C. Single App knock-in mouse models of Alzheimer's disease. *Nat. Neurosci.* **2014**, *17*, 661–663. [CrossRef]
20. Tanokashira, D.; Kurata, E.; Fukuokaya, W.; Kawabe, K.; Kashiwada, M.; Takeuchi, H.; Nakazato, M.; Taguchi, A. Metformin treatment ameliorates diabetes-associated decline in hippocampal neurogenesis and memory via phosphorylation of insulin receptor substrate 1. *FEBS Open Bio* **2018**, *8*, 1104–1118. [CrossRef]
21. Liang, L.; Chen, J.; Zhan, L.; Lu, X.; Sun, X.; Sui, H.; Zheng, L.; Xiang, H.; Zhang, F. Endoplasmic reticulum stress impairs insulin receptor signaling in the brains of obese rats. *PloS ONE* **2015**, *10*, e0126384. [CrossRef] [PubMed]
22. Arnold, S.E.; Lucki, I.; Brookshire, B.R.; Carlson, G.C.; Browne, C.A.; Kazi, H.; Bang, S.; Choi, B.R.; Chen, Y.; McMullen, M.F.; et al. High fat diet produces brain insulin resistance, synaptodendritic abnormalities and altered behavior in mice. *Neurobiol. Dis.* **2014**, *67*, 79–87. [CrossRef] [PubMed]
23. Jiang, T.; Yin, F.; Yao, J.; Brinton, R.D.; Cadenas, E. Lipoic acid restores age-associated impairment of brain energy metabolism through the modulation of Akt/JNK signaling and PGC1alpha transcriptional pathway. *Aging Cell* **2013**, *12*, 1021–1031. [CrossRef] [PubMed]
24. Makinodan, M.; Rosen, K.M.; Ito, S.; Corfas, G. A critical period for social experience-dependent oligodendrocyte maturation and myelination. *Science* **2012**, *337*, 1357–1360. [CrossRef] [PubMed]
25. Tsai, P.T.; Hull, C.; Chu, Y.; Greene-Colozzi, E.; Sadowski, A.R.; Leech, J.M.; Steinberg, J.; Crawley, J.N.; Regehr, W.G.; Sahin, M. Autistic-like behaviour and cerebellar dysfunction in Purkinje cell Tsc1 mutant mice. *Nature* **2012**, *488*, 647–651. [CrossRef] [PubMed]
26. Morrison, C.D.; Pistell, P.J.; Ingram, D.K.; Johnson, W.D.; Liu, Y.; Fernandez-Kim, S.O.; White, C.L.; Purpera, M.N.; Uranga, R.M.; Bruce-Keller, A.J.; et al. High fat diet increases hippocampal oxidative stress and cognitive impairment in aged mice: Implications for decreased Nrf2 signaling. *J. Neurochem.* **2010**, *114*, 1581–1589. [CrossRef]
27. Yang, Y.; Fang, H.; Xu, G.; Zhen, Y.; Zhang, Y.; Tian, J.; Zhang, D.; Zhang, G.; Xu, J. Liraglutide improves cognitive impairment via the AMPK and PI3K/Akt signaling pathways in type 2 diabetic rats. *Mol. Med. Rep.* **2018**, *18*, 2449–2457. [CrossRef]
28. Zhu, B.; Li, Y.; Xiang, L.; Zhang, J.; Wang, L.; Guo, B.; Liang, M.; Chen, L.; Xiang, L.; Dong, J.; et al. Alogliptin improves survival and health of mice on a high-fat diet. *Aging Cell* **2019**, *18*, e12883. [CrossRef]
29. Flood, J.F.; Mooradian, A.D.; Morley, J.E. Characteristics of learning and memory in streptozocin-induced diabetic mice. *Diabetes* **1990**, *39*, 1391–1398. [CrossRef]
30. Nakano, M.; Nagaishi, K.; Konari, N.; Saito, Y.; Chikenji, T.; Mizue, Y.; Fujimiya, M. Bone marrow-derived mesenchymal stem cells improve diabetes-induced cognitive impairment by exosome transfer into damaged neurons and astrocytes. *Sci. Rep.* **2016**, *6*, 24805. [CrossRef]
31. Wang, J.; Wang, L.; Zhou, J.; Qin, A.; Chen, Z. The protective effect of formononetin on cognitive impairment in streptozotocin (STZ)-induced diabetic mice. *Biomed. Pharmacother. Biomed. Pharmacother.* **2018**, *106*, 1250–1257. [CrossRef]
32. Chen, Q.; Mo, R.; Wu, N.; Zou, X.; Shi, C.; Gong, J.; Li, J.; Fang, K.; Wang, D.; Yang, D.; et al. Berberine ameliorates diabetes-associated cognitive decline through modulation of aberrant inflammation response and insulin signaling pathway in DM rats. *Front. Pharmacol.* **2017**, *8*, 334. [CrossRef]
33. Saito, T.; Mihira, N.; Matsuba, Y.; Sasaguri, H.; Hashimoto, S.; Narasimhan, S.; Zhang, B.; Murayama, S.; Higuchi, M.; Lee, V.M.Y.; et al. Humanization of the entire murine Mapt gene provides a murine model of pathological human tau propagation. *J. Biol. Chem.* **2019**. [CrossRef]
34. Minami, Y.; Sonoda, N.; Hayashida, E.; Makimura, H.; Ide, M.; Ikeda, N.; Ohgidani, M.; Kato, T.A.; Seki, Y.; Maeda, Y.; et al. p66Shc signaling mediates diabetes-related cognitive decline. *Sci. Rep.* **2018**, *8*, 3213. [CrossRef]
35. Fukazawa, R.; Hanyu, H.; Sato, T.; Shimizu, S.; Koyama, S.; Kanetaka, H.; Sakurai, H.; Iwamoto, T. Subgroups of Alzheimer's disease associated with diabetes mellitus based on brain imaging. *Dement. Geriatr. Cogn. Disord.* **2013**, *35*, 280–290. [CrossRef]

36. Fukasawa, R.; Hanyu, H.; Shimizu, S.; Kanetaka, H.; Sakurai, H.; Ishii, K. Identification of diabetes-related dementia: Longitudinal perfusion SPECT and amyloid PET studies. *J. Neurol. Sci.* **2015**, *349*, 45–51. [CrossRef]
37. Shah, O.J.; Hunter, T. Turnover of the active fraction of IRS1 involves raptor-mTOR- and S6K1-dependent serine phosphorylation in cell culture models of tuberous sclerosis. *Mol. Cell. Biol.* **2006**, *26*, 6425–6434. [CrossRef]
38. Zhang, J.; Gao, Z.; Yin, J.; Quon, M.J.; Ye, J. S6K directly phosphorylates IRS-1 on Ser-270 to promote insulin resistance in response to TNF-(alpha) signaling through IKK2. *J. Biol. Chem.* **2008**, *283*, 35375–35382. [CrossRef]
39. Wu, J.; Zhou, S.L.; Pi, L.H.; Shi, X.J.; Ma, L.R.; Chen, Z.; Qu, M.L.; Li, X.; Nie, S.D.; Liao, D.F.; et al. High glucose induces formation of tau hyperphosphorylation via Cav-1-mTOR pathway: A potential molecular mechanism for diabetes-induced cognitive dysfunction. *Oncotarget* **2017**, *8*, 40843–40856. [CrossRef]
40. Kang, S.; Kim, C.H.; Jung, H.; Kim, E.; Song, H.T.; Lee, J.E. Agmatine ameliorates type 2 diabetes induced-Alzheimer's disease-like alterations in high-fat diet-fed mice via reactivation of blunted insulin signalling. *Neuropharmacology* **2017**, *113 Pt A*, 467–479. [CrossRef]
41. McNeilly, A.D.; Williamson, R.; Balfour, D.J.; Stewart, C.A.; Sutherland, C. A high-fat-diet-induced cognitive deficit in rats that is not prevented by improving insulin sensitivity with metformin. *Diabetologia* **2012**, *55*, 3061–3070. [CrossRef]
42. O'Donnell, E.; Vereker, E.; Lynch, M.A. Age-related impairment in LTP is accompanied by enhanced activity of stress-activated protein kinases: Analysis of underlying mechanisms. *Eur. J. Neurosci.* **2000**, *12*, 345–352. [CrossRef]
43. Craft, S. Alzheimer disease: Insulin resistance and AD—Extending the translational path. *Nat. Rev. Neurol.* **2012**, *8*, 360–362. [CrossRef]
44. Liu, Y.J.; Chern, Y. AMPK-mediated regulation of neuronal metabolism and function in brain diseases. *J. Neurogenet.* **2015**, *29*, 50–58. [CrossRef]
45. Wang, X.; Zimmermann, H.R.; Ma, T. Therapeutic potential of AMP-activated protein kinase in alzheimer's disease. *J. Alzheimer's Dis. JAD* **2019**, *68*, 33–38. [CrossRef]
46. Tanokashira, D.; Fukuokaya, W.; Taguchi, A. Involvement of insulin receptor substrates in cognitive impairment and Alzheimer's disease. *Neural Regen. Res.* **2019**, *14*, 1330–1334.

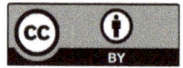

© 2019 by the authors. Licensee MDPI, Basel, Switzerland. This article is an open access article distributed under the terms and conditions of the Creative Commons Attribution (CC BY) license (http://creativecommons.org/licenses/by/4.0/).

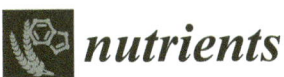

Article

Natural Dietary Supplementation of Curcumin Protects Mice Brains against Ethanol-Induced Oxidative Stress-Mediated Neurodegeneration and Memory Impairment via Nrf2/TLR4/RAGE Signaling

Muhammad Ikram [†], Kamran Saeed [†], Amjad Khan, Tahir Muhammad, Muhammad Sohail Khan, Min Gi Jo, Shafiq Ur Rehman and Myeong Ok Kim *

Division of Applied Life Science (BK 21), College of Natural Sciences, Gyeongsang National University, Jinju 52828, Korea; qazafi417@gnu.ac.kr (M.I.); kamran.biochem@gnu.ac.kr (K.S.); amjadkhan@gnu.ac.kr (A.K.); mtahir.khan@gnu.ac.kr (T.M.); sohail.bannu@gnu.ac.kr (M.S.K.); mingi.cho@gnu.ac.kr (M.G.J.); shafiq12@gnu.ac.kr (S.U.R.)
* Correspondence: mokim@gnu.ac.kr; Tel.: +82-55-772-1345; Fax: +82-55-772-2656
† These authors contributed equally to this paper.

Received: 3 April 2019; Accepted: 14 May 2019; Published: 15 May 2019

Abstract: The aim of the current study was to explore the underlying neuroprotective mechanisms of curcumin (50 mg/kg, for six weeks) against ethanol (5 mg/kg i.p., for six weeks) induced oxidative stress and inflammation-mediated cognitive dysfunction in mice. According to our findings, ethanol triggered reactive oxygen species (ROS), apoptosis, neuroinflammation, and memory impairment, which were significantly inhibited with the administration of curcumin, as assessed by ROS, lipid peroxidation (LPO), and Nrf2/HO-1 (nuclear factor erythroid 2-related factor 2/Heme-oxygenase-1) expression in the experimental mice brains. Moreover, curcumin regulated the expression of the glial cell markers in ethanol-treated mice brains, as analyzed by the relative expression TLR4 (Toll like Receptor 4), RAGE (Receptor for Advanced Glycations End products), GFAP (Glial fibrillary acidic protein), and Iba-1 (Ionized calcium binding adaptor molecule 1), through Western blot and confocal microscopic analysis. Moreover, our results showed that curcumin downregulated the expression of p-JNK (Phospo c-Jun N-Terminal Kinase), p-NF-kB (nuclear factor kappa-light-chain-enhancer of activated B cells), and its downstream targets, as assessed by Western blot and confocal microscopic analysis. Finally, the expression of synaptic proteins and the behavioral results also supported the hypothesis that curcumin may inhibit memory dysfunction and behavioral alterations associated with ethanol intoxication. Altogether, to the best of our knowledge, we believe that curcumin may serve as a potential, promising, and cheaply available neuroprotective compound against ethanol-associated neurodegenerative diseases.

Keywords: neurodegenerative diseases; oxidative stress; neuroinflammation; apoptosis; synaptic dysfunction

1. Introduction

Alcohol is a sedative agent and is pharmacologically similar to other hypnotic drugs, which makes it a potential candidate for abuse worldwide. In Western, European, and North American populations, the percentage of alcoholics among the adult population varies from 2% to 12% [1]. Alcohol and its derivatives promote physiological, behavioral, and cognitive dysfunctions in consumers [2], so worldwide alcohol dependence is considered to be a serious health issue in the modern world [3]. Ethanol has shown strong neurodegenerative consequences in experimental animal brains [4,5]. The neurodegenerative effects are associated with neuroinflammation, apoptotic cell death [6], and synaptic dysfunction [7,8]. Moreover, it has been shown that the consumption of alcohol leads to the generation of free radicals and to the chain reaction of lipid peroxidation that causes damage to the brain and other vital organs [9,10]. To combat the challenges of free radical generation, a potent antioxidant defense mechanism is of crucial importance. In the journey to find a novel, potent, and effective antioxidant system, naturally occurring compounds have always drawn more attention because of their ease of availability, safety, and efficacy. Many natural compounds and their derivatives have shown efficacy in the management of different neurological disorders [11–13], and are under consideration and evaluation for these disorders. Curcumin, a compound known to inhibit neuroinflammation, reduces plaque deposition in AD (Alzheimer's Disease) models and improves vascular dysfunction [14]. It has been shown to antagonize many steps in the inflammatory cascade [15], including the suppression of nuclear factor-B, iNOS (Inducible nitric oxide synthase), and JNK (c-Jun N-terminal kinases) [13,16]. Moreover, it has shown the best antioxidant effects in mice [17]. It has shown effectiveness against the MPTP (1-methyl-4-phenyl-1,2,3,6-tetrahydropyridine) model of Parkinson's disease [18] and the MCAO (middle cerebral artery occlusion) animal model of the ischemic brain [19]. Based on the promising therapeutic potentials of naturally occurring curcumin, we hypothesized that chronic curcumin administration may inhibit ethanol-induced neurodegeneration and memory impairment in mice, by regulating reactive oxygen species (ROS), toll-like receptor-4 (TLR4), and Receptor for advanced glycation end products (RAGE)-mediated neuroinflammation, while p-JNK and p-NF-kB triggered the release of cytokines and synaptic dysfunction. The main target of the current study is oxidative stress, regulated by nuclear factor erythroid-2 (Nrf2; an endogenous antioxidant enzyme), and neuroinflammation, initiated by the activation of the innate immune response, mostly tailored by the activation of TLR4 and RAGE, playing a role in recognizing the microbial-associated molecular patterns initiating and modulating the immune response. The activation of the TLR4 signaling promotes the phosphorylation of NF-kB, thereby promoting the inflammatory effects [20]. The signals generated by both the RAGE and TLR4 receptors funnel to the same pathway of neuroinflammation [21]. Compounds counteracting the abnormal ROS generation, inhibition of TLR4/RAGE, and inhibition of the phosphorylation of JNK/NF-kB signaling may render protection to the brain against the mediators of neurodegeneration. Here, we have made an attempt to explore the underlying neuroprotective mechanisms of chronic curcumin administration against ethanol-induced neurodegeneration and memory impairment, by targeting the oxidative stress, neuroinflammation, and apoptotic cell death.

2. Materials and Methods

2.1. Chemicals and Antibodies

The antibodies used in the Western blot and immunofluorescence studies were anti-Nrf2 (sc-722), anti-HO1 (sc-136,961), anti-synaptosomal-associated protein 23 (SNAP-23) (sc-374,215), anti-PSD-95 (sc-71,933), anti-Syntaxin (sc-12,736), anti-tumor necrosis factor-α (TNF-α) (sc-52,746), anti-PARP-1 (sc-8007), TLR4 (sc-16240), Synaptophysin (sc-17750), anti-interleukin (IL)-1β (sc-32,294), anti-Bax (sc-7480), anti-Bcl2 (sc-7382), anti-p-NF-κB (sc-136,548), anti-Iba-1 (sc-32,725), anti-Glial fibrillary acidic protein (GFAP; sc-33,673), and anti-β- actin (sc-47,778) (Santa Cruz Biotechnology, Dallas, TX, USA). In addition, the anti-Cleaved Caspase-3 (#9664) antibodies were obtained from Cell Signaling Technology (Danvers, MA, USA). For Syntaxin and β-actin, the antibodies were diluted in TBST (1:10000) (Santa Cruz Biotechnology, Dallas, TX, USA). Other primary antibodies were diluted in 1x TBST (1:1000), and Secondary anti-mouse HRP (Horseradish peroxidase) conjugated (Promega Ref# W402) and anti-rabbit HRP conjugated (Promega Ref# W401) were diluted 1:10,000 in 1× TBST and were purchased from Promega, (Fitchburg, WI, USA). TAK242, Resatorvid (CAS 243984-11-4), the specific inhibitor of TLR4. For the confocal microscopic studies, the secondary fluorescent antibodies used were goat anti-mouse (Ref# A11029) and goat anti-rabbit (Ref# 32732) diluted in 1× PBS.

2.2. Animals Grouping and Drugs Administration

Male mice (C57BL/6N, $n = 60$, mice 25 ± 3 g, eight old weeks) were acclimatized to the animal house environment for one week, at 12/12 h light/dark cycles at room temperature. The study was approved and conducted in accordance with the guidelines of the Institutional Animal Care and Use Committee (IACUC) of the Division of Applied Life Science, Gyeongsang National University, South Korea (approval ID: 125). Efforts were made to minimize the number of animals used, as well as their suffering. The mice were randomly divided into three groups. (1) The control group mice were treated with an equal volume of vehicle intraperitoneally (physiological saline 0.1 mL/100 g/day) for six weeks, and the mice were freely allowed water and food ad-libitum. (2) The ethanol group mice were treated with an intraperitoneal injection of ethanol for six weeks (5 g/kg i.p., for six weeks, daily). (3) The ethanol and curcumin group mice were treated with curcumin 50 mg/kg for six weeks, daily. The doses of ethanol and curcumin were purely selected on the bases of previously published papers [22]. After the completion of the treatment and behavioral analysis, the mice were sacrificed.

2.3. Tissues Collections for Molecular and Morphological Analysis

For biochemical studies, the mice (8–10/group) were anesthetized, sacrificed, and the brain sections were separated. Next, the brain tissue was homogenized in a protein extraction solution (PRO-PREP™), according to the instructions (iNtRON Biotechnology, Inc., Sungnam, South Korea). After homogenization, the samples were centrifuged at 13,000 r.p.m. at 4 °C for 25 min. The supernatants were collected and stored at −80 °C.

For the morphological studies, the mice (seven to eight per group) were anesthetized and perfused transcardially with saline at a flow rate of 10 mL/min for 3 min, followed by perfusion with a 4% paraformaldehyde solution for 8 min using a peristaltic pump, as provided [23]. The brains were removed and fixed in 4% cold neutral buffer paraformaldehyde for 48 h, and cryoprotected by immersing into a 30% sucrose phosphate buffer for 48 h at 4 °C [23]. After that, the whole brain was frozen in an OCT (optimal cutting temperature compound) compound (Sakura, Torrance, CA, USA), and 14 μm sections were made in the coronal planes using a microtome (Leica cryostat CM 3050S, Nussloch, Germany). The sections were mounted on the probe-on plus charged slides (Fisher, Pittsburgh, PA, USA), and were stored at −70 °C for further analyses.

2.4. In Vitro Cell Culturing, Drug Treatment, Nuclear Factor-2 Erythroid-2 (Nrf2) Gene Silencing by Small Interfering RNA (siRNA) and Western Blot Analysis

The mouse hippocampal HT22 and murine BV2 microglial cells were cultured in Dulbecco's modified Eagle's medium (DMEM) supplemented with FBS (Fetal bovine serum) (10%) and penicillin/streptomycin (1%) in a 5% CO_2 incubator at 37 °C. After attaining a confluency of 70%, the cells were pretreated for 1 h with ethanol (100 μM), followed by curcumin (2 μM) or Nrf2 siRNA for 24 h, or TAK242 (TLR4 specific inhibitor). The Nrf2 gene was knocked down with Nrf2 siRNA at a concentration of 10 μM per transfection for 36 h, as directed (SC: 37049, Santa Cruz Biotechnology, Inc., Dallas, TX, USA). The transfection was conducted with lipofectamine™2000 reagent (Invitrogen, Waltham, MA, USA) when the cells culture reached to 75–80%. The control group cells were treated with 0.01% Dimethyl sulfoxide (DMSO).

2.5. Western Blot Analysis

Western blot was performed as described previously, with some modifications [24,25]. The proteins were loaded and separated by SDS–PAGE (sodium dodecyl sulfate-polyacrylamide gel electrophoresis), and transferred to a polyvinylidene difluoride (PVDF) membrane (Immobilon-P^{SQ}, Transfer membrane, Merck Millipore, Burlington, MA, USA). The immunoreaction was carried out for 16 h at 4 °C using an appropriate ratio of the primary antibodies. After that, the membranes were washed with 1× TBST three times for 10 min, and reacted with a horseradish peroxidase-conjugated secondary antibody for

2 h, as appropriate. The expression of the respective proteins was detected using an ECL (Enhanced chemiluminescence) -detection reagent, according to the manufacturer's instructions. The expressions of the different proteins were obtained on X-ray films and were scanned, and the optical densities of the bands were analyzed by densitometry, using the computer-based ImageJ software (version 1.50, NIH, https://imagej.nih.gov/ij/, Bethesda, MD, USA).

2.6. Immunofluorescence Staining

The fluorescence assay was performed as mentioned previously [26,27]. The slides were dried overnight at room temperature, washed with PBS (0.01 mM) for 8–10 min (two times), treated with proteinase K for 5 min, rinsed with PBS, and blocked with normal serum (2% goat/rabbit, as appropriate) in PBS, added with 0.1% Triton X-100. After that, the slides were incubated with primary antibodies overnight at 4 °C. The slides were then incubated with tetramethylrhodamine isothiocyanate–fluorescein isothiocyanate (FITC)-labeled secondary antibodies (antirabbit and antimouse, as appropriate), at room temperature for 95 min. The slides were covered using the fluorescent mounting medium. Images were taken using a confocal laser-microscope (FluoView FV 1000 MPE, Olympus, Tokyo, Japan). Integrated density was used for the quantification of the staining intensity and for the amount in the immunofluorescent microscopic image. ImageJ software (wsr@nih.gov., https://imagej.nih.gov/ij/) was used to quantify the integrated density, which represents the sum of the pixel values in an image.

2.7. ROS Assay

To analyze the effects of curcumin against ethanol-induced oxidative stress, we conducted a ROS assay, as described previously [28,29]. The assay is based on the oxidation of 2′,7′-dichlorodihydrofluorescein diacetate (CAS 4091-99-0, Santa Cruz Biotechnology, Dallas, TX, USA) to 2′ 7′ dichlorofluorescein (DCF). The brain homogenates were diluted with cold Lock's buffer at 1:20, to yield the final concentration of 2.5 mg tissue/500 µL. The reaction mixture of Lock's buffer (1 mL; pH ± 7.4), 0.2 mL of homogenate, and 10 mL of DCFH-DA (dichlorodihydrofluorescein diacetate) (5 mM) was incubated at room temperature for 15 min, to convert the DCFH-DA to the fluorescent product DCF. The conversion of DCFH-DA to the DCF was analyzed using a spectrofluorimeter (Promega, Fitchburg, WI, USA), with excitation at 484 nm and emission at 530 nm. For the background fluorescence (conversion of DCFH-DA in the absence of homogenate), parallel blanks were measured. The quantitative expression of ROS has been shown with a histogram.

2.8. Determination of Lipid Peroxidation

Lipid peroxidation (LPO) is used to assess oxidative stress. Free malondialdehyde (MDA), which is an indicator of LPO, was analyzed in the tissue homogenates, by using a lipid peroxidation (MDA) colorimetric/fluorometric assay kit (BioVision, San Francesco, CA, USA, Cat#739-100), according to the manufacturer's instructions.

2.9. Morris Water Maze Test

The behavioral analysis was done by the MWM (Morris Water Maze) and Y-maze test ($n = 12$ mice/group), as performed previously [30,31]. The apparatus used for the analysis was made of a circular tank (100 cm in diameter, 40 cm in height), containing water (23 ± 1 °C) to a depth of 15.5 cm. The water was made opaque by adding a non-toxic white color. A platform made of white plastic was kept 1 cm below the water surface, at one quadrant. For five consecutive days, the mice were trained consecutively. The latency to escape from the water (searching the hidden platform) was calculated for each trial. On the sixth day, the probe test was conducted for the evaluation of the memory effects. The probe test was conducted by removing the platform and allowing the mice to explore the tank freely for one hour. The time spent by the mice in the target quadrant and the number of crossings over the position of the platform were recorded. The time spent in the target quadrant was taken to show the degree of memory changes. The data were recorded using video-tracking software (SMART Panlab, Harvard Apparatus, Holliston, MA, USA).

2.10. Y-Maze Test

The apparatus used for the evaluation of the Y-maze was made of black-painted wood, and the dimensions of the arms were 50 cm long and 20 cm height and 10 cm width, as already used by our group [32] and others [33]. The mice were allowed to move freely in the Y-maze, and for that, the mice were kept in the center of the apparatus for 8 min, three times. The arm entries were visualized and observed carefully. The successive entry of the mice into the arms was defined as spontaneous alternations. The alternation behaviors were considered as (successive triplet sets (entries into three different arms consecutively)/total number of arm entries (2)) × 100. A higher percentage (%) of spontaneous alternations was considered to be an indicator of the improved cognitive performance of the experimental mice, and vice versa.

2.11. Fluoro-Jade B Staining

The Fluoro-Jade B staining was done as described previously [28], and according to the instructions provided (Burlington, MA, USA, Cat #AG310, Lot #2159662). The slides were dried at room temperature for 24 h. Furthermore, the slides were dipped in a solution of 1% sodium hydroxide and 80% ethanol, for five min. After that, the slides were kept in 70% ethanol for 2 min and in D-water for 2 min, transferred into a potassium permanganate solution (0.06%) for 10 min, rinsed with D-water, and kept in 0.1% acetic acid solution and 0.01% Fluoro-Jade B solution for 20 min, washed with D-water, and dried for 10 min. The sections were covered using a DPX mounting medium, and the images were taken using a confocal laser microscope (FV 1000, Olympus, Tokyo, Japan). Integrated density was used for the quantification of the staining intensity and for the amount in the immunofluorescent microscopic image. ImageJ software (wsr@nih.gov, https://imagej.nih.gov/ij/) was used to quantify the integrated density, which represents the sum of the pixel values in an image.

2.12. Nissl Staining

Nissl staining was performed according to the previously used methods [34], so as to visualize the histological changes in the brain. The slides were washed with 0.01 M BPS, twice for 15 min, and stained with 0.5% cresyl violet solution (containing a few drops of glacial acetic acid) for 12 to 15 min. Then, the sections were washed with D-water and dehydrated in ethanols (70%, 95%, and 100%), and xylene was dropped on the slides and covered by using the non-fluorescent mounting medium. The neurodegeneration was visualized by light microscope, and the densities of the cells were counted by using ImageJ software.

2.13. Data Analysis and Statistics

The densities of the bands were analyzed by densitometry using the ImageJ software. We performed one-way ANOVA (Analysis of variance) with Tukey's post-hoc test for comparisons among the different experimental groups. The data are presented as the "mean (SD)" of 7–10 mice per group, and are representative of three independent experiments. The calculations and graphs were generated by using Prism 6 software (GraphPad Software, San Diego, CA, USA). Ω is significantly different from the vehicle-treated, Φ is significantly different from the ethanol-treated group. Significance = Ω, $p < 0.05$, Φ, $p < 0.05$, and Ψ, $p < 0.05$.

3. Results

3.1. Chronic Administration of Curcumin Inhibits Ethanol-Induced Oxidative Stress in Mice Brains and In-Vitro HT22 Cells

Oxidative stress has been a significant player in ethanol [35] and other neurotoxins-induced neurodegenerative disorders [36,37]. To find the potential effects of curcumin against ethanol-induced oxidative stress, we performed ROS and LPO assays. According to our findings, curcumin inhibits the elevated level of LPO and ROS (Figure 1A,B). Similarly, the other main antioxidant genes, Nrf2/HO-1, were also analyzed in the experimental groups. According to our Western blot and confocal findings, the chronic co-administration of curcumin with ethanol inhibited the suppression of Nrf2/HO-1 in the mice brains, thereby preserving the endogenous antioxidant mechanism of the brains (Figure 2C,D). Furthermore, we observed a reduced expression of Nrf2 and its target genes HO-1, in the ethanol (100 µM) exposed HT22 cells, which was markedly reversed by curcumin (2 µM), thereby upregulating the expression of Nrf2 and HO-1 in the cells. Interestingly, curcumin could not upregulate the expression of Nrf2/HO-1 in the ethanol-treated cell lines, where the Nrf2 genes were knocked down by Nrf2 siRNA (Figure 1E), indicating that curcumin abrogated the elevated ROS, by upregulating the Nrf2 genes, and the downstream targets of Nrf2.

3.2. Chronic Administration of Curcumin Attenuates Ethanol-Induced Astrocytes and Microglia Activation in Ethanol-Treated Mouse Brains and In-Vitro Microglial Cells

Previous literature has shown that there is activated microglia and astrocytes with ethanol intoxication [4], which may promote neurological disorders such as AD and dementia [38]. TLR4, a receptor for innate immune response, has been shown to be upregulated with ethanol; another receptor is RAGE, which has been shown to be playing a similar role in the inflammatory signaling. Our findings demonstrate that there was a significant reduction in the activation of both of the receptors in the curcumin-treated group. The Glial fibrillary acidic protein (GFAP) and ionized calcium-binding adaptor 1 (Iba-1) are assigned markers for the activities of astrocytes and microglia, respectively [28]. According to our Western blot and confocal microscopic results, there was an increased expression of GFAP and Iba-1 in the ethanol-treated mice brains, which was significantly rescued with the administration of curcumin (Figure 2). Furthermore, the in vitro findings also showed an enhanced expression of TLR4 and Iba-1 in the ethanol treated BV-2 microglial cells, which were significantly reduced in the curcumin and TAK242 (a specific inhibitor of TLR4) treated cells.

3.3. Chronic Administration of Curcumin Regulated Ethanol-Induced Inflammatory Markers in Mouse Brains

Previous studies have shown that ethanol intoxication is responsible for the activation of stress-markers and inducing inflammatory cytokines [39]. To explore whether these markers may be inhibited with the administration of curcumin, we analyzed the expression of stress and inflammatory markers, such as p-JNK, p-NF-κB, cyclooxygenase-2 (COX-2), interleukin-1β (IL-1β), and tissue necrosis factor-α (TNF-α), in the mice brains. As shown here, treatment with ethanol elevated the expression of p-JNK, p-Nf-κB, IL-1β, COX-2, and TNF-α. However, the mice that were co-administered the curcumin and ethanol had a lower expression of these markers compared with the ethanol-treated group, supporting the hypothesis that curcumin inhibits the expression of inflammatory cytokines, thereby rendering protection to mice brains against ethanol-induced neurodegeneration. The Western blot results were further supported by the confocal microscopic analysis, which showed that curcumin inhibits the effects of ethanol against the activation of p-JNK in mice brains (Figure 3).

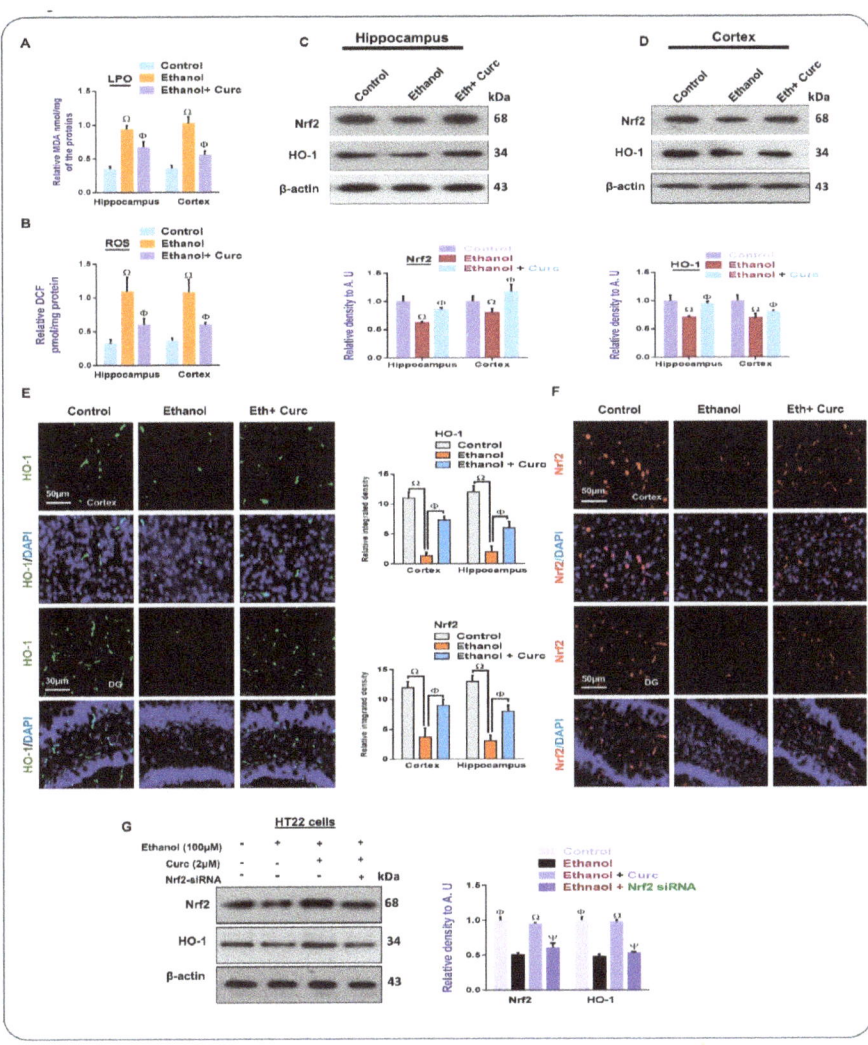

Figure 1. Chronic administration of curcumin inhibits ethanol-induced oxidative stress in mice brain: (**A** & **B**) Results of lipid peroxidation (LPO) and reactive oxygen species (ROS) assays, respectively; (**C** & **D**) Western blot results of nuclear factor erythroid 2-related factor 2 (Nrf2) & heme-oxygenase 1 (HO-1), in the mice brain; (**E** & **F**) Confocal microscopic results of HO-1, and Nrf2 in the experimental groups, with bar graphs, magnification 30×, scale bar 50 µm; (**G**) In vitro HT22 cells treated with ethanol. Curcumin or ethanol + curcumin, and Ω, significantly different from the vehicle-treated, Φ, significantly different from the ethanol-treated group, and Ψ, significantly different from the ethanol + Curc treated group. DG means dentate gyrus, Significance = Φ $p < 0.05$; Ω, $p < 0.05$; Ψ, $p < 0.05$. MDA: malondialdehyde, DCF: 2′ 7′ dichlorofluorescein, eth: ethanol, curc: curcumin.

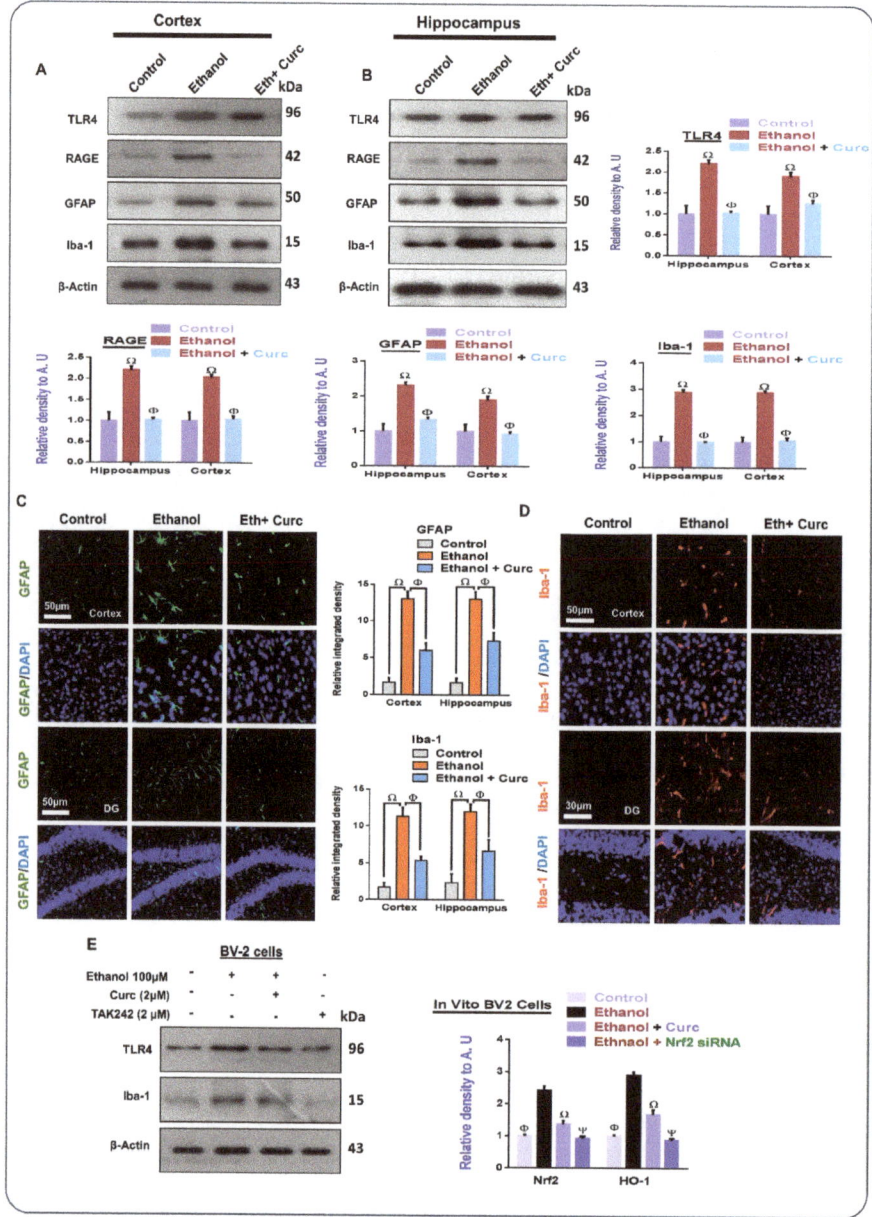

Figure 2. Curcumin Rescued activated Microglia and Astrocytes in the ethanol-treated Mouse Brains: (**A** & **B**) The Western blot results of toll-like receptor 4 (TLR4), Receptor for Advanced Glycations End Product (RAGE), glial fibrillary acidic protein (GFAP), and ionized calcium binding adaptor molecule 1 (Iba-1) in the brains of the experimental groups; (**C**) Immunofluorescence images of the expression of GFAP in the experimental groups; (**D**) Immunofluorescence images of Iba-1 in the experimental groups ($n = 12$ mice per group); (**E**) Immunoblot results of TLR4 and Iba-1 in BV-2 Cells, in different experimental groups. Magnification 30× objective field, scale bar = 50 µm & 30 µm. Ω, significantly different from the vehicle-treated, Φ, significantly different from the ethanol-treated group and Ψ, significantly different from the ethanol + Curc treated group. DG means dentate gyrus, Significance = Φ $p < 0.05$; Ω, $p < 0.05$; Ψ, $p < 0.05$. eth: ethanol, curc: curcumin, DAPI: 4′,6-diamidino-2-phenylindole dihydrochloride.

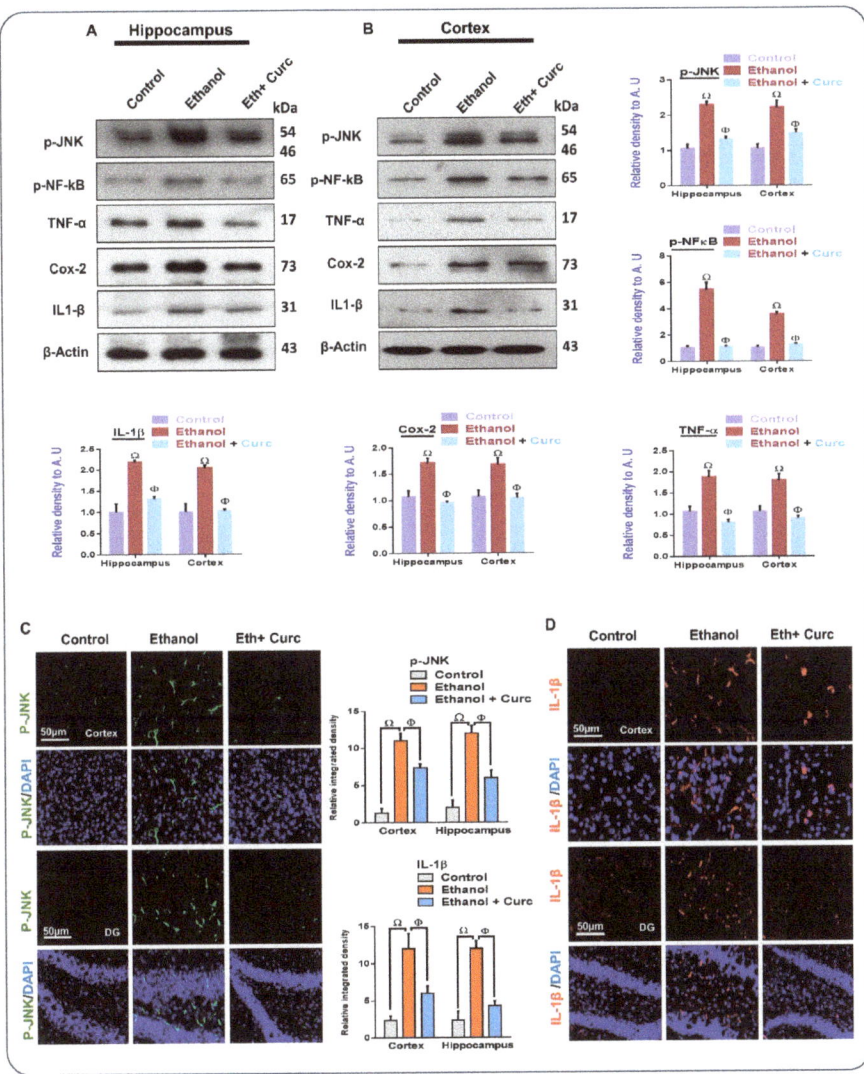

Figure 3. Curcumin Abrogates the Phosphorylation of c-Jun N-Terminal Kinase (JNK) and its Downstream Targets in Ethanol-Treated Mouse Brain: (**A** & **B**) Immunoblot results, showing the expression of active phospho c-Jun N-terminal kinase (p-JNK), nuclear factor kappa-light-chain enhancer of activated B cells (p-NF-kB), tumor necrosis factor alpha (TNF-α), cyclooxygenase-2 (COX-2), and IL-1β and in mice that received saline, ethanol, and ethanol plus Curcumin for 6 weeks ($n = 12$ mice per group), normalized with its β-actin, as a loading control, with its Histograms; (**C** & **D**). Confocal images, showing active JNK and interleukin-1β (IL-1β) in the mouse brain. Magnification 30× objective field, scale bar = 50 μm, Ω, significantly different from the vehicle-treated, Φ, significantly different from the ethanol-treated group. DG means dentate gyrus, Significance = Φ $p < 0.05$, Ω, $p < 0.05$. eth: ethanol, curc: curcumin.

3.4. Chronic Administration of Curcumin Rescued Apoptotic Cell Death and Neurodegeneration

Studies have shown that there is an increased expression of apoptotic markers in ethanol-treated mice brains, which leads to apoptotic cell death and neuronal loss [4,40]. Keeping in mind the role of these apoptotic markers in ethanol-induced neurodegeneration, we analyzed the expression of apoptotic markers, including Bax and Bcl-2, Cleaved Caspase-3, and PARP-1 in mice brains. Per our Western blot results, there was an increased expression of pro-apoptotic markers Caspase-3, Bax, and PARP-1, and a decreased expression of Bcl-2 (anti-apoptotic marker) in the ethanol-treated mice brains. However, curcumin regulated the expression of these markers. Moreover, the immunofluorescence results indicated the increased expression of Caspase-3 and PARP-1 in the ethanol-treated mice brains, which were inhibited with chronic administration of curcumin (Figure 4).

3.5. Chronic Administration of Curcumin Rescued the Neuronal Cell Loss, as Assessed by Fluoro-Jade B and Nissl staining

Overall, the neuroprotective effects of curcumin were further confirmed by visualizing the morphology of hippocampal neurons, by using Nissl and FJB staining on the mice brains, as these staining protocols have extensively been used to visualize the morphology of neurons in different experimental settings [41,42]. According to FJB staining, there were increased FJB stained neurons in the ethanol-treated group, which was significantly inhibited with the administration of curcumin, as shown (Figure 5A). Similarly, in the Nissl staining, there was a decrease in the Nissl stained neurons in the ethanol injected group, which was significantly preserved with the administration of curcumin, as shown (Figure 5B), thereby confirming the hypothesis that curcumin plays a rescuing role against ethanol-induced neurodegeneration and memory impairment.

3.6. Chronic Administration of Curcumin Reversed Synaptic Dysfunction and Memory Impairment in the Ethanol-Treated Mouse Brain

Previous studies have shown that ethanol intoxication contributes to the loss of synaptic protein in animal models [39,43]. To explore the effects of curcumin on synaptic marker ethanol-treated mouse brains, we evaluated the expression of synaptic proteins via Western blot and confocal microscopy. According to our findings, the synaptic proteins, including PSD-95, synaptophysin, and SNAP-25, were significantly downregulated in the ethanol-treated mice brains compared with the control mice. Interestingly, curcumin significantly inhibited these effects. The confocal microscopic results of PSD-95 showed significant fluorescence in the curcumin- and ethanol-treated group compared with the ethanol alone group, showing that curcumin preserves the synaptic markers by regulating oxidative stress, neuroinflammation, and apoptotic cell death in mouse brains (Figure 6). Previously, it has been shown that chronic ethanol intoxication causes abnormalities in motor functions and impaired spatial learning and memory [39]. To show whether curcumin could rescue ethanol-induced memory impairment, we performed the MWM and Y-maze tests. First, we recorded the learning abilities of the mice ($n = 12$ mice/group) with the MWM test. We found that ethanol-treated mice had an enhanced latency to reach to the platform, and the mice that had received curcumin (50 mg/kg, i.p., six weeks) showed a decreased escape latency (Figure 6). Twenty-four hours after the fifth day of training, the platform was removed and the mice were allowed to swim freely. We found that the ethanol-treated mice spent less time in the target quadrant and showed less platform crossings, highlighting that ethanol induces memory impairments. Interestingly, curcumin improved the ethanol-induced memory impairments by increasing the total time spent in the target quadrant, and the number of crossings of the platform (Figure 6F,G). After that, we checked the spontaneous alternation behaviors (showing the spatial working memory or short-term memory) of mice ($n = 12$ mice/group) in the Y-maze test. In the ethanol-treated mice, there was a reduction in the spontaneous alternation behaviors compared with the saline-treated mice, showing a cognition decline in the ethanol treated mice. Interestingly, curcumin significantly increased the spontaneous alternation behaviors in the ethanol-treated mice compared with the ethanol-treated group (Figure 6H). Collectively, our findings showed that the co-administration of curcumin with ethanol significantly prevents cognitive dysfunctions in mice.

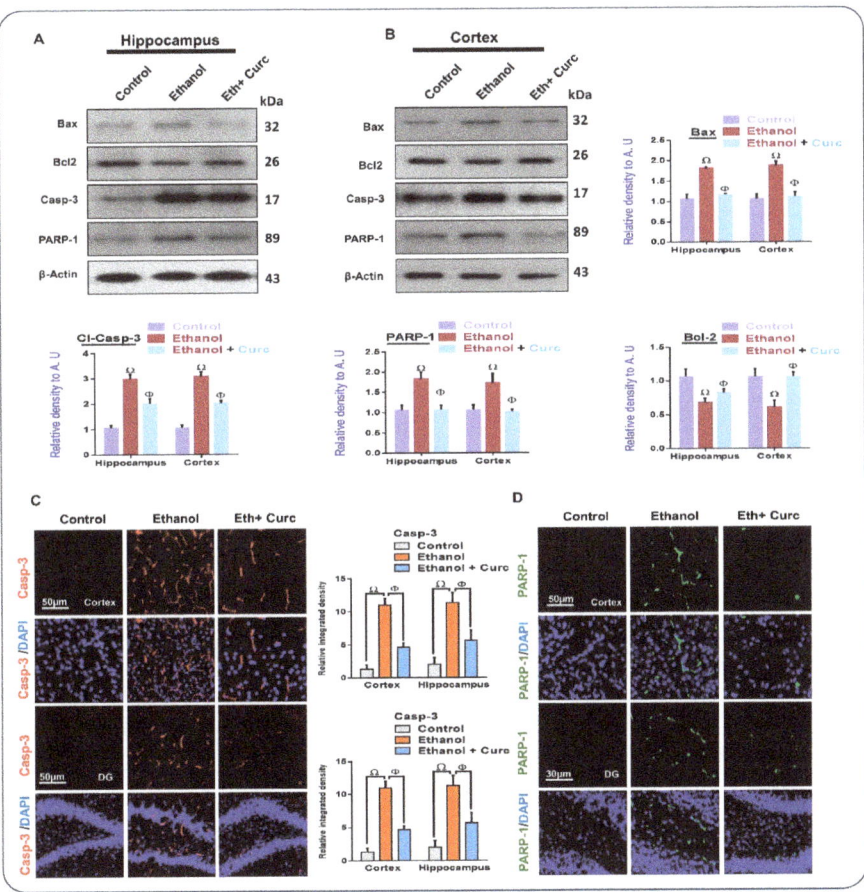

Figure 4. Curcumin Abrogated Ethanol-Induced Apoptotic Cell Death in Mouse Brain: (**A** & **B**) Immunoblot results of B-cell lymphoma 2-associated X (Bax); , B-cell lymphoma 2 (Bcl-2), Caspase-3, and PARP-1 in the brains of the experimental groups, with their relative bra graphs; (**C** & **D**) Immunofluorescence results of activated Caspase-3 and poly (ADP-ribose)polymerase 1 (PARP-1) in the brains of the experimental mice, with their histograms (n = 12 mice/group), Magnification, 40×, scale bar 50 μm & 30 μm. Ω, significantly different from the vehicle-treated, Φ, significantly different from the ethanol-treated group. DG means dentate gyrus, Significance = Φ p < 0.05, Ω, p < 0.05. eth: ethanol, curc: curcumin.

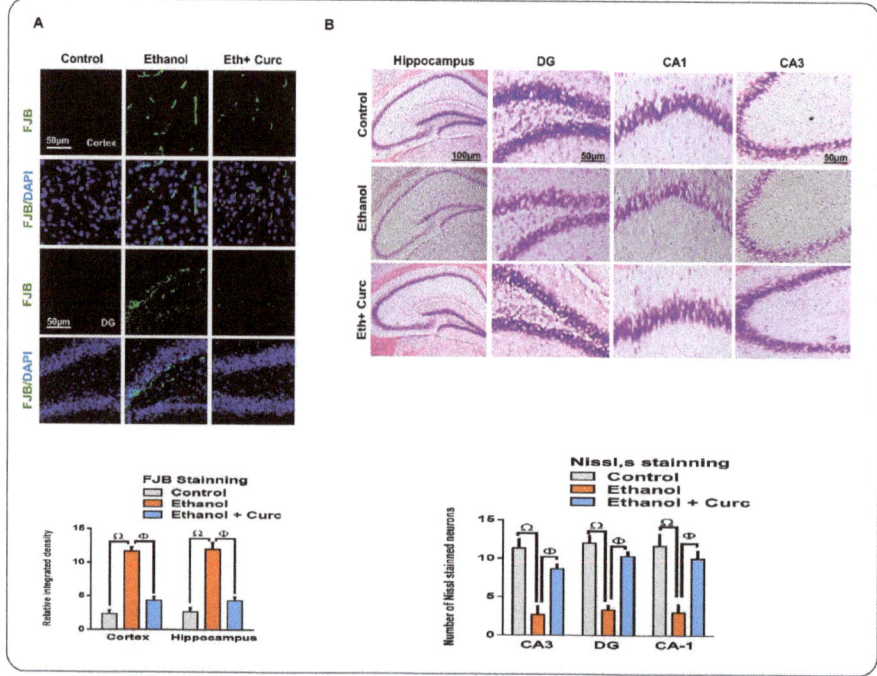

Figure 5. Curcumin Ameliorates Neurodegeneration in Mouse Brains, as visualized by Nissl and FJB staining: (**A**) FJB stained sections from mice hippocampus, co-stained with DAPI and its histogram, the differences have been shown in the histogram; (**B**) Images of the Nissl stained sections (CA1, CA3 and DG) from different experimental groups with histograms, $n = 12$ mice/group, scale bar 50 μm & 100 μm, Ω, significantly different from the vehicle-treated, Φ, significantly different from the ethanol-treated group. DG means dentate gyrus, Significance = Φ, $p < 0.05$, Ω, $p < 0.05$. eth: ethanol, curc: curcumin.

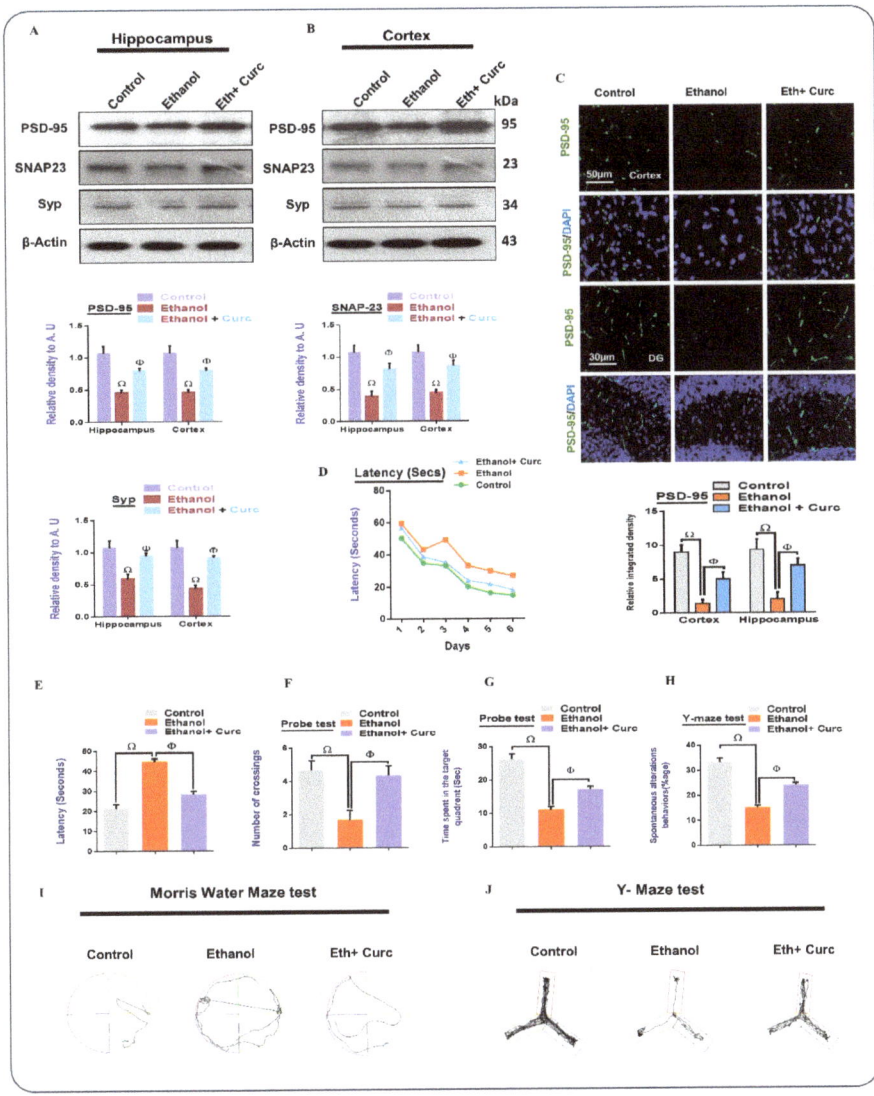

Figure 6. Curcumin Rescued Ethanol-Induced Synaptic Dysfunction and Memory Impairment in Mouse: (**A** & **B**) Immunoblot results of PSD95, SNAP23 and synaptophysin in mice brain ($n = 10$), with histograms; (**C**) Confocal images of PSD-95 in mouse brains, with its bar graph. Magnification, 40×, scale bar up to 50 μm; (**D**). Mean escape latency (shown in seconds) to the platform during a training session, $n = 12$ mice/group; (**E**). Latency on the final day of the probe test; (**F**). Histograms showing the number of platform crossings during the probe test; (**G**) Time spent in the target quadrant during the probe trial; (**H**) Spontaneous alternations (in percent) in the Y-maze test; (**I** & **J**). Trajectories of the MWM tests & Y-maze tests, respectively ($n = 12$ mice/group). Ω, significantly different from the vehicle-treated, Φ, significantly different from the ethanol-treated group. Significance = Φ $p < 0.05$, Ω, $p < 0.05$. eth: ethanol, curc: curcumin.

4. Discussion

The current study has the following main findings. (i) Curcumin has strong anti-oxidant potentials against ethanol-induced oxidative stress, in vivo mouse brains, and in vitro mouse hippocampal HT22 cells, and the antioxidant effects of curcumin are solely dependent on Nrf2. (ii) Curcumin has rescuing effects against ethanol induced activated astrocytes and microglia, in vivo and in vitro, as revealed by the reduced expression of TLR4/RAGE, GFAP, and Iba-1. (iii) Curcumin may rescue the mice brain from ethanol-induced apoptotic cell death, synaptic dysfunction, and memory impairment in mice brains. Several lines of studies have also reported the neuroprotective effects of curcumin against neuroinflammation and apoptotic cell death [44–46]. One study completely focused on oxidative stress mediated neuroinflammation [47]. However, they have not further extended their study to the main antioxidant enzymes, such as Nrf2/HO-1. Curcumin was administered intraperitoneally, and although it is considered a parenteral route of administration, the pharmacokinetics of substances administered intraperitoneally are more similar to those seen after oral administration. In both cases, the primary route of absorption is into the mesenteric vessels, which drain into the portal vein and pass through the liver [48].

Curcumin has long since been reported to be a potent antioxidant, but no studies have yet reported its effects on the endogenous antioxidant mechanisms (Nrf2/HO-1) and TLR4/RAGE mediated neurodegeneration. A wide range of effects are associated with ethanol intoxication, including oxidative stress, apoptotic neurodegeneration, excitotoxicity, and the disruption of cell to cell interactions [40,49]. The production of ROS may cause other serious consequences, such as an altered metabolism, deleterious structural modifications of proteins, DNA mishandlings, and altered mitochondrial homeostasis. Here, we report that ethanol-induced oxidative stress mediated neuroinflammation via Nrf-2/TLR4 signaling. The induction of oxidative stress with the administration of ethanol is in accordance with previous studies [50]. Interestingly, the in vitro findings also support the results, showing antioxidant effects against ethanol induced oxidative stress. For more confirmatory purposes, we used specific Nrf2 siRNA, and the findings showed that curcumin may relieve the elevated ROS level through Nrf2.

The other outcome of our study is that curcumin may inhibit the TLR4/RAGE triggered neuroinflammation in mice brains and in in vitro microglial cells. TLR4, which is mainly expressed in the microglial cells, induces microglial activation and the expression of proinflammatory cytokines, such as TNF-α and p-NF-kB, in response to a variety of stimuli [51]. Besides TLR4, other receptors are also involved in neurodegenerative conditions, such as RAGE. Here, we also evaluated the expression of RAGE in the experimental groups. According to our findings, there was an enhanced expression of TLR4/RAGE and its downstream inflammatory mediators in the ethanol-treated mice brain. Interestingly, these markers were significantly reduced with the administration of curcumin. For more confirmatory purposes, we used a specific TLR4 inhibitor (TAK242). Interestingly, the rescuing effects of curcumin against TLR4/iba-1 in the microglial cells were comparable to TAK 242. GFAP and Iba-1, which are the assigned markers for the activated astrocytes and microglia, were significantly upregulated in the ethanol-treated group, however, there was a significantly lower expression in the curcumin-treated group. The upregulation of GFAP and Iba1 in the ethanol-treated group is in accordance with the previous reports [4]. The inhibition of TLR4 further inhibited the expression of its downstream effectors (Iba-1) in the microglial cells. The upregulation of TLR4, RAGE, and the iba-1 in the ethanol-treated mice brains is in accordance with the previous reported effects of ethanol [52].

The other inducer of the neurodegenerative conditions are as follows: the phosphorylation of MAP kinases, which phosphorylates and translocates the NF-kB to the nucleus, playing a pivotal role in the release of inflammatory mediators [53]. According to our findings, there were enhanced expressions of p-JNK and p-NF-kB, as well as other inflammatory mediators (TNF-α, Cox-2, and IL-1β) in the ethanol treated mice, which is in accordance with previous studies [39]. Another main contributor to the neurodegeneration is apoptotic cell death in neurodegenerative conditions [54], as apoptotic cell death has closely been linked to the oxidative damage [55]. For the evaluation of the effects of curcumin against apoptotic cell death, the expression of proapoptotic (Bax, Caspase-3, and PARP-1) and antiapoptotic (Bcl-2) markers were evaluated; according to our findings, ethanol promoted proapoptotic cell death, which was significantly inhibited with the administration of curcumin. For more confirmatory purposes, we performed Nissl and FJB staining, which showed that curcumin significantly inhibited the neurotoxic effects of ethanol on mice brains. The ultimate consequence of neurodegeneration is synaptic dysfunction and loss of memory, which have been extensively reported with ethanol intoxication [56].

For the evaluation of synaptic dysfunction and memory impairment, we performed behavioral studies in Morris water maze and Y-maze tests, as well as the protein markers related to synaptotoxicity. According to our results, curcumin significantly improved the behavioral alterations and synaptic markers (postsynaptic density protein-95, SNAP-23, and synaptophysin) in the mice brain. The protective effects of curcumin on the behavioral changes and synaptic dysfunction are in accordance with previous studies [43,57].

5. Conclusions

Altogether, our findings support the hypothesis that the chronic administration of curcumin may protect mice brains against the detrimental effects of ethanol, by serving as a strong antioxidant, anti-inflammatory, and antiapoptotic agent in vivo mice brains and in vitro cells.

Author Contributions: M.I designed and conducted the experiments, and wrote manuscript; K.S., and M.S.K. conducted the experiments; A.K., T.M., M.G.J., and S.U.R. conducted the statistical analysis, reviewed and edited the manuscripts; M.O.K. supervised and organized the final version of the manuscript. All of the authors reviewed and approved the paper.

Funding: This research was supported by the Brain Research Program through the National Research Foundation of Korea (NRF), funded by the Ministry of Science—ICT (2016M3C7A1904391).

Conflicts of Interest: The authors declare no competing financial interests.

References

1. Kohnke, M.D. Approach to the genetics of alcoholism: A review based on pathophysiology. *Biochem. Pharmacol.* **2008**, *75*, 160–177. [CrossRef] [PubMed]
2. Lee, J.W.; Lee, Y.K.; Lee, B.J.; Nam, S.Y.; Lee, S.I.; Kim, Y.H.; Kim, K.H.; Oh, K.W.; Hong, J.T. Inhibitory effect of ethanol extract of Magnolia officinalis and 4-O-methylhonokiol on memory impairment and neuronal toxicity induced by β-amyloid. *Pharmacol. Biochem. Behav.* **2010**, *95*, 31–40. [CrossRef] [PubMed]
3. Badshah, H.; Kim, T.H.; Kim, M.J.; Ahmad, A.; Ali, T.; Yoon, G.H.; Naseer, M.I.; Kim, M.O. Apomorphine attenuates ethanol-induced neurodegeneration in the adult rat cortex. *Neurochem. Int.* **2014**, *74*, 8–15. [CrossRef] [PubMed]
4. Saito, M.; Chakraborty, G.; Hui, M.; Masiello, K.; Saito, M. Ethanol-induced neurodegeneration and glial activation in the developing brain. *Brain Sci.* **2016**, *6*. [CrossRef]
5. Naseer, M.I.; Ullah, I.; Narasimhan, M.L.; Lee, H.Y.; Bressan, R.A.; Yoon, G.H.; Yun, D.J.; Kim, M.O. Neuroprotective effect of osmotin against ethanol-induced apoptotic neurodegeneration in the developing rat brain. *Cell Death Dis.* **2014**, *5*, e1150. [CrossRef] [PubMed]
6. von Haefen, C.; Sifringer, M.; Menk, M.; Spies, C.D. Ethanol enhances susceptibility to apoptotic cell death via down-regulation of autophagy-related proteins. *Alcohol. Clin. Exp. Res.* **2011**, *35*, 1381–1391. [CrossRef]
7. Menetski, J.; Mistry, S.; Lu, M.; Mudgett, J.S.; Ransohoff, R.M.; Demartino, J.A.; Macintyre, D.E.; Abbadie, C. Mice overexpressing chemokine ligand 2 (CCL2) in astrocytes display enhanced nociceptive responses. *Neuroscience* **2007**, *149*, 706–714. [CrossRef] [PubMed]
8. Lucas, S.M.; Rothwell, N.J.; Gibson, R.M. The role of inflammation in CNS injury and disease. *Br. J. Pharmacol.* **2006**, *147* (Suppl. 1), S232–S240. [CrossRef]
9. Manoharan, J.P.S.; Subramaniyan, A.V.D. Neuroprotective Effects of pterois volitans venom against alcohol induced oxidative dysfunction in Rats. *J. Environ. Anal. Toxicol.* **2015**, *5*. [CrossRef]
10. Ojala, J.; Sutinen, E. The role of interleukin-18, oxidative stress and metabolic syndrome in Alzheimer's disease. *J. Clin. Med.* **2017**, *6*, 55. [CrossRef] [PubMed]

11. Bent, S. Herbal medicine in the United States: Review of efficacy, safety, and regulation: Grand rounds at University of California, San Francisco Medical Center. *J. Gen. Intern. Med.* **2008**, *23*, 854–859. [CrossRef]
12. Jun, Y.L.; Bae, C.H.; Kim, D.; Koo, S.; Kim, S. Korean Red Ginseng protects dopaminergic neurons by suppressing the cleavage of p35 to p25 in a Parkinson's disease mouse model. *J. Ginseng Res.* **2015**, *39*, 148–154. [CrossRef] [PubMed]
13. Begum, A.N.; Jones, M.R.; Lim, G.P.; Morihara, T.; Kim, P.; Heath, D.D.; Rock, C.L.; Pruitt, M.A.; Yang, F.; Hudspeth, B.; et al. Curcumin structure-function, bioavailability, and efficacy in models of neuroinflammation and Alzheimer's disease. *J. Pharmacol. Exp. Ther.* **2008**, *326*, 196–208. [CrossRef]
14. Sompamit, K.; Kukongviriyapan, U.; Nakmareong, S.; Pannangpetch, P.; Kukongviriyapan, V. Curcumin improves vascular function and alleviates oxidative stress in non-lethal lipopolysaccharide-induced endotoxaemia in mice. *Eur. J. Pharmacol.* **2009**, *616*, 192–199. [CrossRef] [PubMed]
15. Ng, Q.; Soh, A.; Loke, W.; Venkatanarayanan, N.; Lim, D.; Yeo, W.-S. A meta-analysis of the clinical use of curcumin for irritable bowel syndrome (IBS). *J. Clin. Med.* **2018**, *7*, 298. [CrossRef] [PubMed]
16. Weber, W.M.; Hunsaker, L.A.; Gonzales, A.M.; Heynekamp, J.J.; Orlando, R.A.; Deck, L.M.; Vander Jagt, D.L. TPA-induced up-regulation of activator protein-1 can be inhibited or enhanced by analogs of the natural product curcumin. *Biochem. Pharmacol.* **2006**, *72*, 928–940. [CrossRef]
17. Ataie, A.; Sabetkasaei, M.; Haghparast, A.; Moghaddam, A.H.; Kazeminejad, B. Neuroprotective effects of the polyphenolic antioxidant agent, Curcumin, against homocysteine-induced cognitive impairment and oxidative stress in the rat. *Pharmacol. Biochem. Behav.* **2010**, *96*, 378–385. [CrossRef] [PubMed]
18. Venkatesan, R.; Ji, E.; Kim, S.Y. Phytochemicals that regulate neurodegenerative disease by targeting neurotrophins: A comprehensive review. *BioMed Res. Int.* **2015**, *2015*, 814068. [CrossRef]
19. Thiyagarajan, M.; Sharma, S.S. Neuroprotective effect of curcumin in middle cerebral artery occlusion induced focal cerebral ischemia in rats. *Life Sci.* **2004**, *74*, 969–985. [CrossRef] [PubMed]
20. Nakano, Y.; Shimazawa, M.; Ojino, K.; Izawa, H.; Takeuchi, H.; Inoue, Y.; Tsuruma, K.; Hara, H. Toll-like receptor 4 inhibitor protects against retinal ganglion cell damage induced by optic nerve crush in mice. *J. Pharmacol. Sci.* **2017**, *133*, 176–183. [CrossRef]
21. Frasnelli, S.C.; de Medeiros, M.C.; Bastos Ade, S.; Costa, D.L.; Orrico, S.R.; Rossa Junior, C. Modulation of immune response by RAGE and TLR4 signalling in PBMCs of diabetic and non-diabetic patients. *Scand. J. Immunol.* **2015**, *81*, 66–71. [CrossRef] [PubMed]
22. Sorrenti, V.; Contarini, G.; Sut, S.; Dall'Acqua, S.; Confortin, F.; Pagetta, A.; Giusti, P.; Zusso, M. Curcumin prevents acute neuroinflammation and long-term memory impairment induced by systemic lipopolysaccharide in mice. *Front. Pharmacol.* **2018**, *9*, 183. [CrossRef] [PubMed]
23. Jackson-Lewis, V.; Przedborski, S. Protocol for the MPTP mouse model of Parkinson's disease. *Nat. Protoc.* **2007**, *2*, 141–151. [CrossRef] [PubMed]
24. Badshah, H.; Ullah, I.; Kim, S.E.; Kim, T.H.; Lee, H.Y.; Kim, M.O. Anthocyanins attenuate body weight gain via modulating neuropeptide Y and GABAB1 receptor in rats hypothalamus. *Neuropeptides* **2013**, *47*, 347–353. [CrossRef] [PubMed]
25. Khan, A.; Ali, T.; Rehman, S.U.; Khan, M.S.; Alam, S.I.; Ikram, M.; Muhammad, T.; Saeed, K.; Badshah, H.; Kim, M.O. Neuroprotective effect of quercetin against the detrimental effects of LPS in the adult mouse brain. *Front. Pharmacol.* **2018**, *9*, 1383. [CrossRef]
26. Badshah, H.; Kim, T.H.; Kim, M.O. Protective effects of anthocyanins against amyloid β-induced neurotoxicity in vivo and in vitro. *Neurochem. Int.* **2015**, *80*, 51–59. [CrossRef]
27. Lee, Y.; Chun, H.J.; Lee, K.M.; Jung, Y.S.; Lee, J. Silibinin suppresses astroglial activation in a mouse model of acute Parkinson's disease by modulating the ERK and JNK signaling pathways. *Brain Res.* **2015**, *1627*, 233–242. [CrossRef]
28. Amin, F.U.; Shah, S.A.; Kim, M.O. Vanillic acid attenuates Aβ1-42-induced oxidative stress and cognitive impairment in mice. *Sci. Rep.* **2017**, *7*, 40753. [CrossRef] [PubMed]
29. Ikram, M.; Muhammad, T.; Rehman, S.U.; Khan, A.; Jo, M.G.; Ali, T.; Kim, M.O. Hesperetin confers neuroprotection by regulating Nrf2/TLR4/NF-κB signaling in an Aβ mouse model. In *Molecular Neurobiology*; Springer: Berlin, Germany, 2019.
30. Khan, M.; Shah, S.A.; Kim, M.O. 17β-Estradiol via SIRT1/Acetyl-p53/NF-kB signaling pathway rescued postnatal rat brain against acute ethanol intoxication. *Mol. Neurobiol.* **2017**. [CrossRef] [PubMed]

31. Lin, Y.-T.; Wu, Y.-C.; Sun, G.-C.; Ho, C.-Y.; Wong, T.-Y.; Lin, C.-H.; Chen, H.-H.; Yeh, T.-C.; Li, C.-J.; Tseng, C.-J. Effect of resveratrol on reactive oxygen species-induced cognitive impairment in rats with angiotensin II-induced early alzheimer's disease. *J. Clin. Med.* **2018**, *7*, 329. [CrossRef] [PubMed]
32. Rehman, S.U.; Ahmad, A.; Yoon, G.-H.; Khan, M.; Abid, M.N.; Kim, M.O. Inhibition of c-Jun N-Terminal kinase protects against brain damage and improves learning and memory after traumatic brain injury in adult mice. *Cereb. Cortex* **2017**. [CrossRef] [PubMed]
33. Ayaz, M.; Junaid, M.; Ullah, F.; Subhan, F.; Sadiq, A.; Ali, G.; Ovais, M.; Shahid, M.; Ahmad, A.; Wadood, A.; et al. Anti-Alzheimer's studies on β-Sitosterol isolated from *Polygonum hydropiper* L. *Front. Pharmacol.* **2017**, *8*, 697. [CrossRef]
34. Muhammad, T.; Ali, T.; Ikram, M.; Khan, A.; Alam, S.I.; Kim, M.O. Melatonin rescue oxidative stress-mediated neuroinflammation/neurodegeneration and memory impairment in scopolamine-induced amnesia mice model. *J. Neuroimmune Pharmacol.* **2018**. [CrossRef] [PubMed]
35. Bauer, A.K.; Fitzgerald, M.; Ladzinski, A.T.; Lenhart Sherman, S.; Maddock, B.H.; Norr, Z.M.; Miller, R.R., Jr. Dual behavior of N-acetylcysteine during ethanol-induced oxidative stress in embryonic chick brains. *Nutr. Neurosci.* **2017**, *20*, 478–488. [CrossRef]
36. Jo, M.G.; Ikram, M.; Jo, M.H.; Yoo, L.; Chung, K.C.; Nah, S.Y.; Hwang, H.; Rhim, H.; Kim, M.O. Gintonin mitigates MPTP-induced loss of nigrostriatal dopaminergic neurons and accumulation of alpha-synuclein via the Nrf2/HO-1 pathway. *Mol. Neurobiol.* **2018**. [CrossRef]
37. Ali, T.; Kim, T.; Rehman, S.U.; Khan, M.S.; Amin, F.U.; Khan, M.; Ikram, M.; Kim, M.O. Natural dietary supplementation of anthocyanins via PI3K/Akt/Nrf2/HO-1 pathways mitigate oxidative stress, neurodegeneration, and memory impairment in a mouse model of alzheimer's disease. *Mol. Neurobiol.* **2018**, *55*, 6076–6093. [CrossRef] [PubMed]
38. Fernandez-Lizarbe, S.; Pascual, M.; Guerri, C. Critical role of TLR4 response in the activation of microglia induced by ethanol. *J. Immunol.* **2009**, *183*, 4733–4744. [CrossRef]
39. Shah, S.A.; Yoon, G.H.; Kim, M.O. Protection of the developing brain with anthocyanins against ethanol-induced oxidative stress and neurodegeneration. *Mol. Neurobiol.* **2015**, *51*, 1278–1291. [CrossRef] [PubMed]
40. Crews, F.T.; Nixon, K. Mechanisms of neurodegeneration and regeneration in alcoholism. *Alcohol. Alcohol.* **2009**, *44*, 115–127. [CrossRef] [PubMed]
41. Damjanac, M.; Rioux Bilan, A.; Barrier, L.; Pontcharraud, R.; Anne, C.; Hugon, J.; Page, G. Fluoro-Jade B staining as useful tool to identify activated microglia and astrocytes in a mouse transgenic model of Alzheimer's disease. *Brain Res.* **2007**, *1128*, 40–49. [CrossRef]
42. Ullah, N.; Naseer, M.I.; Ullah, I.; Kim, T.H.; Lee, H.Y.; Kim, M.O. Neuroprotective profile of pyruvate against ethanol-induced neurodegeneration in developing mice brain. *Neurol. Sci.* **2013**, *34*, 2137–2143. [CrossRef]
43. Muhammad, T.; Ikram, M.; Ullah, R.; Rehman, S.U.; Kim, M.O. Hesperetin, a citrus flavonoid, attenuates lps-induced neuroinflammation, apoptosis and memory impairments by modulating TLR4/NF-κB signaling. *Nutrients* **2019**, *11*. [CrossRef] [PubMed]
44. Fan, C.; Song, Q.; Wang, P.; Li, Y.; Yang, M.; Yu, S.Y. Neuroprotective effects of curcumin on IL-1β-induced neuronal apoptosis and depression-like behaviors caused by chronic stress in rats. *Front. Cell. Neurosci.* **2018**, *12*, 516. [CrossRef]
45. Xu, L.; Ding, L.; Su, Y.; Shao, R.; Liu, J.; Huang, Y. Neuroprotective effects of curcumin against rats with focal cerebral ischemia-reperfusion injury. *Int. J. Mol. Med.* **2019**. [CrossRef]
46. Cole, G.M.; Teter, B.; Frautschy, S.A. Neuroprotective effects of curcumin. In *The Molecular Targets and Therapeutic Uses of Curcumin in Health and Disease*; Springer: Boston, MA, USA, 2007; pp. 197–212.
47. Tiwari, V.; Chopra, K. Protective effect of curcumin against chronic alcohol-induced cognitive deficits and neuroinflammation in the adult rat brain. *Neuroscience* **2013**, *244*, 147–158. [CrossRef]
48. Turner, P.V.; Brabb, T.; Pekow, C.; Vasbinder, M.A. Administration of substances to laboratory animals: Routes of administration and factors to consider. *J. Am. Assoc. Lab. Anim. Sci.* **2011**, *50*, 600–613. [PubMed]
49. Goldowitz, D.; Lussier, A.A.; Boyle, J.K.; Wong, K.; Lattimer, S.L.; Dubose, C.; Lu, L.; Kobor, M.S.; Hamre, K.M. Molecular pathways underpinning ethanol-induced neurodegeneration. *Front. Genet.* **2014**, *5*, 203. [CrossRef]
50. Comporti, M.; Signorini, C.; Leoncini, S.; Gardi, C.; Ciccoli, L.; Giardini, A.; Vecchio, D.; Arezzini, B. Ethanol-induced oxidative stress: Basic knowledge. *Genes Nutr.* **2010**, *5*, 101–109. [CrossRef] [PubMed]

51. McColl, B.W.; Allan, S.M.; Rothwell, N.J. Systemic infection, inflammation and acute ischemic stroke. *Neuroscience* **2009**, *158*, 1049–1061. [CrossRef] [PubMed]
52. Crews, F.T.; Vetreno, R.P. Mechanisms of neuroimmune gene induction in alcoholism. *Psychopharmacology* **2016**, *233*, 1543–1557. [CrossRef]
53. Saha, R.N.; Jana, M.; Pahan, K. MAPK p38 regulates transcriptional activity of NF-κB in primary human astrocytes via acetylation of p65. *J. Immunol.* **2007**, *179*, 7101–7109. [CrossRef] [PubMed]
54. Radi, E.; Formichi, P.; Battisti, C.; Federico, A. Apoptosis and oxidative stress in neurodegenerative diseases. *J. Alzheimers Dis.* **2014**, *42* (Suppl. 3), S125–S152. [CrossRef]
55. Khan, A.; Ikram, M.; Muhammad, T.; Park, J.; Kim, M.O. Caffeine modulates cadmium-induced oxidative stress, neuroinflammation, and cognitive impairments by regulating Nrf-2/HO-1 in vivo and in vitro. *J. Clin. Med.* **2019**, *8*, 680. [CrossRef]
56. Wang, P.; Luo, Q.; Qiao, H.; Ding, H.; Cao, Y.; Yu, J.; Liu, R.; Zhang, Q.; Zhu, H.; Qu, L. The neuroprotective effects of carvacrol on ethanol-induced hippocampal neurons impairment via the antioxidative and antiapoptotic pathways. *Oxid. Med. Cell. Longev.* **2017**, *2017*, 4079425. [CrossRef] [PubMed]
57. Wang, X.S.; Zhang, Z.R.; Zhang, M.M.; Sun, M.X.; Wang, W.W.; Xie, C.L. Neuroprotective properties of curcumin in toxin-base animal models of Parkinson's disease: A systematic experiment literatures review. *BMC Complement. Altern. Med.* **2017**, *17*, 412. [CrossRef] [PubMed]

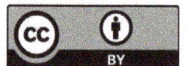

© 2019 by the authors. Licensee MDPI, Basel, Switzerland. This article is an open access article distributed under the terms and conditions of the Creative Commons Attribution (CC BY) license (http://creativecommons.org/licenses/by/4.0/).

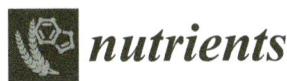

Article

The Chinese Herbal Formula PAPZ Ameliorates Behavioral Abnormalities in Depressive Mice

Huiling Chen [1], Qing Huang [1,2], Shunjia Zhang [1,3], Kaiqiang Hu [1], Wenxiang Xiong [1], Lingyun Xiao [4], Renhuai Cong [4], Qingfei Liu [1,*] and Zhao Wang [1,*]

1. MOE Key Laboratory of Protein Science, School of Pharmaceutical Sciences, Tsinghua University, Beijing 100084, China; chenhl16@mails.tsinghua.edu.cn (H.C.); qinghuangfgh@163.com (Q.H.); shunjia.zhang@yale.edu (S.Z.); hkq15@mails.tsinghua.edu.cn (K.H.); xiongwxiang@163.com (W.X.)
2. School of Life Science and Technology, Tokyo Institute of Technology, Yokohama 2668501, Japan
3. Environmental Health Science, School of Public Health, Yale University, New Haven, CT 06520, USA
4. Research & Development Centre, Infinitus (China) Company Ltd., Guangzhou 510663, China; xiaolingyun12@126.com (L.X.); Renhuai.Cong@infinitus-int.com (R.C.)
* Correspondence: liuqf@tsinghua.edu.cn (Q.L.); zwang@tsinghua.edu.cn (Z.W.); Tel: +86-10-62772241 (Q.L. & Z.W.)

Received: 11 March 2019; Accepted: 12 April 2019; Published: 16 April 2019

Abstract: Major depressive disorder (MDD) is a chronic mental disorder characterized by mixed symptoms and complex pathogenesis. With long history of practical application, traditional Chinese medicine (TCM) offers many herbs for the treatment and rehabilitation of chronic disease. In this study, we developed a modified Chinese herbal formula using *Panax ginseng*, *Angelica Sinensis*, *Polygala tenuifolia* Willd, and *Ziziphi spinosae* Semen (PAPZ), based on an ancient TCM prescription. The antidepressant effects of PAPZ were investigated with a corticosterone (CORT) model of depression in mice. Our results showed that administration of PAPZ ameliorated depression-like phenotypes in the CORT model. An anatomic study showed that chronic PAPZ administration upregulated the protein expression of brain-derived neurotrophic factor (BDNF) in hippocampal tissue. The enzyme activity of superoxide dismutase was enhanced in hippocampal tissue, in line with a decreased malondialdehyde level. Taken together, these findings suggested that PAPZ has therapeutic effects in a mice depression model through increasing protein expression of BDNF and improving the anti-oxidation ability of the brain.

Keywords: major depressive disorder; Chinese herbal formula; corticosterone; BDNF; oxidative stress

1. Introduction

Major depressive disorder (MDD) or depression, which has an estimated global prevalence of 4.7%, is a mental disorder that affects human thoughts, mood, and physical health. It can occur at as early as 3 years of age, and appears across all world regions [1,2]. The global burden of disease (GBD) in 2010 identified MDD as a leading contributor to the global disease burden [3]. Similar to anxiety disorder, MDD has been reported to cause brain injury, especially damaging the hippocampus region of the brain, causing neuronal dysfunction or affecting neural plasticity [4]. Brain-derived neurotrophic factor (BDNF) plays a critical neurotrophic role in neural plasticity [5,6]. In prior studies, *bdnf* has been identified as a target gene in depression treatment [5,7,8]. Adachi et al. [9] reported that the loss of BDNF in the hippocampal tissue contributed to increasing vulnerability to depression, whereas upregulation mediated antidepressant efficacy.

MDD has been thought to be a heterogeneous disease with diverse etiological and multifactorial pathogenesis [10,11]. Modern medicine has primarily focused on symptomatic treatment, and drugs are mainly applied in single-target and single-factor therapy. Traditional Chinese medicine (TCM), whose treatments are designed systematically based upon the constitution of patients, has a long history and the potential to treat many diseases including depressive-like syndromes [10,12]. Chinese herbal medicine is the major form of prescription of TCM. Chinese herbal formulas (CHFs), which aim to help patients re-achieve the Yin–Yang balance of the body, usually consist of multiple herbs that synchronize with one other when administered. Considerable progress has occurred not only in basic research, but also in clinical research, with a better understanding of the underlying neurobiological basis of CHFs. It is believed that a multi-component and multi-target mechanism may be the essential mechanism through which CHF achieve holistic effects [13].

The most common traditional method of preparing CHFs is through the water decocting method. In brief, prepared slices of medical herbs are boiled in hot water, and the decoction administrated orally [14]. Aiming to seek CHFs that have the potential to serve as alternatives for MDD treatment, Infinitus (China) Co., Ltd. offered 22 modified CHFs for regulating mood. We then explored whether the decoction of them had protective effects on hippocampal neuronal cell line (HT22) against corticosterone (CORT)-induced apoptosis (Supplementary Table S1). We found that the formula WXJ-17-001, which comprises *Panax ginseng, Angelica ginensis, Polygala tenuifolia* Willd, and *Ziziphi spinosae* Semen, had the best protection effect among them. We then renamed the formula according to its composing as PAPZ.

Each single herb of PAPZ is beneficial for central nervous system disorders and widely used in an Asian-medicated diet. *P. ginseng* is a widely-used medicinal plant in Asian countries; it has various pharmacological effects such as neuroprotection, endocrine modulation, cardiovascular protection, and immunoregulation [10]. Many research articles have reported that *P. ginseng* or its components are beneficial to the central nervous system, and have therapeutic effects on neuropsychiatric disorders [15]. *A. sinensis*, known as *Dong-Gui*, is served as a healthy food and is also a common traditional medicine used for the treatment of cerebrovascular diseases [16,17]. A study showed that the formula *Dang-Gui-Shao-Yao-San*, of which the major active component is *A. sinensis*, had pharmaceutical effects on depression [18]. *P. tenuifolia* Willd is used as an expectorant, tonic, tranquillizer, or antipsychotic agent in TCM [19]. *Senegenin*, extracted from *P. tenuifolia* Willd, shows an antidepressant effect by inhibiting the nuclear factor κ-light-chain-enhancer of activated B cells (NF-κB) pathway [20]. *Z. spinosae* Semen is the mature seed of sour jujube, and is used as a sedative agent in TCM [21–23]. *Z. spinosae* Semen could improve learning and memory of mice [24]. It has been reported to have an antidepressant effect in a rat depressive model [25]. However, whether a formula of these herbs would have antidepressant effects, and the underlying molecular mechanism, remains unclear.

In the present study, chronic treatment with corticosterone (CORT), which is a common inducer of depression-related behavior both in rats and mice [26,27], was used to establish a depressive-like mice model. A hippocampus-derived HT22 cell line was applied to in vitro experiments. Our results showed that administration of PAPZ ameliorated depressive-like phenotypes by improving the protein expression of BDNF and the activity of superoxide dismutase (SOD) of hippocampal tissue in mice. PAPZ also attenuated CORT-induced apoptosis in HT22 cell in vitro. Taken together, the results demonstrated the neuroprotective effect of PAPZ, which suggested PAPZ is a good candidate for treatment of depressive disorders.

2. Materials and Methods

2.1. Materials

CORT was purchased from Takyo Chemical Industry Co., Ltd. (Shanghai, China). The Chinese herbs *P. ginseng, A. sinensis, P. tenuifolia* Willd, and *Z. spinosae* Semen were purchased from Beijing Tong Ren Tang Guangzhou Pharmaceutical chain Co., Ltd. (Guangzhou, China). The HT22 cell line was purchased from Tong Pai Biotechnology Co., Ltd. (Shanghai, China). Dulbecco's Modified Eagle Medium (DMEM) and penicillin/streptomycin were obtained from Corning Incorporated (Corning, NY, USA). Fetal bovine serum (FBS) was purchased from Invitrogen Corporation (Carlsbad, CA, USA). The cell counting kit-8 (CCK-8) and fluorescein isothiocyanate (FITC)-Annexin V apoptosis detection kit were purchased from Beyotime Biotechnology (Shanghai, China). Real-time quantitative polymerase chain reaction (qPCR)-related kits, the FastQuant RT kit, and Super Real PreMix Plus were purchased from Tiangen Biotech CO., Ltd. (Beijing, China). The SOD assay kit and malondialdehyde (MDA) assay kit were obtained from Nanjing Jiancheng Biotechnology Co., Ltd. (Nanjing, China). Anti-BDNF and anti-β-tubulin were purchased from Cell Signaling Technology (Danvers, MA, USA). All other chemicals were of analytical grade and used as received.

2.2. Preparation of CHFs and CORT

All CHFs used in this study were prepared using the water decocting method from dried medical herbs purchased in the form of prepared slices. Water was added to the mixture of prepared slices of the herbs in a 1:10 (g/mL) ratio of materials to liquid and boiled for 2 h. The decoction was collected and the same amount of water was added to the residue. Then, the mixture was boiled for another 2 h. Next, the decoctions were combined and concentrated to a constant volume. The water extract was centrifuged (13,000 rpm, 10 min, 4 °C) to separate any insoluble materials, and then the supernatant was filtered through a 0.2 μm syringe filter before use. The prepared water extract was frozen at −20 °C for storage. Four Chinese medicine herbs, *P. ginseng*, *A. sinensis*, *P. tenuifolia* Willd, and *Z. spinosae* Semen, were included in PAPZ (Table 1). The dosage of PAPZ described in this paper was in the form of equivalent dry herb amount.

Corticosterone (CORT) powder was suspended in 0.9% (w/v) physiological saline with 0.1% dimethyl sulfoxide (DMSO) acting as a cosolvent

Table 1. Chinese herbs included in PAPZ.

Scientific Name	Family Name	Source	Proportion of PAPZ
Panax ginseng C.A. Meyer	Araliaceae	Beijing, China	25%
Angelica sinensis (Oliv.) Diels	Umbelliferae	Gansu, China	25%
Polygala tenuifolia Willd	Polygalaceae	Shanxi, China	25%
Ziziphi spinosae Semen	Rhamnaceae	Hebei, China	25%

2.3. Animals and Treatment

Male C57BL/6J mice weighing 18–22 g were obtained from the laboratory animal center of Tsinghua University (Beijing, China) and were housed in cages with free access to food and water in a room with an ambient temperature of 22 ± 2 °C and a 12 h light/dark cycle. All animal experiments were conducted according to the relevant guidelines and regulations and with the approval of the Institutional Ethical Committee of China.

After an adaptive phase of 3 days, the mice were randomly divided into the control, CORT, and PAPZ+CORT group ($n = 10$/group). The dose of CORT (40 mg/kg) was selected based on data from the literature [28,29] and PAPZ (1000 mg/kg) treatment was calculated by extrapolating the human recommended daily dosage of the single herb according to the Chinese Pharmacopoeia. For the control group and CORT group, normal saline was administrated to mice by oral gavage first, and 30 min later, the mice were subcutaneously injected with saline or CORT. For the PAPZ+CORT group, the mice were administrated with PAPZ by oral gavage 30 min prior to CORT supplement. All drugs were administrated at a volume of 10 mL/kg. During behavioral assessments, the administration of all drugs continued.

2.4. Open Field Test

An open field test (OFT) was conducted 24 h after the 21 days of CORT treatment. An open box (60 × 60 × 50 cm) was used in the OFT. At the beginning of the test period, mice were placed in the center of the box to adapt for 3 min. The experimental parameters were set, and the test time was set to 10 min. The locomotor activity (movement distance, movement speed, and other indicators) was monitored and traced with an automated video-tracking system. Between one mouse and the next one, the apparatus was thoroughly cleaned with 75% ethanol, followed by distilled water and dried before using.

2.5. Novel Object Recognition Test

A novel object recognition (NOR) test was conducted after OFT. NOR is a commonly used behavioral assay for the investigation of various aspects of learning and memory level in mice. NOR is fairly simple and can be completed over 5 days: habituation (3 days), training (day 4), and testing day (day 5). During training, the mouse was allowed to explore two identical objects in the open field area (50 × 50 cm). On testing day, one of the training objects was replaced with a novel object. The exploring time of the novel object and familiar object was recorded within 5 min. The discrimination index (DI) was used to evaluate the learning and memory ability of animals. The DI calculation formula is as follows:

$$DI = (N - F) / (N + F) \times 100\%,$$

where N is the time spent on novel location/object exploration and F is the time spent on familiar location/object exploration.

2.6. Tail Suspension Test

A tail suspension test (TST) was conducted after NOR. Briefly, mice were individually suspended 5 cm above the bottom of the TST box. The tip of the tail was stuck with adhesive tape. Immobility time was detected during the last 4 min of total 6 min test.

2.7. Morris Water Maze Experiment

A Morris water maze (MWM) experiment was conducted in submerged platform following standard procedures and it was conducted after TST. The hidden-platform was fixed in the center of one of quadrants and 1.5 cm below the water surface. Mice underwent three trials each day for 6 days. Each time, mice were placed into the water from other three quadrants. Before and after each test, mice were placed on the platform to adapt for 20 s. Mice that remained on the platform for more than 5 s were considered to have searched platform successfully during the 90 s of detection. The mice were deeply anesthetized and sacrificed by cervical dislocation after MWM test was finished.

Once the mice were sacrificed, the hippocampal tissues were quickly dissected and immersed immediately in liquid nitrogen and then transferred to refrigerator at −80 °C until being used.

2.8. Real-time Quantitative PCR and Western Blotting

For qPCR analysis, total RNA from hippocampal tissues were extracted using trizol regent according to the manufacturer's instructions. Complementary deoxyribonucleic acid (cDNA) was obtained by using a FastQuant RT Kit and real-time PCR analysis was used with SuperReal PreMix Plus according to the 2-step reaction program. qPCR analysis was conducted using primers as follows: *gapdh* forward 5′-CATGGCCTTCCGTGTTCCTA-3′, reverse 5′-CCTGCTTCACCACCTTCTTGAT-3′, *bdnf* forward 5′-GCCTTCATGCAACCGAAGTA-3′, reverse 5′-TGAGTCTCCAGGACAGCAAA-3′.

For immunoblot analysis, hippocampal tissues were resuspended with lysis buffer. The protein was extracted and samples were resolved on 10% sodium dodecyl sulfonate–polyacrylamide gel (SDS-PAGE) and then transferred to polyvinylidene fluoride (PVDF) membranes. Antibodies against the following proteins were used: BDNF and β-tubulin goat anti-rabbit immunoglobulin G (IgG).

2.9. SOD and MDA Assay

The supernatant of hippocampal tissues was used to detect SOD activity and MDA level using SOD assay kit and MDA assay kit, respectively, following the manufacturer's instructions.

2.10. Determination of Cell Viability

HT22 cells were seeded into 10-cm dishes and cultured in DMEM supplemented with 10% FBS and 1% penicillin-streptomycin at 37 °C in a humidified incubator containing 5% CO_2.

Cell viability was measured by CCK-8 assay. Briefly, the cells were cultured at a density of 5×10^3 cells per well into 96-well plates. When the cells reached 70–80% confluence, they were pre-treated with 400 μM CORT for 24 h, and then treated with PAPZ with concentrations of 0.5, 5.0, and 10.0 mg/mL for 24 h in the presence of CORT. In this study, 400 μM CORT was determined as the optimal dose of cell damage model through preliminary experiments (Supplementary Figure S1). The absorbance at 450 nm was measured in an enzyme standard instrument.

2.11. Determination of Cell Apoptosis by Flow Cytometry

The apoptotic cells were measured using the FITC-Annexin V Apoptosis Detection Kit. After drug treatment as a cell viability experiment, cells were harvested and then washed with 1 mL PBS. Next, cells were resuspended in 195 μL FITC-Annexin V binding buffer, and then 5 μL of FITC-Annexin V and 10 μL propidium iodide (PI) incubation buffer were added according to the manufacturer's instructions. The cells were incubated for 15 min at room temperature and protected from light. Samples were not stored, but analyzed immediately. Samples were analyzed with an imaging flow cytometer.

2.12. Statistical Analysis

Results are presented as mean ± SEM. For the in vitro experiments, all results reported were formed at least three independent experiments ($n = 6$ for each group). For the in vivo animal experiments, each group contained 10 mice. Data were analyzed with Graph-Pad Prism 5.0 software (GraphPad Software Inc., San Diego, CA, USA). Two-tailed, unpaired t-tests were used to compare two groups. Differences were considered significant when $p < 0.05$. To directly compare the effect of PAPZ treatment, data from the CORT group and PAPZ+CORT group were normalized to the control group.

3. Results

3.1. Antidepressant Effects of PAPZ

To investigate the effect of PAPZ on depressive-like behavior, we chose the chronic CORT model of depression, which has been widely used in depression-related research (Figure 1). Mice were administrated subcutaneously with CORT once daily for 21 consecutive days, and PAPZ were administered by oral gavage 30 minutes prior to the CORT injection. Behavioral tests were performed after the treatments had finished (Figure 1a). The chronic CORT injection resulted in a significant prolonged immobility time in the TST when compared with the control group (Figure 1b). The PAPZ+CORT treated group exhibited a significantly decreased immobility time compared with the model group, which suggested that PAPZ could protect against the CORT-induced depressive-like behavior in the TST test. An OFT was conducted to assess the influence of PAPZ on the locomotor activities of mice. PAPZ administration had no significant impact on the total distance and movement speed of mice spent in the zone in the OFT (Figure 1c,d).

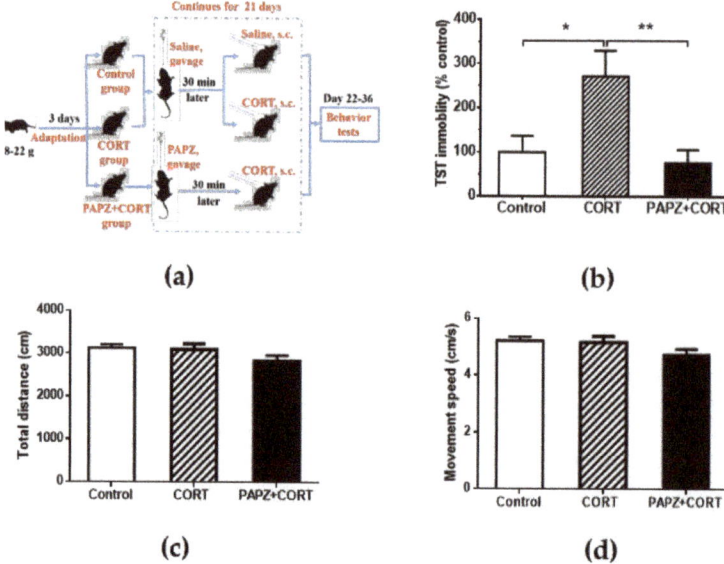

Figure 1. PAPZ ameliorated depressive-like behavior induced by corticosterone (CORT) in mice. (**a**) Schematic representation of the treatment protocol. (**b**) The immobility time in the tail suspension test (TST). (**c**) Total distance travelled in the open field test (OFT). (**d**) Movement speed during bouts of walking in the OFT. Data from the CORT group and PAPZ+CORT group were normalized to the control group and data are expressed as mean ± SEM. * $p < 0.05$, ** $p < 0.01$ represent significant differences. s.c.: sub-cutaneous.

3.2. Effects of PAPZ on Learning and Memory Capacity

We evaluated the effect of PAPZ on cognitive capacity in CORT-induced mice using the NOR test and learning, and memory ability using the MWM test, respectively (Figure 2). The discrimination index (DI), representing cognitive ability, was determined from the NOR task. CORT induced a significant decrease in the DI score for the novel object when compared with the control group. As expected, we found a significant increase in the DI score for the novel object in the PAPZ+CORT treated group when compared to the group treated with CORT alone. The DI score for the novel location in the CORT-treated group demonstrated a decreasing tendency, although there was no significant difference when compared with the control group (Figure 2a). Treatment with PAPZ significantly increased the DI score for the novel location when compared with the CORT group (Figure 2b). In the MWM test, latency refers to the time spent by the mouse to find the platform. There was a relative increasing tendency of latency in the chronic CORT-treated group when compared with the control group. PAZA treatment significantly decreased the latency when compared with the CORT-treated group, especially on the fifth and sixth day (Figure 2c). All these results indicated that PAPZ could ameliorate depressive-like behavior and improve cognitive capacity and learning ability in depressive-like mice induced by the chronic administration of CORT.

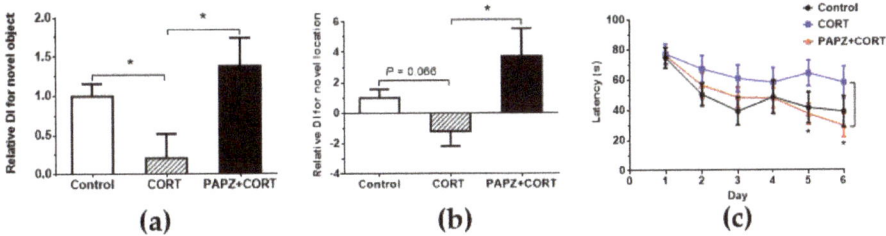

Figure 2. PAPZ ameliorated learning and memory impairment induced by CORT in mice. (a,b) The relative discrimination index (DI) for the novel object, (a) for novel location and (b) in the novel object recognition (NOR) test. (c) The total latency in the Morris water maze (MWM) test. Data from the CORT group and PAPZ+CORT group were normalized to the control group and data are expressed as mean ± SEM. * $p < 0.05$ represents a significant difference.

3.3. Molecular Mechanism of the Cerebral Protection Effect of PAPZ

To investigate the underlying molecular mechanism of PAPZ in CORT-induced depressive-like mice, we examined the effect of PAPZ on the expression of *bdnf* on hippocampal tissue in mice (Figure 3). The real-time qPCR result demonstrated that the mRNA level of *bdnf* significantly decreased by almost 50% when compared with the non-treated control group. Treatment with PAPZ showed that the *bdnf* values were significantly increased when compared with the CORT group, which indicated that the PAPZ could promote the expression of *bdnf* at the level of transcription (Figure 3a). We next detected the expression of BDNF protein. The immunoblot result was consistent with the qPCR result (Figure 3b) and revealed that the expression of BDNF protein in the model group significantly decreased after treatment with CORT, and PAPZ could enhance the expression of BDNF protein, which indicates that PAPZ could ameliorate the damage of CORT to hippocampus tissues.

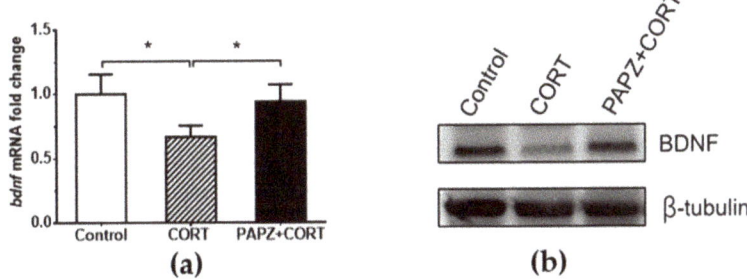

Figure 3. PAPZ enhanced the expression of brain-derived neurotrophic factor BDNF in hippocampal tissue. (a) Real-time quantitative polymerase chain reaction (qPCR) analysis of *bdnf* gene in the hippocampal tissues in mice. (b) Representative Western blots show the difference of BDNF protein expression in hippocampal tissue. Data from the CORT group and PAPZ+CORT group were normalized to the control group and data are expressed as mean ± SEM. * $p < 0.05$ represents a significant difference.

3.4. PAPZ Enhanced Cerebral Antioxidant Ability of Tested Mice

Oxidative stress has been shown to cause neuronal degeneration and to play a role in the pathogenesis of anxiety and depression [30,31]. We hypothesized that PAPZ exerted neuroprotective effects by reducing cerebral oxidative stress and verified the hypothesis by SOD and MDA assays (Figure 4). Reactive oxygen species (ROS) are a kind of free radical that can damage cells through enzyme inactivation, lipid peroxidation, DNA modification, and other pathways [32]. Studies have reported that SOD is an important endogenous antioxidant enzyme and an important part of the first-line defense system against ROS [33,34]. Therefore, the SOD viability of hippocampal tissue was detected in mice. CORT treatment significantly deceased the SOD viability when compared with the control group, and PAPZ treatment significantly increased the SOD viability when compared with the CORT-treated group (Figure 4a). These results indicate that PAPZ could improve the SOD viability of mice in vivo.

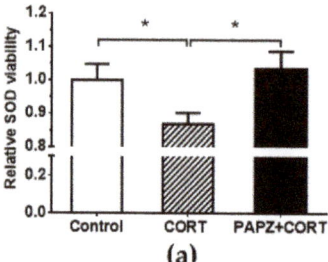 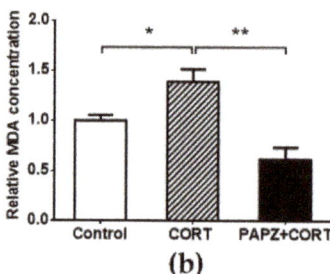

Figure 4. PAPZ enhanced superoxide dismutase (SOD) viability and decreased malondialdehyde (MDA) level in depressive-like mice. (**a**) The SOD activity of hippocampal tissue in mice was measured by the SOD assay kit. (**b**) The MDA activity of hippocampal tissue in mice was measured by the MDA assay kit. Data from the CORT group and PAPZ+CORT group were normalized to the control group and data are expressed as mean ± SEM. * $p < 0.05$, ** $p < 0.01$ represent significant differences.

MDA is a metabolite of lipid peroxidation, and its content can indirectly reflect the degree of damage of lipid peroxidation. Studies have reported that MDA concentrations in depressed patients increased when compared with healthy control groups [35,36]. The concentration of MDA in the hippocampal tissue in the CORT group significantly increased after treatment with CORT when compared with that in the control group. The change in MDA content in the PAPZ+CORT group was, as opposed to SOD, markedly decreased when compared with that in the CORT group (Figure 4b). All the results indicated that PAPZ could enhance the cerebral antioxidant ability in mice treated with CORT.

3.5. PAPZ Protected Neurons In Vitro

The HT22 cell line is a widely used model to evaluate the pharmacological effects of potential antidepressant drugs [37,38]. To detect the effect of PAPZ on CORT-induced HT22 cells death (Figure 5), we selected 400 µM CORT, which decreased the viability of the HT22 cells by 30% (Supplementary Figure S1), as the optimal dose of the cell model to detect the effect of PAPZ on CORT-induced HT22 cells death. At these experimental conditions, the viability of the HT22 cells was significantly reduced in the CORT group when compared to the control group. Co-treatment with PAPZ increased the viability of HT22 cells in a dose-dependent manner when compared with CORT-only treated HT22 cells. The viability of HT22 cells in the PAPZ+CORT treated group was significantly higher than that in the CORT group, which indicated that PAPZ promoted the cell proliferation of HT22 cells (Figure 5a).

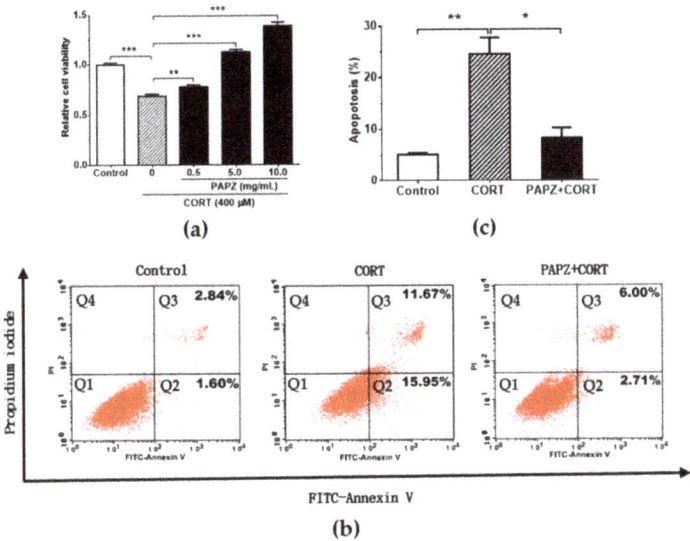

Figure 5. PAPZ attenuated CORT-induced apoptosis in HT22 cells. (**a**) Effects of different concentrations of PAPZ on CORT-induced HT22 cell viability determined by cell counting kit-8 (CCK-8 assay). (**b**) Fluorescein isothiocyanate (FITC)-Annexin V and propidium iodide (PI) staining followed by flow cytometry was performed to evaluate cell apoptosis of the HT22 cells. Living cells can be categorized as double negative (Q1). Early apoptotic cells can be classified as single positive or FITC-Annexin V positive (Q2). Late apoptotic cells are double positive (Q3). Dead cells can be categorized as single positive or PI positive (Q4). (**c**) The statistical analysis of total apoptosis in flow cytometry test. Data from the CORT group and PAPZ+CORT group were normalized to the control group and data are presented as mean ± SEM. * $p < 0.05$, ** $p < 0.01$, *** $p < 0.001$ represent significant differences.

Flow cytometry analysis using conventional FITC-Annexin V and PI staining was performed to characterize three types of neuronal death. Total apoptosis in HT22 cells treated with CORT showed a significant increase when compared with the control group. PAPZ treatment decreased the percentage of both early and late apoptosis in HT22 cells when compared to the CORT group (Figure 5b). The statistical analysis of total apoptosis is provided in Figure 5c. The results suggested that HT22 cells were likely to undergo apoptotic rather than necrotic death when treated with CORT. Treatment with PAPZ could prevent against apoptosis induced by CORT. Our results suggested that PAPZ exerted a neuroprotective effect through inhibiting the apoptosis of HT22 cells induced by CORT.

4. Discussion

Given its long history usage in Asia, a reliable amount of clinical experience with TCM has been accumulated, forming a comprehensive and vital medical and cultural system. Chinese herbal medicine is the fundamental of TCM, which includes several medicinal herbs. The typical characteristics of TCM treatments are "multi-component, multi-channel, and multi-target", which is a requirement for treating complex diseases including depression or MDD [39].

Repeated CORT injection in rodents have been considered as a reliable animal model for evaluating chronic stress depressive disorder [27]. The TST test is one of the classic experiments used to evaluate the anti-depression pharmacology of drugs and has often been used to observe the anti-depression effect of drugs by causing behavioral despair in animals [40,41]. In the present study, compared with the control group, a significant prolonged immobility time in the TST test was observed in the CORT-treated group mice. As expected, the mice treated with PAPZ+CORT exhibited a significant decrease in immobility time as compared to the CORT group (Figure 1b). PAPZ showed minor side effects on locomotor activities at the indicated dose (Figure 1c,d). Depression is often accompanied by cognitive impairment, and especially obvious learning and memory impairment [42]. In this study, the NOR test and MWM test were used to evaluate the learning and memory ability of mice. A significant increase in the DI score for new objects and new locations was shown in the PAPZ+CORT-treated group compared with the CORT-only treated group (Figure 2a,b). From the MWM results (Figure 2c), we found that the latency period of escape increased in the model group even though there was no statistical difference, whereas treatment with PAPZ significantly decreased the latency. These results demonstrated that PAPZ slightly decreased the progression of the chronic treatment of CORT-induced mild stress-mediated depressive-like behaviors as observed by the TST, NOR, and MWM tests.

Studies have shown that various pathophysiological mechanisms are involved in depression and cognitive impairment. Synaptic dysfunction and structural damage have become the focus of research. BDNF functions as an endogenous growth factor within the central nervous system [43], playing a key role in processes such as neuronal differentiation and growth, synapse formation and synaptic plasticity, and higher cognitive functions [44,45]. BDNF has also been implicated in a number of psychiatric disorders, including schizophrenia, and the development of mood disorders such as MDD and its treatment [46]. Many experiments have shown that chronic stress can down-regulate the expression of BDNF protein in the hippocampus, and this phenomenon can be effectively reversed by antidepressant therapy [47–49]. Neto et al. [49] found that up-regulation of neurotrophic factor expression and its signaling pathway activity could be a common pathway of antidepressant action. Therefore, we speculated that PAPZ may promote neurogenesis or change neuroplasticity by increasing the level of BDNF protein, and thus play an antidepressant role in reversing hippocampal atrophy and cell damage. According to the results of the qPCR and Western blot tests, we found that the expression of hippocampal BDNF protein in the repeated CORT injection group significantly decreased when compared with the control group. Treatment with PAPZ showed significantly increased the expression of BDNF in the hippocampal tissue when compared to the CORT group (Figure 3). Therefore, we concluded that PAPZ might exert an antidepressant role by up-regulating the expression of BDNF.

The antioxidant defense system is comprised of a series of enzymatic and non-enzymatic components. SOD is a critical antioxidant enzyme that can remove oxygen free radicals produced by the body and protect tissues from damage. Maes et al. [50] revealed that the pathogenesis of MDD might primarily or secondarily be related to oxidative stress. Antidepressant drugs function by affecting the oxidative or antioxidative systems [51], and are partly connected with their effects on the immune system [52]. Many reports have shown that disturbances in SOD activity are generally dysregulated in depressed populations. For example, the SOD activity of a red blood cell was reported to be lower in MDD patients [53]. Freitas et al. [2] reported that acute restraint stress can increase SOD activity and this effect can be abrogated by treatment with agmatine; however, no changes were observed in the unstressed animals. These disagreements in the data on SOD activity could be explained by means of variations in different drugs or a different administration period.

The results of our study showed that the SOD activity of hippocampal tissue in the CORT group mice significantly decreased, indicating that the function of the oxygen free radical defense system of depressed mice was significantly reduced, and the oxygen free radicals could not be effectively removed. PAPZ administration could reverse the trend of SOD activity. The increased SOD activity was in line with a decreased MDA level (Figure 4). Therefore, we concluded that the role of PAPZ in anti-depression could be related to the involvement of SOD and MDA. The results (Figure 5) demonstrated that PAPZ significantly attenuated CORT-induced neuroexcitotoxicity in HT22 cells, which was indicated that PAPZ could protect HT22 cells in vitro. However, the complex mechanism of PAPZ are not yet completely clear, which need to be explored in further study. In future studies, we will pay more attention to the exploration of the relevant herb of PAPZ under the guidance of the theory and practice of TCM, and clarify the role of each herb and the relationship and influences among them.

5. Conclusions

In summary, a modified TCM formula (PAPZ) protected HT22 cells from CORT-induced apoptosis. PAPZ ameliorated behavioral changes induced by chronic CORT injections in the TST, NOR, and MWM tests. The essential mechanism involved in the protective effects of PAPZ in vivo included augmentation of the BDNF level and SOD activity in the hippocampal tissue. These findings provide scientific evidence for the neuroprotective and antidepressant effects of PAPZ, which suggest potential benefits of using PAPZ in the treatment or rehabilitation of MDD patients.

Supplementary Materials: The following are available online at http://www.mdpi.com/2072-6643/11/4/859/s1. Figure S1: Effects of different concentrations of CORT on TH22 cell viability determined by CCK-8 assay; Table S1: Effects of different concentrations of CHFs on CORT-induced HT22 cell viability determined by CCK-8 assay.

Author Contributions: H.C., W.X., and Q.L. designed the experiments; Q.H. and S.Z. performed the experiments; R.C. and L.X. analyzed references and traditional medical literature; and H.C., K.H., and Z.W. wrote the manuscript.

Acknowledgments: This study was financially supported by grants from the National Key R&D Program of China (2018YFD0400204), the Key International S&T Cooperation Program of China (2016YFE113700), the National Key R&D Program of China (2018YFC2000304), the European Union's Horizon 2020 Research and Innovation Program (633589), and the National Natural Science Foundation of China (81471396, 81871095).

Conflicts of Interest: The authors declare no conflict of interest.

References

1. Charlson, F.J.; Ferrari, A.J.; Flaxman, A.D.; Whiteford, H.A. The epidemiological modelling of dysthymia: Application for the Global Burden of Disease Study 2010. *J. Affect. Disord.* **2013**, *151*, 111–120. [CrossRef] [PubMed]
2. Ferrari, A.J.; Somerville, A.J.; Baxter, A.J.; Norman, R.; Patten, S.B.; Vos, T.; Whiteford, H.A. Global variation in the prevalence and incidence of major depressive disorder: A systematic review of the epidemiological literature. *Psychol. Med.* **2013**, *43*, 471–481. [CrossRef] [PubMed]
3. Ferrari, A.J.; Charlson, F.J.; Norman, R.E.; Patten, S.B.; Freedman, G.; Murray, C.J.; Vos, T.; Whiteford, H.A. Burden of depressive disorders by country, sex, age, and year: Findings from the global burden of disease study 2010. *PLoS Med.* **2013**, *10*, e1001547. [CrossRef] [PubMed]
4. Liu, W.; Ge, T.; Leng, Y.; Pan, Z.; Fan, J.; Yang, W.; Cui, R. The Role of Neural Plasticity in Depression: From Hippocampus to Prefrontal Cortex. *Neural Plast.* **2017**, *2017*, 6871089. [CrossRef] [PubMed]
5. Duman, R.S.; Monteggia, L.M. A neurotrophic model for stress-related mood disorders. *Biol. Psychiatry* **2006**, *59*, 1116–1127. [CrossRef]
6. Numakawa, T.; Suzuki, S.; Kumamaru, E.; Adachi, N.; Richards, M.; Kunugi, H. BDNF function and intracellular signaling in neurons. *Histol. Histopathol.* **2010**, *25*, 237–258.
7. Mendez-David, I.; Tritschler, L.; Ali, Z.E.; Damiens, M.H.; Pallardy, M.; David, D.J.; Kerdine-Romer, S.; Gardier, A.M. Nrf2-signaling and BDNF: A new target for the antidepressant-like activity of chronic fluoxetine treatment in a mouse model of anxiety/depression. *Neurosci. Lett.* **2015**, *597*, 121–126. [CrossRef]
8. Nibuya, M.; Morinobu, S.; Duman, R.S. Regulation of BDNF and trkB mRNA in rat brain by chronic electroconvulsive seizure and antidepressant drug treatments. *J. Neurosci.* **1995**, *15*, 7539–7547. [CrossRef]
9. Adachi, M.; Barrot, M.; Autry, A.E.; Theobald, D.; Monteggia, L.M. Selective loss of brain-derived neurotrophic factor in the dentate gyrus attenuates antidepressant efficacy. *Biol. Psychiatry* **2008**, *63*, 642–649. [CrossRef]
10. Chen, G.; Guo, X. Neurobiology of Chinese Herbal Medicine on Major Depressive Disorder. *Int. Rev. Neurobiol.* **2017**, *135*, 77–95.
11. Miyata, S.; Hattori, T.; Shimizu, S.; Ito, A.; Tohyama, M. Disturbance of oligodendrocyte function plays a key role in the pathogenesis of schizophrenia and major depressive disorder. *Biomed. Res. Int.* **2015**, *2015*, 492367. [CrossRef] [PubMed]
12. Gao, X.; Sun, P.; Qiao, M.; Wei, S.; Xue, L.; Zhang, H. Shu-Yu capsule, a Traditional Chinese Medicine formulation, attenuates premenstrual syndrome depression induced by chronic stress constraint. *Mol. Med. Rep.* **2014**, *10*, 2942–2948. [CrossRef] [PubMed]

13. Ding, F.; Zhang, Q.; Ung, C.O.; Wang, Y.; Han, Y.; Hu, Y.; Qi, J. An analysis of chemical ingredients network of Chinese herbal formulae for the treatment of coronary heart disease. *PLoS ONE* **2015**, *10*, e0116441. [CrossRef] [PubMed]
14. Sheridan, H.; Krenn, L.; Jiang, R.; Sutherland, I.; Ignatova, S.; Marmann, A.; Liang, X.; Sendker, J. The potential of metabolic fingerprinting as a tool for the modernisation of TCM preparations. *J. Ethnopharmacol.* **2012**, *140*, 482–491. [CrossRef] [PubMed]
15. Kim, H.J.; Kim, P.; Shin, C.Y. A comprehensive review of the therapeutic and pharmacological effects of ginseng and ginsenosides in central nervous system. *J. Ginseng Res.* **2013**, *37*, 8–29. [CrossRef] [PubMed]
16. Wu, Y.C.; Hsieh, C.L. Pharmacological effects of Radix Angelica Sinensis (Danggui) on cerebral infarction. *Chin. Med.* **2011**, *6*, 32–36. [CrossRef]
17. Yeh, J.C.; Cindrova-Davies, T.; Belleri, M.; Morbidelli, L.; Miller, N.; Cho, C.W.; Chan, K.; Wang, Y.T.; Luo, G.A.; Ziche, M.; et al. The natural compound n-butylidenephthalide derived from the volatile oil of Radix Angelica sinensis inhibits angiogenesis in vitro and in vivo. *Angiogenesis* **2011**, *14*, 187–197. [CrossRef]
18. Shen, J.; Zhang, J.; Deng, M.; Liu, Y.; Hu, Y.; Zhang, L. The Antidepressant Effect of Angelica sinensis Extracts on Chronic Unpredictable Mild Stress-Induced Depression Is Mediated via the Upregulation of the BDNF Signaling Pathway in Rats. *Evid. Based Complement. Alternat. Med.* **2016**, *2016*, 7434692. [CrossRef]
19. Hu, Y.; Liu, M.; Liu, P.; Guo, D.H.; Wei, R.B.; Rahman, K. Possible mechanism of the antidepressant effect of 3,6′-disinapoyl sucrose from Polygala tenuifolia Willd. *J. Pharm. Pharmacol.* **2011**, *63*, 869–874. [CrossRef]
20. Li, H.; Lin, S.; Qin, T.; Li, H.; Ma, Z.; Ma, S. Senegenin exerts anti-depression effect in mice induced by chronic un-predictable mild stress via inhibition of NF-kappaB regulating NLRP3 signal pathway. *Int. Immunopharmacol.* **2017**, *53*, 24–32. [CrossRef]
21. Zhang, M.; Zhang, Y.; Xie, J. Simultaneous determination of jujuboside A, B and betulinic acid in semen Ziziphi spinosae by high performance liquid chromatography-evaporative light scattering detection. *J. Pharm. Biomed. Anal.* **2008**, *48*, 1467–1470. [CrossRef]
22. Jeong, E.J.; Lee, H.K.; Lee, K.Y.; Jeon, B.J.; Kim, D.H.; Park, J.H.; Song, J.H.; Huh, J.; Lee, J.H.; Sung, S.H. The effects of lignan-riched extract of Shisandra chinensis on amyloid-beta-induced cognitive impairment and neurotoxicity in the cortex and hippocampus of mouse. *J. Ethnopharmacol.* **2013**, *146*, 347–354. [CrossRef]
23. Liu, Z.; Zhao, X.; Liu, B.; Liu, A.J.; Li, H.; Mao, X.; Wu, B.; Bi, K.S.; Jia, Y. Jujuboside A, a neuroprotective agent from semen Ziziphi Spinosae ameliorates behavioral disorders of the dementia mouse model induced by Abeta 1-42. *Eur. J. Pharmacol.* **2014**, *738*, 206–213. [CrossRef]
24. Li, B.; Fu, Z.; Hu, R.U.I.; Chen, Y.; Zhang, Z. Semen Ziziphi Spinosae and Fructus Gardeniae extracts synergistically improve learning and memory of a mouse model. *Biomed. Rep.* **2013**, *1*, 247–250. [CrossRef]
25. Wang, Y.; Huang, M.; Lu, X.; Wei, R.; Xu, J. Ziziphi spinosae lily powder suspension in the treatment of depression-like behaviors in rats. *BMC Complement. Altern. Med.* **2017**, *17*, 238. [CrossRef]
26. Huston, J.P.; Komorowski, M.; de Souza Silva, M.A.; Lamounier-Zepter, V.; Nikolaus, S.; Mattern, C.; Muller, C.P.; Topic, B. Chronic corticosterone treatment enhances extinction-induced depression in aged rats. *Horm. Behav.* **2016**, *86*, 21–26. [CrossRef]
27. Mei, L.; Mochizuki, M.; Hasegawa, N. Pycnogenol ameliorates depression-like behavior in repeated corticosterone-induced depression mice model. *Biomed. Res. Int.* **2014**, *2014*, 942927. [CrossRef]
28. Ali, S.H.; Madhana, R.M.; Kv, A.; Kasala, E.R.; Bodduluru, L.N.; Pitta, S.; Mahareddy, J.R.; Lahkar, M. Resveratrol ameliorates depressive-like behavior in repeated corticosterone-induced depression in mice. *Steroids* **2015**, *101*, 37–42. [CrossRef]
29. Wang, S.S.; Mu, R.H.; Li, C.F.; Dong, S.Q.; Geng, D.; Liu, Q.; Yi, L.T. microRNA-124 targets glucocorticoid receptor and is involved in depression-like behaviors. *Prog. Neuropsychopharmacol. Biol. Psychiatry* **2017**, *79*, 417–425. [CrossRef]
30. Cheng, J.; Dong, S.; Yi, L.; Geng, D.; Liu, Q. Magnolol abrogates chronic mild stress-induced depressive-like behaviors by inhibiting neuroinflammation and oxidative stress in the prefrontal cortex of mice. *Int. Immunopharmacol.* **2018**, *59*, 61–67. [CrossRef]
31. Lindqvist, D.; Dhabhar, F.S.; James, S.J.; Hough, C.M.; Jain, F.A.; Bersani, F.S.; Reus, V.I.; Verhoeven, J.E.; Epel, E.S.; Mahan, L.; et al. Oxidative stress, inflammation and treatment response in major depression. *Psychoneuroendocrinology* **2017**, *76*, 197–205. [CrossRef]
32. Singh, M.; Kapoor, A.; Bhatnagar, A. Oxidative and reductive metabolism of lipid-peroxidation derived carbonyls. *Chem. Biol. Interact.* **2015**, *234*, 261–273. [CrossRef]

33. Alscher, R.G.; Erturk, N.; Heath, L.S. Role of superoxide dismutases (SODs) in controlling oxidative stress in plants. *J. Exp. Bot.* **2002**, *53*, 1331–1341. [CrossRef]
34. Wang, Q.; Dong, X.; Li, N.; Wang, Y.; Guan, X.; Lin, Y.; Kang, J.; Zhang, X.; Zhang, Y.; Li, X.; et al. JSH-23 prevents depressive-like behaviors in mice subjected to chronic mild stress: Effects on inflammation and antioxidant defense in the hippocampus. *Pharmacol. Biochem. Behav.* **2018**, *169*, 59–66. [CrossRef]
35. Lopresti, A.L.; Maker, G.L.; Hood, S.D.; Drummond, P.D. A review of peripheral biomarkers in major depression: The potential of inflammatory and oxidative stress biomarkers. *Prog. Neuropsychopharmacol. Biol. Psychiatry* **2014**, *48*, 102–111. [CrossRef]
36. Gałecki, P.; Szemraj, J.; Bieńkiewicz, M.; Florkowski, A.; Gałecka, E. Lipid peroxidation and antioxidant protection in patients during acute depressive episodes and in remission after fluoxetine treatment. *Pharmacol. Rep.* **2009**, *61*, 436–447. [CrossRef]
37. Olianas, M.C.; Dedoni, S.; Onali, P. LPA1 is a key mediator of intracellular signalling and neuroprotection triggered by tetracyclic antidepressants in hippocampal neurons. *J. Neurochem.* **2017**, *143*, 183–197. [CrossRef]
38. Tavares, M.K.; Dos Reis, S.; Platt, N.; Heinrich, I.A.; Wolin, I.A.V.; Leal, R.B.; Kaster, M.P.; Rodrigues, A.L.S.; Freitas, A.E. Agmatine potentiates neuroprotective effects of subthreshold concentrations of ketamine via mTOR/S6 kinase signaling pathway. *Neurochem. Int.* **2018**, *118*, 275–285. [CrossRef]
39. Hu, R.-F.; Sun, X.-B. Design of new traditional Chinese medicine herbal formulae for treatment of type 2 diabetes mellitus based on network pharmacology. *Chin. J. Nat. Med.* **2017**, *15*, 436–441. [CrossRef]
40. Cryan, J.F.; Mombereau, C.; Vassout, A. The tail suspension test as a model for assessing antidepressant activity: Review of pharmacological and genetic studies in mice. *Neurosci. Biobehav. Rev.* **2005**, *29*, 571–625. [CrossRef]
41. Liu, K.F.; Li, Y.; Cheng, K.C.; Hsu, C.C.; Cheng, J.T.; Peng, W.H. Changes in PPARdelta expression in a rat model of stress-induced depression. *Clin. Exp. Pharmacol. Physiol.* **2017**, *44*, 664–670. [CrossRef] [PubMed]
42. Mcintyre, R.S.; Xiao, H.X.; Syeda, K.; Vinberg, M.; Carvalho, A.F.; Mansur, R.B.; Maruschak, N.; Cha, D.S. The prevalence, measurement, and treatment of the cognitive dimension/domain in major depressive disorder. *CNS Drugs* **2015**, *29*, 577–589. [CrossRef] [PubMed]
43. Leal, G.; Comprido, D.; Duarte, C.B. BDNF-induced local protein synthesis and synaptic plasticity. *Neuropharmacology* **2014**, *76 Pt C*, 639–656. [CrossRef]
44. Bjorkholm, C.; Monteggia, L.M. BDNF—A key transducer of antidepressant effects. *Neuropharmacology* **2016**, *102*, 72–79. [CrossRef] [PubMed]
45. Park, H.; Poo, M.M. Neurotrophin regulation of neural circuit development and function. *Nat. Rev. Neurosci.* **2013**, *14*, 7–23. [CrossRef]
46. Autry, A.E.; Monteggia, L.M. Brain-Derived Neurotrophic Factor and Neuropsychiatric Disorders. *Pharmacol. Rev.* **2012**, *64*, 238–258. [CrossRef]
47. Masi, G.; Brovedani, P. The hippocampus, neurotrophic factors and depression: Possible implications for the pharmacotherapy of depression. *CNS Drugs* **2011**, *25*, 913–931. [CrossRef]
48. Liu, Z.; Qi, Y.; Cheng, Z.; Zhu, X.; Fan, C.; Yu, S.Y. The effects of ginsenoside Rg1 on chronic stress induced depression-like behaviors, BDNF expression and the phosphorylation of PKA and CREB in rats. *Neuroscience* **2016**, *322*, 358–369. [CrossRef]
49. Neto, F.L.; Borges, G.; Torres-Sanchez, S.; Mico, J.A.; Berrocoso, E. Neurotrophins role in depression neurobiology: A review of basic and clinical evidence. *Curr. Neuropharmacol.* **2011**, *9*, 530–532. [CrossRef]
50. Maes, M.; De Vos, N.; Pioli, R.; Demedts, P.; Wauters, A.; Neels, H.; Christophe, A. Lower serum vitamin E concentrations in major depression. Another marker of lowered antioxidant defenses in that illness. *J. Affect. Disord.* **2000**, *58*, 241–246. [CrossRef]
51. Khanzode, S.D.; Dakhale, G.N.; Khanzode, S.S.; Saoji, A.; Palasodkar, R. Oxidative damage and major depression: The potential antioxidant action of selective serotonin re-uptake inhibitors. *Redox Rep.* **2003**, *8*, 365–370. [CrossRef]

52. Ravindran, A.V.; Griffiths, J.; Merali, Z.; Anisman, H. Lymphocyte subsets associated with major depression and dysthymia: Modification by antidepressant treatment. *Psychosom. Med.* **1995**, *57*, 555–563. [CrossRef]
53. Rybka, J.; Kedziora-Kornatowska, K.; Banas-Lezanska, P.; Majsterek, I.; Carvalho, L.A.; Cattaneo, A.; Anacker, C.; Kedziora, J. Interplay between the pro-oxidant and antioxidant systems and proinflammatory cytokine levels, in relation to iron metabolism and the erythron in depression. *Free Radic. Biol. Med.* **2013**, *63*, 187–194. [CrossRef]

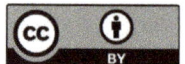

© 2019 by the authors. Licensee MDPI, Basel, Switzerland. This article is an open access article distributed under the terms and conditions of the Creative Commons Attribution (CC BY) license (http://creativecommons.org/licenses/by/4.0/).

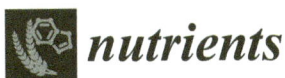

Article

Palatability of Goat's versus Cow's Milk: Insights from the Analysis of Eating Behavior and Gene Expression in the Appetite-Relevant Brain Circuit in Laboratory Animal Models

Anica Klockars [1,†], Erin L. Wood [1,†], Sarah N. Gartner [1], Laura K. McColl [1], Allen S. Levine [2], Elizabeth A. Carpenter [3], Colin G. Prosser [3] and Pawel K. Olszewski [1,2,*]

1. Faculty of Science and Engineering, University of Waikato, Hamilton 3240, New Zealand; anica.klockars@waikato.ac.nz (A.K.); elw14@students.waikato.ac.nz (E.L.W.); snm10@students.waikato.ac.nz (S.N.G.); laura.mccoll@waikato.ac.nz (L.K.M.)
2. Department of Food Science and Nutrition, University of Minnesota, St. Paul, MN 55113, USA; aslevine@umn.edu
3. Dairy Goat Cooperative (NZ) Ltd., Hamilton 3206, New Zealand; Liz.Carpenter@dgc.co.nz (E.A.C.); Colin.Prosser@dgc.co.nz (C.G.P.)
* Correspondence: pawel@waikato.ac.nz
† The authors contributed equally to the finished manuscript.

Received: 11 February 2019; Accepted: 25 March 2019; Published: 28 March 2019

Abstract: Goat's (GM) and cow's milk (CM) are dietary alternatives with select health benefits shown in human and animal studies. Surprisingly, no systematic analysis of palatability or preference for GM vs. CM has been performed to date. Here, we present a comprehensive investigation of short-term intake and palatability profiles of GM and CM in laboratory mice and rats. We studied consumption in no-choice and choice scenarios, including meal microstructure, and by using isocaloric milks and milk-enriched solid diets. Feeding results are accompanied by qPCR data of relevant genes in the energy balance-related hypothalamus and brain stem, and in the nucleus accumbens, which regulates eating for palatability. We found that GM and CM are palatable to juvenile, adult, and aged rodents. Given a choice, animals prefer GM- to CM-based diets. Analysis of meal microstructure using licking patterns points to enhanced palatability of and, possibly, greater motivation toward GM over CM. Most profound changes in gene expression after GM vs. CM were associated with the brain systems driving consumption for reward. We conclude that, while both GM and CM are palatable, GM is preferred over CM by laboratory animals, and this preference is driven by central mechanisms controlling eating for pleasure.

Keywords: milk; hypothalamus; nucleus accumbens; reward; appetite; palatability

1. Introduction

Milk is a widely consumed, affordable, and highly nutritive food, which serves as a key source of, among others, protein, calcium, potassium, magnesium, and vitamins (especially A and D) in industrialized countries [1–6]. In Western societies, cow's milk (CM) products represent the largest share of dairy available on the market, and cow's skim milk varieties have become common. However, recent years have generated interest in milk from other species, such as goat's milk (GM). The use of GM as an alternative to CM has been driven by the findings in humans and laboratory animals showing potential beneficial nutritive consequences of GM intake and differences in physiological responses to GM or CM consumption, (for review, see [7]). For example, Bellioni-Businco et al. reported that individuals with a CM allergy were able to drink five times more GM than CM before the symptoms of an allergic response appeared [8]. In studies utilizing rodent models, Barrionuevo et al. demonstrated that GM increases utilization of copper, zinc, and selenium [9]. Bioavailability of iron and copper was found to be improved in GM-fed rodents suffering from malabsorptive syndrome and in healthy controls [9,10]. Finally, GM improved bone turnover in iron-deficient rats compared to rats fed CM [11,12].

Surprisingly, little is known about GM's acceptance and preference relative to the main dairy product in today's food environment in the Western world. There is no systematic analysis of propensity to ingest GM and CM or relative palatability of GM vs. CM in either humans or in laboratory animal models. Consequently, our understanding of acceptance and palatability of GM compared to CM is still mainly based on anecdotal evidence and on market availability, both heavily influenced by local cultural or environmental aspects (such as in Western vs. Asian countries) and habituation-driven intake of a specific milk type [13]. This is a major gap in knowledge as palatability affects, among others, the amount of food eaten in a single meal, the rate of consumption, food anticipation, and satiety. It has a profound effect on activity of brain circuits responsible for processing energy intake (including the hypothalamus (HYP) and brain stem (BS)) and reward (such as the nucleus accumbens; NAcc) [14–16]. These parameters can, in turn, impact a plethora of mechanisms outside the central nervous system (CNS), via neural and hormonal interactions linking the brain and peripheral tissues [17–19].

Here, we present for the first time a comprehensive investigation of short-term intake and palatability profiles of GM and CM in laboratory rodent models (mice and rats) using skim milks. We report consumption data on the acceptance (no-choice) and preference (choice) scenarios of calorie-matched milks and milk-enriched solid diets. Consumption data are accompanied by the analysis of expression of appetite-related genes in the HYP and BS, two brain regions predominantly involved in energy balance control, and in the NAcc, a key site that regulates eating for palatability [15,16]. We examined mRNA levels of genes involved in promoting consumption, such as those encoding neuropeptide Y (NPY), Agouti-related protein (AgRP), ghrelin receptor, orexin, opioid peptides/receptors, and gap junction protein, connexin 36 (Cx36). The analysis also included transcripts related to decreased appetite and termination of consumption, such as oxytocin, melanocortin receptors 3 (MC3R) and 4 (MC4R), and proopiomelanocortin (POMC). Typically, presentation of tastants that differ in palatability and composition, among other traits, evokes some changes in expression within this subset of genes, reflecting a different propensity of an animal to ingest specific diets [16,20]. A number of physiological functions by the brain vary with age, including appetite. Weight is typically gained throughout early and middle age, followed by gradual, age-associated anorexia. In line with that, a drive to consume food (and responsiveness to palatability) is high during the earlier stages of life, whereas in aged animals, anhedonia and decreased responsiveness to rewarding diets and to drugs that promote eating for pleasure ensue (e.g., see [21–23]). Therefore, in our feeding experiments, we studied rodents that belong to three distinct age groups: adolescents, adults, and aged animals. It should also be noted that rats and most mammals, other than select groups of humans, poorly digest lactose post-weaning. Though lactase activity in adult rats is residual, rats fed as much as 30% lactose in their daily diet from post-weaning to day 98 had normal body growth or body weight course (their body weight was somewhat lower) [24]. Taking it into consideration, however, in this current study we focused on short-term rather than long-term exposure to milk or milk containing chow.

2. Materials and Methods

2.1. Animals

Male Sprague-Dawley rats and C57Bl mice (all weaned on day 21) used in these studies were single-housed in a temperature-controlled (22 °C) animal facility with a 12:12-h LD cycle (lights on at 07:00). Standard chow (Diet 86, Sharpes Stock Feed, Wairarapa, New Zealand) and water were available ad libitum unless indicated otherwise. The University of Waikato animal ethics committee had approved the procedures (ethics approval numbers: 1020, 1043, and 1057), and they are compliant with the NIH Guide for the Care and Use of Laboratory Animals (NIH Publ., no. 80–23, rev. 1996). Feeding experiments were performed in separate cohorts of animals unless specified otherwise. The age of animals included in the adolescent (5–6 weeks), adult (3–5 months), and aged (25–27 months) categories was based on previous publications pertaining to the aging process in rodents [25]. It should be noted that despite poor digestibility of lactose post-weaning, we did not observe any signs of gastrointestinal discomfort or sickness, which is in line with previous studies showing that rats fed as much as 30% lactose in their daily diet (thus, more than given here) for several weeks displayed good tolerance of the carbohydrate [24].

2.2. Episodic Intake of Individually Presented GM and CM in Sated Adult Mice and Rats

We based the protocol on previous studies assessing episodic intake of palatable tastants [26–28]. Individually housed mice and rats were accustomed (in homecages) to receiving one of the four isocaloric (0.6 kcal/g) solutions for 2 h/day on 2 days (10:00–12:00) prior to the experiments using their usual 250 mL sized water bottles (used for all bottle scenarios) to avoid neophobia(mice: n = 8–9/group; rats: 8–10/group): GM, CM, an energy-equivalent 15% sucrose solution (a reference palatable solution), or a 15% cornstarch (CS) suspension (a negative control for palatability; as CS is insoluble in water, 0.3% xanthan gum was added to this liquid in this experiment as described previously in [29]). On the experimental day, bottles with the solutions (at room temperature) were placed in the cages and water and chow were removed for the 2-h experimental session. Spillage (g) from each individual bottle was recorded before placement into cage. Intakes were measured after 2 h using a digital scale and expressed in grams per gram of body weight. This feeding experiment was conducted in a separate cohort of animals. Composition of the milks are shown in Table 1.

Table 1. CM and GM milk powder composition.

Sample	Protein	Fat	Carbohydrate (Lactose)	Ash	Moisture
CM	37.1	1.1	51	6.5	4.3
GM	36.1	0.9	49.9	9.5	3.6

2.3. Energy Deprivation-Induced Intake of Individually Presented GM and CM in Mice and Rats

Mice and rats previously exposed in their homecages to GM, CM, cornstarch, and sucrose were deprived of standard chow overnight (food taken away at 16:00). On the next day (10:00), water bottles were removed and replaced with bottles (at room temperature) containing one of the four treatments (mice: n = 8–10/group; rats: 7–8/group). Spillage (g) from each individual bottle was recorded before placement into cage. Intakes were measured using a digital scale after 2 h and expressed in grams per gram of body weight. This feeding experiment was conducted in a separate cohort of animals.

2.4. Episodic Intake of Individually Presented GM- and CM-Enriched Chow in Sated Adult Mice and Rats

Rats and mice were given episodic access to the chow enriched with GM or CM according to the protocol described above, where, instead of GM or CM, a GM- or CM-enriched chow (see Table 2 for composition of GM and CM chow) was presented for 2 h (10:00). Standard chow pellets were removed during this 2-h meal, but water was left in the cages. Intake of chow pellets (at room temperature) was measured using a digital scale after 2 h and expressed in grams per gram of body weight. In order to assess baseline intake, a control group of animals had a fresh batch of the standard chow placed in the hopper for 2 h (n = 7–8/group for both mice and rats). This feeding experiment was conducted in a separate cohort of animals.

Table 2. Composition of CM- and GM-enriched chow.

Base Skim Milk Powder Composition (1% Milk Fat)	Goat Skim Milk Powder (SMP)		Cow SMP	
	%	g/kg	%	g/kg
Protein	37.8	120	37.1	120
Fat	1.7	5.40	0.86	2.78
Ash	9.4	29.84	7.3	23.61
Moisture	4.1	13.02	4.2	13.58
Lactose	47	149.21	50.54	163.47
Total	100	317.46	100	323.45
	Goat SMP		Cow SMP	
Skim Milk Chow—Ingredient	g/kg		g/kg	
Goat SMP—to supply 12% protein	317.46			
Cow SMP—to supply 12% protein			323.45	
Vitamin mix	50.00		50.00	
Salt mix	50.00		50.00	
Corn oil (added to make 5% fat)	44.60		47.22	
Starch	447.15		452.80	
Lactose (added to make 16.5%)	15.79		1.53	
Cellulose	75.00		75.00	
Moisture				
	1000.00		1000.00	
Target Dietary Content				
Protein	12%		12%	
Fat	5%		5%	
Lactose	16.50%		16.50%	
Fiber	7.50%		7.50%	
Starch	44.7%		45.3%	
Calories				
Protein (4 cal/g)	48		48	
Fat (9 cal/g)	45		45	
Lactose (4 cal/g)	66		66	
Fiber (2 cal/g)	15		15	
Starch (4 cal/g)	179		181	
Calories/100 g	353		355	
% calories				
Protein	14%		14%	
Fat	13%		13%	
Lactose	19%		19%	
Fiber	4%		4%	
Starch	51%		51%	
Skim Milk Powder (1% Milk Fat)	Goat SMP		Cow SMP	
Ingredients	g/kg		g/kg	
Goat SMP	317.46			
Cow SMP			323.45	
Vitamin mix	50.00		50.00	
Salt mix	50.00		50.00	
Corn oil	44.60		47.22	
Starch	447.15		452.80	
Lactose	15.79		1.53	
Cellulose	75.00		75.00	
Moisture				
	1000.00		1000.00	

Table 2. Cont.

Base Skim Milk Powder Composition (1% Milk Fat)	Goat Skim Milk Powder (SMP)	Cow SMP
Target Dietary Content		
Protein	12%	12%
Fat	5%	5%
Lactose	16.50%	16.50%
Fiber	7.50%	7.50%
Starch	44.7%	45.3%
Calories		
Protein (4 cal/g)	48	48
Fat (9 cal/g)	45	45
Lactose (4 cal/g)	66	66
Fiber (2 cal/g)	15	15
Starch (4 cal/g)	179	181
Calories/100 g	353	355
% calories		
Protein	14%	14%
Fat	13%	13%
Lactose	19%	19%
Fiber	4%	4%
Starch	51%	51%

2.5. Energy Deprivation-Induced Intake of Individually Presented GM- and CM-Enriched Chow in Sated Adult Mice and Rats

Rats and mice previously exposed to GM- and CM-enriched chow (pre-exposure to both chow types was simultaneous) were deprived of standard chow overnight (food taken away at 16:00). On the next day (10:00), animals received either standard chow, GM- or CM-enriched pellets (mice: $n = 7$–8/group; rats: $n = 8$–9/group) at room temperature. Intakes were measured using a digital scale after 2 h and expressed in grams per gram of body weight. This feeding experiment was conducted in a separate cohort of animals.

2.6. Episodic Intake of Individually Presented GM and CM in Sated Adolescent and Aged Rodents

Mice and rats aged 5–6 weeks ($n = 9$–11/group for each species) were used in the study on adolescent animals, whereas 25-month old mice and 26-month old rats ($n = 8$–9/group for each species) were used as the aged cohorts. The feeding experiments utilizing individually presented cornstarch, sucrose, GM, and CM solutions followed the protocol described above for the relevant studies in adult sated rodents that received one of the four solutions for 2 h. This feeding experiment was conducted in a separate cohort of animals.

2.7. Episodic Intake of GM and CM Presented Simultaneously in Sated Adolescent, Adult, and Aged Rodents

Mice ($n = 20$) and rats ($n = 21$) aged 5–6 weeks were used in the study on adolescent animals, 16–18-week old mice ($n = 10$) and rats ($n = 12$) were included in the study on adults, whereas 25-month old mice ($n = 12$) and 26-month old rats ($n = 11$) were used as the aged cohorts. Adult and adolescent rats and mice had been previously exposed to GM and CM (pre-exposure to both milk types was simultaneous). The aged animals came from the cohorts described above (pt. 2.6), however, a week-long 'washout' period was allowed between the previous experiment and this study. First, the animals were accustomed to simultaneously receiving GM and CM as a two-bottle choice (bottles placed next to each other; random order) for circa 1 h per day on two days in their homecage. Then, on the experimental day, chow and water were removed from cages and GM and CM (at room temperature) were given to the animals for 2 h (11:00–13:00). Spillage (g) from each individual bottle was recorded before placement into cage. Intakes were measured using a digital scale after 2 h and expressed in grams per gram of body weight. This feeding experiment was conducted in a separate cohort of adolescent and adult animals.

2.8. Episodic Intake of GM- and CM-Enriched Chow Presented Simultaneously in Sated Adult and Aged Rodents

Mice and rats aged 18–20 weeks old mice ($n = 8$) and rats ($n = 8$) were included in the study on adults, whereas 25-month old mice ($n = 9$) and 27-month old rats ($n = 10$) were used as the aged cohorts. Adult rats and mice had been previously exposed to GM and CM chow (pre-exposure to both chow types was simultaneous). The aged animals came from the same cohort as in the GM/CM chow experiment described above (Section 2.5), however, a two-week-long 'washout' period was allowed between the previous experiment and this study. First, the animals were accustomed to receiving simultaneously CM- and GM-enriched chow in a subdivided hopper in their homecages (placement of GM/CM pellets was random; standard chow was removed) for circa 1 h per day on two days. Then, on the experimental day, after removal of standard chow, CM- and GM-enriched pellets (at room temperature) were given to the animals for 2 h (10:00–12:00). Intakes were measured using a digital scale after 2 h and expressed in grams per gram of body weight. This feeding experiment was conducted in a separate cohort of adult animals.

2.9. Lickometer-Assessed Preference for Simultaneously Presented GM and CM in Sated Adult Rats

Six 12-week old male rats were housed individually in cages equipped with bottles attached to lickometers (Lafayette Instruments, Lafayette, IN, USA). The animals were previously given GM and CM to prevent neophobia (the pre-exposure was simultaneous). They were accustomed to receiving a choice between GM and CM on two separate days for 30 min (random order of bottles) in lickometer cages. On the experimental day, standard chow and water were removed from the cages and animals were given simultaneous access to GM and CM (room temperature) for 30 min. The number of licks on each bottle was counted and analyzed (Scurry Activity Monitoring software, Lafayette, IN, USA), both as total number of licks as well as number of licks per 5-minute interval. We also assessed the cluster number (number of bouts of licking—each bout was defined as continuous licking interspaced by no more than 0.5 s between each other) and an average cluster length (bout duration measured in seconds) of GM vs. CM. This feeding experiment was conducted in a separate cohort of animals.

2.10. 72-h Cumulative Intake of Simultaneously Presented CM- and GM-Enriched Chow in Adult Rats

First, the animals were accustomed to receiving two types of chow pellets (room temperature) simultaneously in a subdivided hopper in their homecage (placement of pellets was random) for circa 2 h per day on two days. On the experimental day 1 (17:00), animals received a choice of either standard/CM chow ($n = 9$), standard/GM chow ($n = 10$), or GM/CM chow for 72 h (pellets were exchanged daily; $n = 16$). Cumulative 72-h intakes were recorded in grams. This feeding experiment was conducted in a separate cohort of animals.

2.11. Effect of 24-h CM vs. GM Consumption on Feeding-Related Gene Expression in the Brain Circuit

In order to assess the effect of 24-h intake of GM and CM solutions on the expression of feeding-related genes in the brain, mice were given CM or GM (at room temperature) as the only tastant (starting at 10:00). Animals given water served as baseline controls. At 10:00 on the subsequent day (thus, 24 h after milk presentation), the animals were sacrificed via cervical dislocation. Brains were dissected out and the hypothalamus, nucleus accumbens, and brain stem excised and stored in RNAlater at $-80\,^\circ$C until further processing. This experiment was conducted in a separate cohort of animals.

Tissues were homogenized in Trizol (Ambien), 1 mL per 0.1 g tissue. 0.2 mL chloroform was added and samples were centrifuged at room temperature for 10 min at $10,000\times g$. The clear phase containing RNA was isolated and 0.5 mL of isopropanol was added. RNA was precipitated in an ice bath for 10 min then centrifuged at 4 °C for 20 min at 10,000× g. Aqueous phase was removed from the pellets, which were then resuspended in 0.3 mL of ethanol and centrifuged at 4 °C for 10 min at 10,000× g. Liquid was removed and pellets were air-dried.

Pellets were dissolved in 8 µL DEPC water and 1 µL DNAse buffer (dNature). Samples were then incubated with 1 µL DNAse (dNature) at 37 °C for 30 min. DNAse was inactivated via addition of stop buffer (dNature) and incubation at 67 °C for 10 min. Removal of DNA was confirmed via PCR using HOT FIREPol Blend Master Mix (dNature), followed with agarose gel electrophoresis. Concentrations of RNA were measured with a nanodrop.

cDNA was synthesized from RNA samples with iScript Advanced cDNA synthesis kit (BioRad). Synthesis of cDNA was confirmed with PCR followed by agarose gel electrophoresis.

Quantitative RT-PCR (qPCR) was used to determine relative expression levels of housekeeping genes (ActB, GAPDH, β-tubulin) and of genes of interest. Reactions contained 4 µL of 25 ng/µL sample cDNA, 1 µL of each forward and reverse primers (5 µM), 10 µL iTaq Universal SYBR Green Supermix (BioRad) and 4 µL MilliQ water. qPCR experiments were performed in duplicates alongside negative controls of MilliQ water for each primer pair. Amplification protocol was initiated at 95 °C for 15 min, followed by 45 cycles of 15 s at 95 °C, 15 s at the primer-specific annealing temperature and 30 s at 72 °C. Primers used: GADPH F: 5′-AAGGTCATCCCAGAGC TGAA-3′, R: 5′-CTGCTTCACCACCTTCTTGA-3′; ActB F: 5′-AGTGTGACGTTGACATCCGT-3′, R: 5′-TGCTAGGAGCCAGAGCAGTA-3′; POMC F: 5′-GACACTGGCTGCTCTCCAG-3′, R: 5′-AGCAGCCTCCCGAGACA-3′; Agrp F: 5′-GGATCTGTTGCAGGAGGCTCAG-3′, R: 5′-TGAAGAAGCGGCAGTAGCACGT-3′; NPY F: 5′-GGTCTTCAAGCCGAGTTCTG-3′, R: 5′-AACCTCATCACCAGGCAGAG-3′; MC4R F: 5′-CTTATGATGATCCCAACCCG-3′, R: 5′-GTAGCTCCTTGCTTGCATCC-3′; β-tubulin F: 5′-CGGAAGGAGGCGGAGAGC-3′, R: 5′-AGGGTGCCCATGCCAGAGC-3′; GHSR F: 5′-TCCGATCTGCTCATCTTCCT-3′, R: 5′- GGAAGCAGATGGCGAAGTAG-3′; ORX F: 5′-GCCGTCTCTACGAACTGTTGC-3′, R: 5′-CGCTTTCCCAGAGTCAGGATA-3′; OXT F: 5′-CCTACAGCGGATCTCAGACTG-3′, R: 5′-TCAGAGCCAGTAAGCCAAGCA-3′; OXTR F: 5′-TCTTCTTCGTGCAGATGTGG-3′, R: 5′-CCTTCAGGTACCGAGCAGAG-3′; PENK F: 5′-CGACATCAATTTCCTGGCGT-3′, R: 5′-AGATCCTTGCAGGTCTCCCA-3′; DYN F: 5′-GACAGGAGAGGAAGCAGA-3′, R: 5′-AGCAGCACACAAGTCACC-3′; GHRL F: 5′-CCATCTGCAGTTTGCTGCTA-3′, R: 5′-GCTTGTCCTCTGTCCTCTGG-3′; MOR F: 5′-CCTGCCGCTCTTCTCTGG-3′, R: 5′-CGGACTCGGTAGGCTGTAAC-3′; KOR F: 5′-CACCTTGCTGATCCCAAAC-3′, R: 5′-TTCCCAAGTCACCGTCAG-3′; PNOC F: 5′-AGCACCTGAAGAGAATGCCG-3′, R: 5′-CATCTCGCACTTGCACCAAG-3′; ORLP F: 5′-ATGACTAGGCGTGGACCTGC-3′, R: 5′-GATGGGCTCTGTGGACTGACA-3′; GLP1R F: 5′-ATGGCCAGCACCCCAAGCCTCC-3′, R: 5′-TCAGCTGTAGGAACTCTGG-3′; Cx36 F: 5′-CCAGTAAGGAGACAGAACCAGAT-3′, R: 5′-GATGATGTAGAAGCGGGAGATAC-3′.

2.12. Data Analysis

Analyses of qPCR data utilized BioRad CFX Manager software (BioRad); one-way ANOVA followed by Bonferroni's test with the correction for multiple comparisons was used, with $p < 0.05$ set as criterion of statistical significance. Feeding data from studies comparing two groups were analyzed using a *t*-test, whereas comparisons between three or more groups were done with ANOVA followed by Bonferroni's post-hoc test, with differences considered significant when $p < 0.05$.

3. Results

In the non-choice acceptance tests, sated adult mice and rats showed very low levels of consumption of a 'bland' cornstarch emulsion, whereas intakes of the GM (mice, $F(3,30) = 62.8$, $p < 0.001$; rats, $F(3,32) = 25.5$, $p < 0.001$) and CM (mice, $p < 0.001$; rats, $p < 0.001$), as well as of the sucrose solution (mice, $p < 0.001$; rats, $p < 0.001$), were several times higher than of cornstarch. Energy-deprived animals had a higher baseline intake of cornstarch, but consumed significantly more sucrose (mice, $F(3,32) = 9.77$, $p \leq 0.001$; rats, $F(3,26) = 5.5$, $p = 0.039$), GM (mice, $p < 0.001$; rats, $p = 0.0023$), and CM (mice, $p = 0.034$; rats, $p = 0.0083$; Figure 1A–D). Similarly, both deprived and sated adult individuals ate more GM- and CM-enriched pellets than standard chow (sated mice: $F(2,19) = 5.9$, GM, $p = 0.029$ and CM, $p = 0.011$; sated rats: $F(2,19) = 20.5$, GM, $p < 0.001$ and CM, $p = 0.0011$; deprived mice: $F(2,19) = 6.5$, GM, $p = 0.0058$ and CM, $p = 0.034$; deprived rats: $F(2,22) = 10.8$, GM, $p < 0.001$ and CM, $p = 0.0442$; Figure 1E–H). Adolescent and aged sated mice and rats (Figure 2A,B,E,F) given episodic 2-h access to one of the solutions, consumed more GM (adolescent mice, $F(3,35) = 42.7$, $p < 0.001$; rats, $F(3,36) = 16.9$, $p < 0.001$; aged mice, $F(3,29) = 31.2$, $p < 0.001$; rats, $F(3,29) = 18.9$, $p < 0.001$), CM (adolescent mice, $p < 0.001$; rats, $p < 0.001$; aged mice, $p < 0.001$; rats, $p < 0.001$) and sucrose (adolescent mice, $p < 0.001$; rats, $p < 0.001$; aged mice, $p < 0.001$; rats, $p < 0.001$) than cornstarch.

When given a 2-h episodic choice between GM and CM, all age cohorts of rats (adolescent, $p < 0.001$; adult, $p < 0.001$; aged, $p < 0.001$) and adult and aged mice ($p = 0.012$ and 0.011, respectively) preferred GM (Figure 2C,D,G,H and Figure 3A,B). During a brief, 30-min exposure to both GM and CM in cages equipped with lickometers, adult rats exhibited a more robust response to GM cumulatively over that period ($p = 0.01$) as well as during the first ($p = 0.037$) and second ($p = 0.05$) 5-min time interval of the meal (Figure 3C,D). There was a trend approaching significance ($p = 0.088$) toward an increase in the cluster number (number of licking bouts) of GM over CM, and a significantly greater cluster length of each GM than CM bout ($p = 0.022$; Figure 3E,F). In choice experiments involving GM- and CM-enriched chow, adult and aged rats ($p = 0.009$ and 0.023, respectively) and adult mice ($p = 0.028$) preferred GM chow, whereas in aged mice, a trend toward GM preference was detected ($p = 0.059$) (Figure 4A,B). Adult rats given a 72-h uninterrupted access to a choice between GM and CM chow preferred GM chow ($p < 0.001$), while both GM ($p = 0.015$) and CM pellets ($p < 0.001$) were preferred over standard food during a similar time of exposure (Figure 4C).

Real-time PCR analysis after consumption of the two milk formulations (GM: $19.27 +/- 0.18$ g; CM: $18.44 +/- 0.17$ g) revealed that GM upregulated in the nucleus accumbens PNOC ($p = 0.0164$), ORL1 ($p = 0.0042$), Cx36 ($p = 0.0017$), GLP1R ($p = 0.0015$), MC4R ($p = 0.002$), OXT ($p < 0.001$), and GHSR ($p < 0.001$) genes, whereas mRNA levels of PENK were lower (though it did not reach significance with a p value of 0.01), compared with CM consumption. In the hypothalamus, MOR ($p = 0.045$) and KOR ($p = 0.017$) transcript levels were higher after GM consumption, and in the brain stem there was a trend toward upregulation of the MC4R ($p = 0.099$) and the MC3R was upregulated ($p = 0.0275$; Figure 5). Compared to water controls, in the nucleus accumbens, GM affected expression of ORL1 ($p = 0.012$), Cx36 ($p = 0.0052$), GLP1R ($p = 0.0042$), MC4R ($p = 0.0053$), OXT ($p = 0.0149$), and GHSR ($p < 0.001$); in the hypothalamus, ORX ($p = 0.0164$), KOR ($p = 0.0399$), and MC4R ($p = 0.0403$). On the other hand, hypothalamic expression of the MC4R gene was elevated by CM intake ($p = 0.041$; Figure 5).

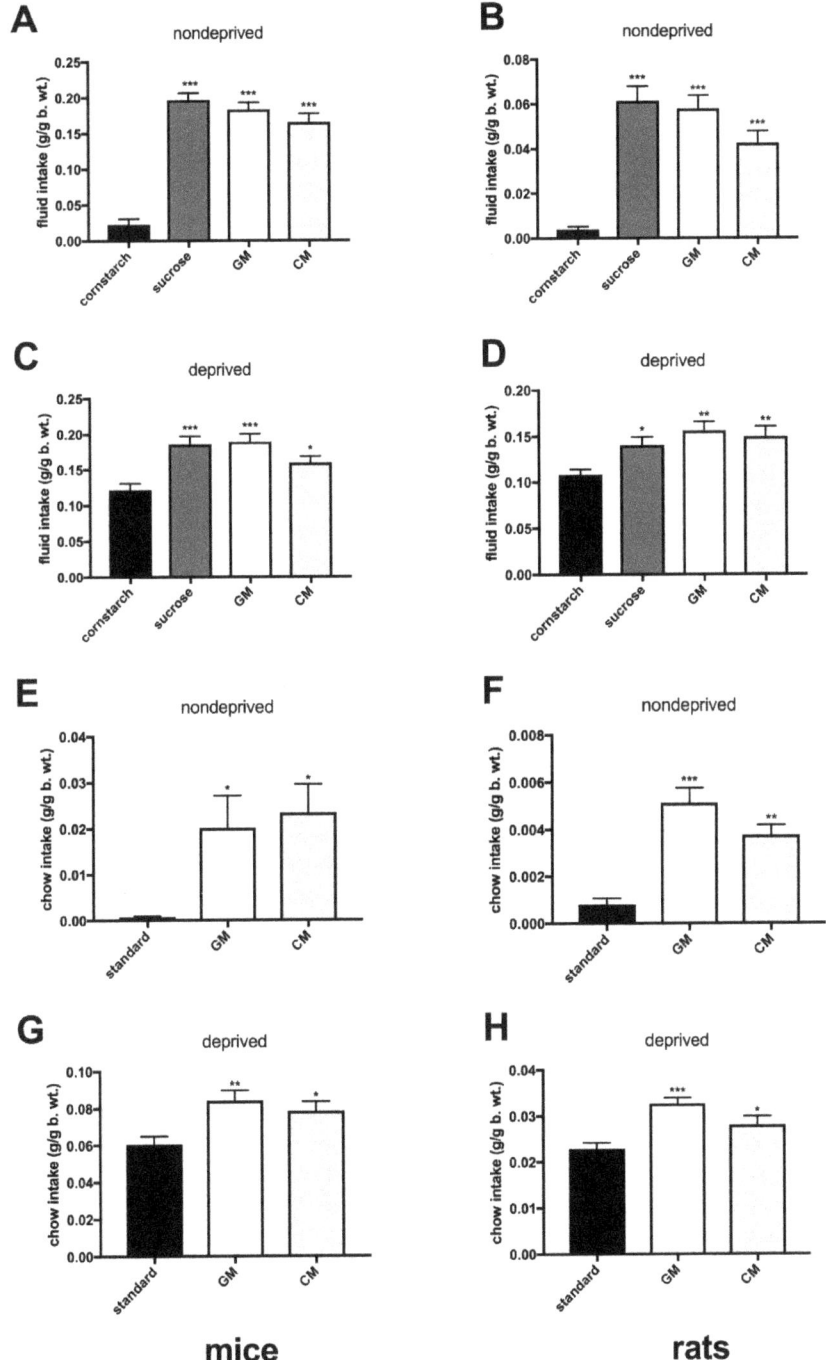

Figure 1. Episodic 2-h consumption of individually presented (acceptance) cornstarch, sucrose, GM, and CM isocaloric solutions (**A–D**), and of standard, GM- and CM-enriched chow (**E–H**) in sated (nondeprived) and energy-deprived mice (left panel) and rats (right panel).*, $p \leq 0.05$; **, $p \leq 0.01$; ***, $p \leq 0.001$.

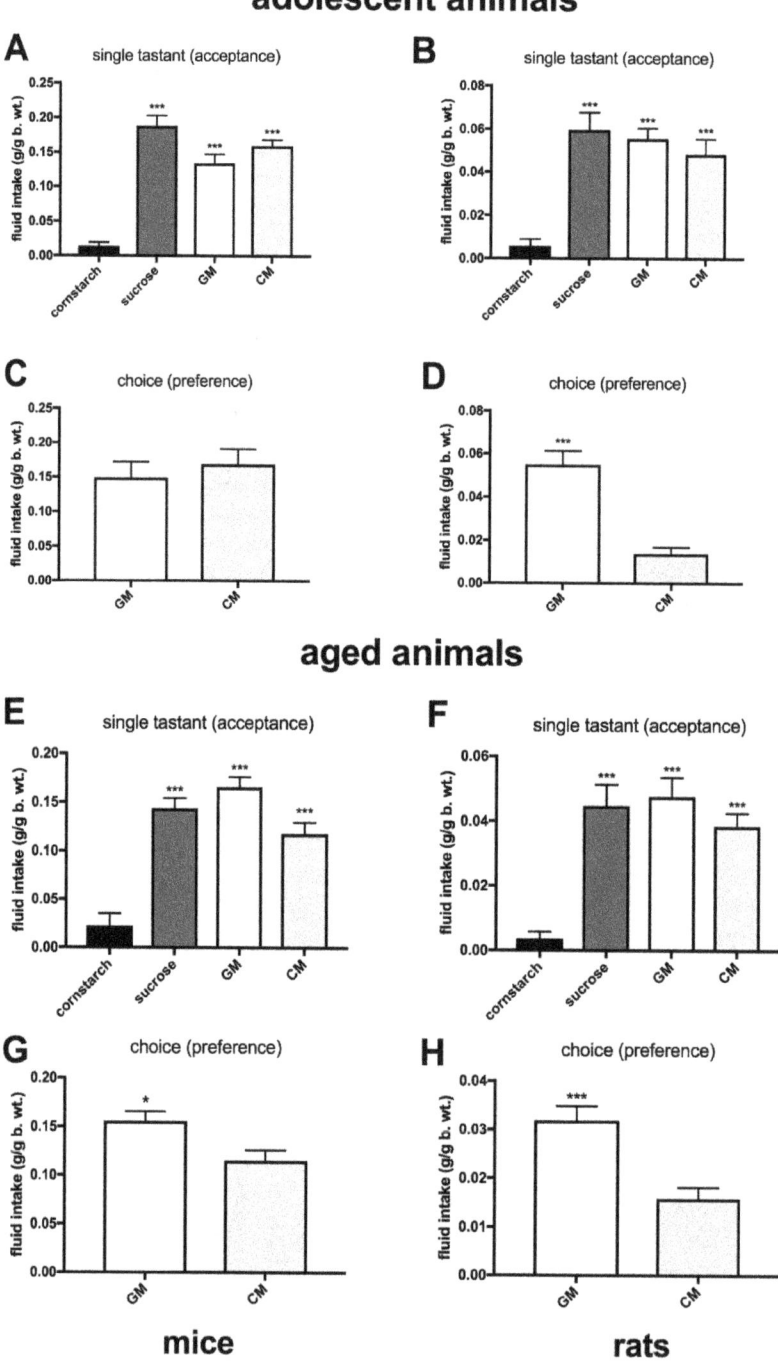

Figure 2. Episodic 2-h consumption of individually presented cornstarch, sucrose, GM, and CM isocaloric solutions (**A,B,E,F**: acceptance) and simultaneously given GM and CM (**C,D,G,H**: preference) in adolescent and aged sated mice (left panel) and rats (right panel). *, $p \leq 0.05$; ***, $p \leq 0.001$.

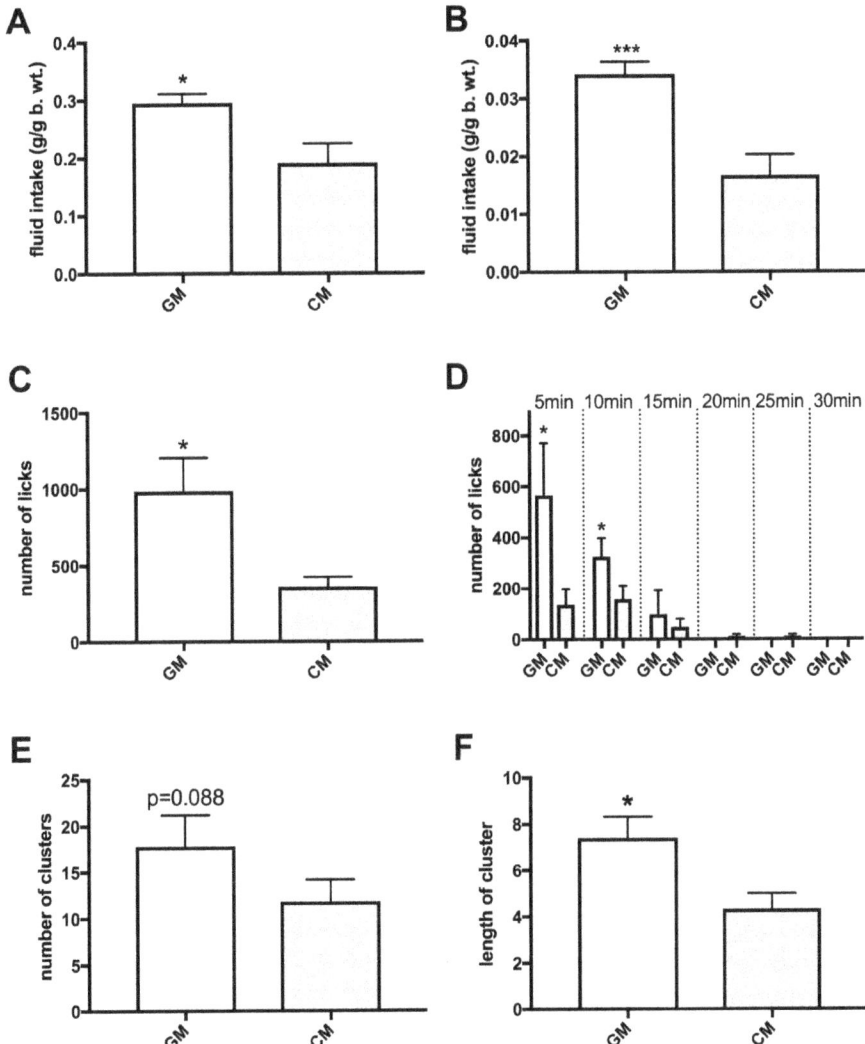

Figure 3. Episodic consumption of simultaneously presented GM and CM over 2-h in sated mice (**A**) and rats (**B**), lickometer activity during a 30-min exposure ((**C**): 0–30 min; (**D**): 5-min intervals), the number of GM over CM licking bouts (cluster number) (**E**), and the cluster length(s) of each GM and CM bout (**F**) in sated rats. *, $p \leq 0.05$; ***, $p \leq 0.001$.

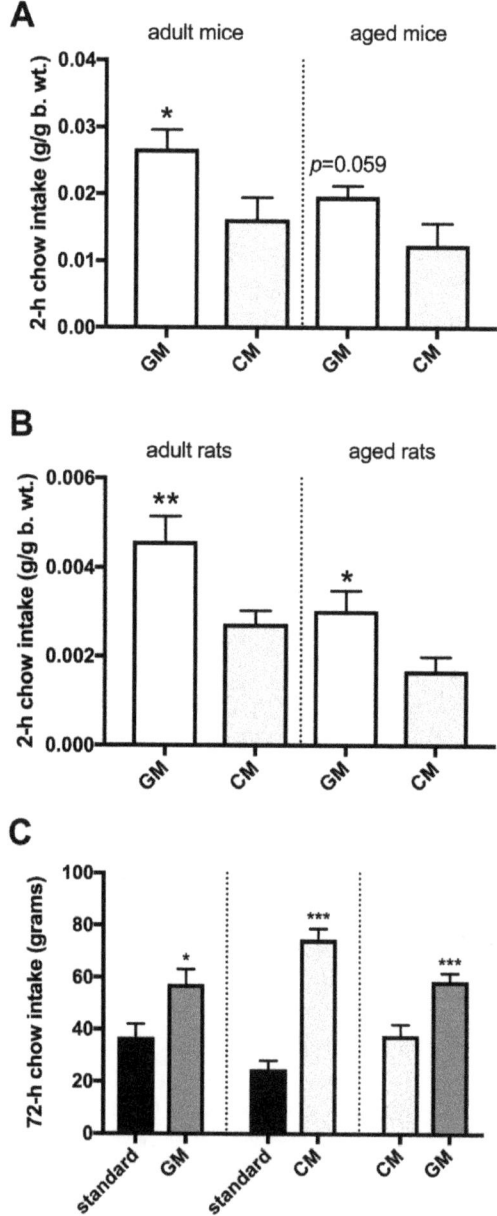

Figure 4. Consumption of simultaneously presented GM- and CM-enriched chow in adult and aged sated mice (**A**) and rats (**B**) over 2 h and simultaneously presented pellets (standard vs. GM; standard vs. CM, and GM vs. CM) over 72 h in adult rats (**C**).*, $p \leq 0.05$; **, $p \leq 0.01$; ***, $p \leq 0.001$.

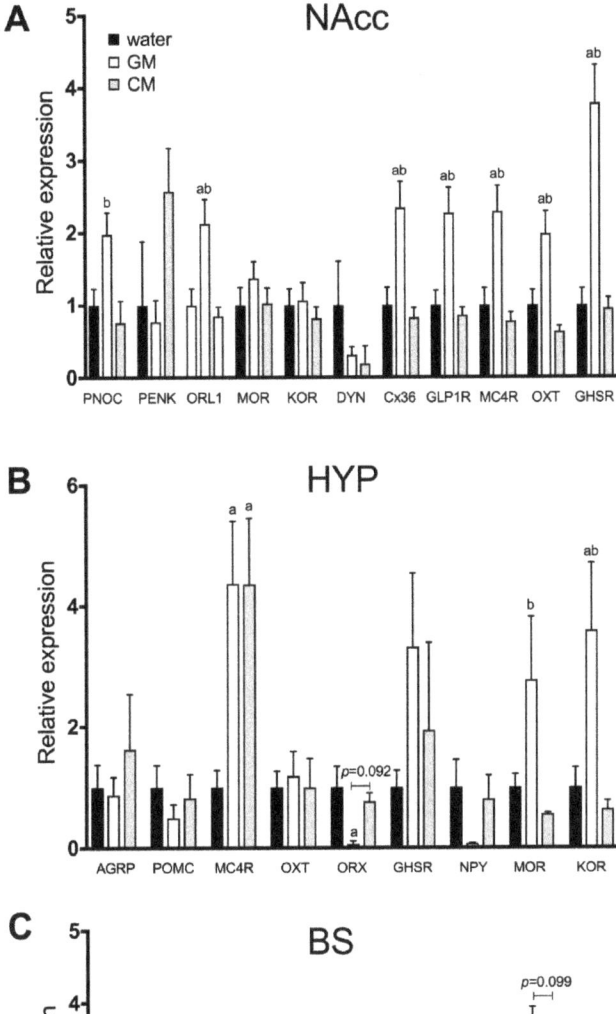

Figure 5. Relative expression of feeding-related genes in the nucleus accumbens (**A**), hypothalamus (**B**), and brain stem (**C**) of mice maintained for 24 h on GM or CM. Water served as a baseline tastant. [a]—significantly different from the water group; [b]—significantly different from the CM group. Analysis performed with ANOVA followed by Bonferroni's test and corrected for multiple comparisons.

4. Discussion

Enhanced motivation to eat in the absence of an immediate need to replenish calories or continuation of a meal beyond levels that restore energy balance typically occur when an individual is given access to food that is highly palatable. In laboratory animal models, similarly to what is observed in humans, a variety of tastants are perceived as palatable. Those include ingestants whose palatability is derived mainly from the flavor and/or postabsorptive effects of either a single macronutrient (e.g., sucrose-sweetened solutions) or from the complex contribution of multiple nutritive components (e.g., in meat rich in protein and fat) [30–32]. Calorie density of food (especially when coupled with high energy needs of an organism) is an additional factor that affects the liking of and preference for a given food [15,33].

The current set of studies show that both GM and CM and milk-enriched solid diets are highly palatable. In no-choice acceptance paradigms, energy non-deprived rats and mice of all age groups (adolescent, adult, and aged) consumed GM and CM as avidly as the calorie-matched 15% sucrose solution (used here as a positive control for a highly palatable tastant in rodents (for review, see [30])), while ingesting only minimal amounts of the 'bland' cornstarch. A similar phenomenon was observed in energy-deprived animals, although the amount by which GM, CM, and sucrose intakes exceeded that of cornstarch was not as pronounced as in sated rodents. That was due to the vigorous energy deficit-driven consumption of cornstarch and a 'ceiling effect' that prevents ingestion of large amounts of the solutions during the brief refeeding period. Importantly, GM and CM enrichment of laboratory chow stimulated intake in both hungry and sated animals well above the level of standard pellets. It indicates that both GM- and CM-derived palatability is a generalized phenomenon, not limited to liquid milks, but extending to solid foods that contain milk powder. This is in concert with the ability of other palatable tastants (including, but not limited to, fat, sucrose, and select amino acids) to have a positive gustatory effect when presented as a component of both liquid and solid foods [34]. The fact that not only adolescent and adult animals, but also the aged ones, readily consume GM and CM suggests that age-related decline in hedonic processing [22,35–37] does not completely abolish a drive to eat milk-based diets. Instead, a slightly depressed intake of GM and CM at an old age parallels that reported for sweet solutions, as shown here and by other authors [38–40]. This finding is particularly relevant from the standpoint of being able to use palatable GM or CM as nutritionally superior alternatives to, e.g., sucrose-sweetened tastants in aged individuals [23]. That adolescent rodents also consume large quantities of both milk types indicates that prolonged dietary habituation is not required to develop the liking of either GM or CM. In fact, the amounts of GM and CM ingested by juveniles were as high as the volume of sucrose (readily consumed in large quantities by young animals, e.g., see [41]) even though the individuals had had only two brief exposures to these solutions prior to the experiment.

The single-tastant scenarios above strongly suggest a high acceptance level for both GM and CM indicating they are palatable, but as these no-choice paradigms produced fairly similar feeding responses, choice studies were needed to define relative preference for these two milk types. Simultaneous 2-h exposure to two bottles containing GM and CM showed that adult and aged mice and rats as well as adolescent rats exhibit a marked preference for GM (adolescent mice were the only cohort in which GM and CM were iso-palatable). The preference for GM did not appear to be related to whether the animals' pre-exposure to the specific diets was simultaneous (such as in adolescents and adults) or sequential (aged rodents). This finding was further expanded by employing the 30-min lickometer analysis in adult rats. It showed approximately four times as many licks at the bottle containing GM compared to CM during the first 5 min of the meal, and twice as many licks at the GM bottle in the subsequent 5-min interval. Overall, the licking activity at both bottles occurred within the same timeframe with neither milk type being ingested in a prolonged fashion. It increases our confidence in that motivation to consume palatable GM rather than maintenance of a meal (due to, e.g., delayed satiation [42]) is the main reason for avid intake of GM. The analysis of the licking bouts provides additional support for this notion. The cluster number (total number of bouts) neared significance for GM, possibly reflecting the incentive motivational properties of the food stimulus; importantly, the relationship of motivation and this measure reflects post-ingestive negative feedback [43–47]. On the other hand, the average cluster length—significantly greater for the GM formulation—typically parallels the hedonic properties (mainly, orosensory pleasure) of ingestive stimuli (as reviewed, e.g., in [45]). In this case, it is the length of clusters that appears to be the main driver for the preference for GM. A good example of the significance of licking bout length versus number in the context of neural regulation of food intake comes from studies on the endogenous opioid system. Ostlund et al. found that mu opioid receptor (MOR) knockout (KO) mice show alterations in sucrose licking: while energy-deprived wild-type mice increased burst length, relative to the nondeprived condition, this aspect of licking was insensitive to changes in food deprivation in MOR KOs. The rate of sucrose and sucralose licking in KOs was lower than in wildtype animals, providing evidence that the MOR was involved in processing palatability [48]. Mendez and colleagues reported that proenkephalin (PENK) KOs given a sucrose solution exhibited fewer bouts of licking (though the length did not differ) than wild type controls, indicating a diminished motivation to eat [46]. Finally, studies on the involvement of nociceptin/orphanin FQ (NOC) revealed that NOC administration initiates new bouts of licking for sweet solutions, which is in line with the notion of its potential relationship to motivational aspects of feeding. Interestingly, energy-deprived NOP KO mice given sucrose showed longer bouts of licking than wild types, suggesting that, under hungry conditions, NOC may also affect hedonics of consumption [49].

The notion that satiety is not delayed by GM intake is supported by the experimental work exploring satiating effects of a CM- versus GM-based meal in humans. In their study, Rubio-Martín et al. presented healthy adults with GM-based or CM-based breakfast after an overnight fast and obtained blood samples and appetite ratings from the subjects just before and up to 5 h after completion of the meal. They found that that the 'desire to eat' rating was significantly lower and hunger rating tended to be lower after the GM breakfast. Interestingly, the area under the curve (AUC) for a satiety hormone GLP-1 was inversely associated with the AUChunger and AUCdesire-to-eat after the GM meal [50].

The aforementioned data obtained in human observations combined with the current results of our experiments in animal models suggest that even though composition differences between GM and CM are relatively minor, they are sufficient to significantly affect appetite-related parameters. It remains to be elucidated whether these effects are produced by a specific macronutrient component, a combination of nutritive components, and/or some physico-chemical characteristics of each milk type (e.g., micelle structures in GM vs. CM differ in diameter, hydration, and mineralization) [51].

The analysis of mRNA levels of feeding-related genes sheds more light on neural processing underlying enhanced preference for GM over CM. One of the most striking outcomes is the fact that, unlike in the NAcc, which showed an increase in multiple mRNA profiles after GM over CM, there are relatively few significant differences in gene expression in the hypothalamus and brain stem. Those two brain areas serve as the foundation for the control of energy homeostasis and consumption-related changes in the internal milieu associated with plasma osmolality, stomach distension, and defense from exposure to food-borne toxins [52]. In this network, the brain stem acts as the relay station between the periphery and the central nervous system, whereas the hypothalamus plays a endocrine role (by releasing, e.g., anorexigenic hormones, such as oxytocin (OXT) via the neurohypophysis) and innervates a number of central target sites (it includes the reciprocal connectivity with the brain stem, as well as multiple pathways with, among others, nigrostriatal and hippocampal structures). It is noteworthy that, despite the same level of intake of GM and CM over the 24-h period, the hypothalamic expression of NPY and orexin (ORX) was lower in the GM group. Both ORX and NPY in the hypothalamus enhance consumption chiefly by increasing hunger and motivating intake of energy-dense tastants [53,54]. Thus, these data suggest that enhanced preference for GM over CM does not stem from the stimulation of neural mechanisms that lead to hunger-driven feeding. In line with the aforementioned conclusion from feeding experiments that the increased preference for GM vs.

CM in choice scenarios is unlikely to be related to suppressed satiety signaling, we found that the brain stem expression of satiation promoting melanocortin receptors [55,56] is elevated after consumption of GM (it remained the same in the hypothalamus). This change in the receptor mRNA level coupled with the lack of a difference in the melanocortin ligand precursor gene expression (proopiomelanocortin, POMC) as well as in the anorexigenic OXT gene [28,57] suggests the lack of impairment in central satiety processing after GM (and, surprisingly, even a somewhat greater sensitivity of the molecular network promoting satiety in response to GM consumption).

Interestingly, the hypothalamic genes whose expression was elevated by GM intake were those encoding the MOR and kappa (KOR) opioid receptors (MOR and KOR brain stem and accumbal mRNA levels were also higher, though the difference did not reach statistical significance). Furthermore, in the NAcc, we found overexpression of genes coding for opioid-related NOC and this peptide's receptor, ORL1. Opioid receptors are directly implicated in the regulation of feeding for reward [14,42]. They are part of a dispersed network that includes the NAcc as one of the key sites mediating hedonic aspects of eating behavior. They are also expressed throughout the 'homeostatic' components of the feeding-related circuit [16], including the hypothalamus and brain stem, where they are theorized to promote excessive consumption of palatable tastants by delaying meal termination. The magnitude at which opioid receptor agonists, such as butorphanol tartrate, dynorphin and beta-endorphin, stimulate consumption parallels the relative palatability of foods [14,58]. Conversely, opioid receptor antagonists, e.g., naltrexone and naloxone, are particularly effective at reducing intake of tasty ingestants [59]. Hence, higher expression of the MOR and KOR mRNA after GM is in line with the observed preference for the GM over CM. Changes in expression of additional NAcc genes that underscore the functional relationship between GM intake and reward processing include upregulation of Cx36 mRNA, as Cx36 ensures proper synchrony of dopaminergic pathways [60], and of the growth hormone secretagogue receptor (GHSR) mRNA, considering that the GHSR in the NAcc has been found to mediate hedonics of ingestive behavior [61]. Again, as in the case of the hypothalamic gene expression analysis, genes encoding molecules that promote satiety—such as OXT, melanocortin receptor 4, and glucagon-like peptide-1 receptor [62]—were upregulated after GM, which points to the heightened reward processing rather than impaired satiation as the factor propelling preference toward GM over CM.

5. Conclusions

We conclude that, in laboratory animal models, GM and CM are highly palatable when presented as liquids and as components of solid diets. Diet choice paradigms reveal preference for GM over CM in mice and rats belonging to different age groups. Feeding studies and analyses of gene expression in the feeding-relevant brain circuit point to feeding reward as the main factor underlying preference for GM. While the current studies draw on the laboratory animal experimental approaches, they have a translational impact relevant to our understanding of the consequences of GM consumption in humans. This outcome is particularly important as, globally, likely more people drink GM than CM. GM owes its popularity to the fact that goats can thrive in diverse and changing environmental conditions, and that GM-based products are regarded as a gourmet food and health benefits of consuming GM have been defined [13]. Here we show that acceptance of GM is high and that GM is even slightly preferred over CM. Therefore, GM can be considered as both a nutritious and palatable choice for individuals at various age groups that incorporate milk in their diets.

Author Contributions: A.K., C.G.P., A.S.L. and P.K.O. designed the studies. A.K., E.L.W., S.N.G. and L.K.M. conducted feeding studies and analyzed the data. A.K. and E.L.W. performed PCR studies and analyzed the results. A.S.L., E.A.C., C.G.P. and P.K.O. aided in interpretation of results. A.K., E.L.W., A.S.L., E.A.C., C.G.P. and P.K.O. co-wrote the manuscript. All authors read and approved the final manuscript.

Funding: This research received support from Callaghan Innovation, New Zealand.

Conflicts of Interest: C.G.P. and E.A.C. are employees of Dairy Goat Co-operative Ltd., and A.K.'s fellowship is supported by the Dairy Goat Co-operative Ltd.

References

1. Drewnowski, A.; Specter, S.E. Poverty and obesity: The role of energy density and energy costs. *Am. J. Clin. Nutr.* **2004**, *79*, 6–16. [CrossRef] [PubMed]
2. Huth, P.J.; Fulgoni, V.L.; Keast, D.R.; Park, K.; Auestad, N. Major food sources of calories, added sugars, and saturated fat and their contribution to essential nutrient intakes in the U.S. diet: Data from the National Health and Nutrition Examination Survey (2003–2006). *Nutr. J.* **2013**, *12*, 116. [CrossRef] [PubMed]
3. Drewnowski, A. The contribution of milk and milk products to micronutrient density and affordability of the U.S. diet. *J. Am. Coll. Nutr.* **2011**, *30* (Suppl. 1), 422S–428S. [CrossRef]
4. Vissers, P.A.; Streppel, M.T.; Feskens, E.J.; de Groot, L.C. The contribution of dairy products to micronutrient intake in the Netherlands. *J. Am. Coll. Nutr.* **2011**, *30* (Suppl. 1), 415S–421S. [CrossRef]
5. Feskanich, D.; Willett, W.C.; Colditz, G.A. Calcium, vitamin D, milk consumption, and hip fractures: A prospective study among postmenopausal women. *Am. J. Clin. Nutr.* **2003**, *77*, 504–511. [CrossRef]
6. Chevalley, T.; Bonjour, J.P.; Ferrari, S.; Rizzoli, R. High-protein intake enhances the positive impact of physical activity on BMC in prepubertal boys. *J. Bone Miner. Res.* **2008**, *23*, 131–142. [CrossRef] [PubMed]
7. Haenlein, G.F.W. Goat milk in human nutrition. *Small Rumin. Res.* **2007**, *51*, 155–163. [CrossRef]
8. Bellioni-Businco, B.; Paganelli, R.; Lucenti, P.; Giampietro, P.G.; Perborn, H.; Businco, L. Allergenicity of goat's milk in children with cow's milk allergy. *J. Allergy Clin. Immunol.* **1999**, *103*, 1191–1194. [CrossRef]
9. Barrionuevo, M.; Lopez Aliaga, I.; Alferez, M.J.; Mesa, E.; Nestares, T.; Campos, M.S. Beneficial effect of goat milk on bioavailability of copper, zinc and selenium in rats. *J. Physiol. Biochem.* **2003**, *59*, 111–118. [CrossRef]
10. Barrionuevo, M.; Alferez, M.J.; Lopez, A.I.; Sanz, S.M.; Campos, M.S. Beneficial effect of goat milk on nutritive utilization of iron and copper in malabsorption syndrome. *J. Dairy Sci.* **2002**, *85*, 657–664. [CrossRef]
11. Díaz-Castro, J.; López-Frías, M.R.; Campos, M.S.; López-Frías, M.; Alférez, M.J.; Nestares, T.; Ojeda, M.L.; López-Aliaga, I. Severe nutritional iron-deficiency anaemia has a negative effect on some bone turnover biomarkers in rats. *Eur. J. Nutr.* **2012**, *51*, 241–247. [CrossRef] [PubMed]
12. Díaz-Castro, J.; Lopez-Frias, M.R.; Campos, M.S.; Lopez-Frias, M.; Alférez, M.J.; Nestares, T.; Ortega, E.; Lopez-Aliaga, I. Goat milk during iron repletion improves bone turnover impaired by severe iron deficiency. *J. Dairy Sci.* **2011**, *94*, 2752–2761. [CrossRef] [PubMed]
13. Silanikove, N.; Leitner, G.; Merin, U.; Prosser, C.G. Recent advances in exploiting goat's milk: Quality, safety and production aspects. *Small Rumin. Res.* **2010**, *89*, 110–124. [CrossRef]
14. Gosnell, B.A.; Levine, A.S. Reward systems and food intake: Role of opioids. *Int. J. Obes.* **2009**, *33* (Suppl. 2), S54–S58. [CrossRef] [PubMed]
15. Olszewski, P.K.; Alsio, J.; Schioth, H.B.; Levine, A.S. Opioids as facilitators of feeding: Can any food be rewarding? *Physiol. Behav.* **2011**, *104*, 105–110. [CrossRef] [PubMed]
16. Olszewski, P.K.; Cedernaes, J.; Olsson, F.; Levine, A.S.; Schiöth, H.B. Analysis of the network of feeding neuroregulators using the Allen Brain Atlas. *Neurosci. Biobehav. Rev.* **2008**, *32*, 945–956. [CrossRef] [PubMed]
17. Agustí, A.; García-Pardo, M.P.; López-Almela, I.; Campillo, I.; Maes, M.; Romaní-Pérez, M.; Sanz, Y. Interplay Between the Gut-Brain Axis, Obesity and Cognitive Function. *Front. Neurosci.* **2018**, *12*, 155. [CrossRef] [PubMed]
18. Schwartz, G.J. Roles for gut vagal sensory signals in determining energy availability and energy expenditure. *Brain Res.* **2018**, *1693*, 151–153. [CrossRef]
19. De Kloet, A.D.; Herman, J.P. Fat-brain connections: Adipocyte glucocorticoid control of stress and metabolism. *Front. Neuroendocrinol.* **2018**, *48*, 50–57. [CrossRef]
20. Olszewski, P.K.; Shaw, T.J.; Grace, M.K.; Höglund, C.E.; Fredriksson, R.; Schiöth, H.B.; Levine, A.S. Complexity of neural mechanisms underlying overconsumption of sugar in scheduled feeding: Involvement of opioids, orexin, oxytocin and NPY. *Peptides* **2009**, *30*, 226–233. [CrossRef]
21. Zink, A.N.; Perez-Leighton, C.E.; Kotz, C.M. The orexin neuropeptide system: Physical activity and hypothalamic function throughout the aging process. *Front. Syst. Neurosci.* **2014**, *8*, 211. [CrossRef] [PubMed]
22. Gosnell, B.A.; Levine, A.S.; Morley, J.E. The effects of aging on opioid modulation of feeding in rats. *Life Sci.* **1983**, *32*, 2793–2799. [CrossRef]
23. Morley, J.E. Pathophysiology of the anorexia of aging. *Curr. Opin. Clin. Nutr. Metab. Care* **2013**, *16*, 27–32. [CrossRef] [PubMed]

24. Van de Heijning, B.J.; Kegler, D.; Schipper, L.; Voogd, E.; Oosting, A.; van der Beek, E.M. Acute and Chronic Effects of Dietary Lactose in Adult Rats Are not Explained by Residual Intestinal Lactase Activity. *Nutrients* **2015**, *7*, 5542–5555. [CrossRef] [PubMed]
25. McCutcheon, J.E.; Marinelli, M. Age matters. *Eur. J. Neurosci.* **2009**, *29*, 997–1014. [CrossRef] [PubMed]
26. Herisson, F.M.; Brooks, L.L.; Waas, J.R.; Levine, A.S.; Olszewski, P.K. Functional relationship between oxytocin and appetite for carbohydrates versus saccharin. *Neuroreport* **2014**, *25*, 909–914. [CrossRef]
27. Herisson, F.M.; Waas, J.R.; Fredriksson, R.; Schioth, H.B.; Levine, A.S.; Olszewski, P.K. Oxytocin Acting in the Nucleus Accumbens Core Decreases Food Intake. *J. Neuroendocrinol.* **2016**, *28*. [CrossRef] [PubMed]
28. Olszewski, P.K.; Klockars, A.; Olszewska, A.M.; Fredriksson, R.; Schioth, H.B.; Levine, A.S. Molecular, immunohistochemical, and pharmacological evidence of oxytocin's role as inhibitor of carbohydrate but not fat intake. *Endocrinology* **2010**, *151*, 4736–4744. [CrossRef] [PubMed]
29. Bonacchi, K.B.; Ackroff, K.; Touzani, K.; Bodnar, R.J.; Sclafani, A. Opioid mediation of starch and sugar preference in the rat. *Pharmacol. Biochem. Behav.* **2010**, *96*, 507–514. [CrossRef] [PubMed]
30. Levine, A.S.; Kotz, C.M.; Gosnell, B.A. Sugars: Hedonic aspects, neuroregulation, and energy balance. *Am. J. Clin. Nutr.* **2003**, *78*, 834S–842S. [CrossRef]
31. Martire, S.I.; Holmes, N.; Westbrook, R.F.; Morris, M.J. Altered feeding patterns in rats exposed to a palatable cafeteria diet: Increased snacking and its implications for development of obesity. *PLoS ONE* **2013**, *8*, e60407. [CrossRef] [PubMed]
32. Martire, S.I.; Maniam, J.; South, T.; Holmes, N.; Westbrook, R.F.; Morris, M.J. Extended exposure to a palatable cafeteria diet alters gene expression in brain regions implicated in reward, and withdrawal from this diet alters gene expression in brain regions associated with stress. *Behav. Brain Res.* **2014**, *265*, 132–141. [CrossRef]
33. Drewnowski, A. Energy density, palatability, and satiety: Implications for weight control. *Nutr. Rev.* **1998**, *56*, 347–353. [CrossRef] [PubMed]
34. Moran, T.H.; Ladenheim, E.E. Physiologic and Neural Controls of Eating. *Gastroenterol. Clin. N. Am.* **2016**, *45*, 581–599. [CrossRef]
35. Landi, F.; Calvani, R.; Tosato, M.; Martone, A.; Ortolani, E.; Savera, G.; Sisto, A.; Marzetti, E. Anorexia of Aging: Risk Factors, Consequences, and Potential Treatments. *Nutrients* **2016**, *8*, 69. [CrossRef] [PubMed]
36. Tenk, J.; Rostás, I.; Füredi, N.; Mikó, A.; Solymár, M.; Soós, S.; Gaszner, B.; Feller, D.; Székely, M.; Pétervári, E.; et al. Age-related changes in central effects of corticotropin-releasing factor (CRF) suggest a role for this mediator in aging anorexia and cachexia. *Geroscience* **2017**, *39*, 61–72. [CrossRef]
37. Tomm, R.J.; Tse, M.T.; Tobiansky, D.J.; Schweitzer, H.R.; Soma, K.K.; Floresco, S.B. Effects of aging on executive functioning and mesocorticolimbic dopamine markers in male Fischer 344 x brown Norway rats. *Neurobiol. Aging* **2018**, *72*, 134–146. [CrossRef]
38. Inui-Yamamoto, C.; Yamamoto, T.; Ueda, K.; Nakatsuka, M.; Kumabe, S.; Inui, T.; Iwai, Y. Taste preference changes throughout different life stages in male rats. *PLoS ONE* **2017**, *12*, e0181650. [CrossRef]
39. Sakai, M.; Kazui, H.; Shigenobu, K.; Komori, K.; Ikeda, M.; Nishikawa, T. Gustatory Dysfunction as an Early Symptom of Semantic Dementia. *Dement. Geriatr. Cogn. Dis. Extra* **2017**, *7*, 395–405. [CrossRef]
40. Shin, Y.K.; Cong, W.N.; Cai, H.; Kim, W.; Maudsley, S.; Egan, J.M.; Martin, B. Age-related changes in mouse taste bud morphology, hormone expression, and taste responsivity. *J. Gerontol. A Biol. Sci. Med. Sci.* **2012**, *67*, 336–344. [CrossRef]
41. Naneix, F.; Darlot, F.; Coutureau, E.; Cador, M. Long-lasting deficits in hedonic and nucleus accumbens reactivity to sweet rewards by sugar overconsumption during adolescence. *Eur. J. Neurosci.* **2016**, *43*, 671–680. [CrossRef]
42. Glass, M.J.; Grace, M.K.; Cleary, J.P.; Billington, C.J.; Levine, A.S. Naloxone's effect on meal microstructure of sucrose and cornstarch diets. *Am. J. Physiol. Regul. Integr. Comp. Physiol.* **2001**, *281*, R1605–R1612. [CrossRef] [PubMed]
43. Higgs, S.; Cooper, S.J. Evidence for early opioid modulation of licking responses to sucrose and intralipid: A microstructural analysis in the rat. *Psychopharmacology* **1998**, *139*, 342–355. [CrossRef] [PubMed]
44. D'Aquila, P.S. Dopamine on D2-like receptors "reboosts" dopamine D1-like receptor-mediated behavioural activation in rats licking for sucrose. *Neuropharmacology* **2010**, *58*, 1085–1096. [CrossRef] [PubMed]
45. Dwyer, D.M. EPS Prize Lecture. Licking and liking: The assessment of hedonic responses in rodents. *Q. J. Exp. Psychol.* **2012**, *65*, 371–394. [CrossRef]

46. Mendez, I.A.; Ostlund, S.B.; Maidment, N.T.; Murphy, N.P. Involvement of Endogenous Enkephalins and beta-Endorphin in Feeding and Diet-Induced Obesity. *Neuropsychopharmacology* **2015**, *40*, 2103–2112. [CrossRef] [PubMed]
47. Davis, J.D.; Smith, G.P. Analysis of the microstructure of the rhythmic tongue movements of rats ingesting maltose and sucrose solutions. *Behav. Neurosci.* **1992**, *106*, 217–228. [CrossRef] [PubMed]
48. Ostlund, S.B.; Kosheleff, A.; Maidment, N.T.; Murphy, N.P. Decreased consumption of sweet fluids in mu opioid receptor knockout mice: A microstructural analysis of licking behavior. *Psychopharmacology* **2013**, *229*, 105–113. [CrossRef] [PubMed]
49. Mendez, I.A.; Maidment, N.T.; Murphy, N.P. Parsing the hedonic and motivational influences of nociceptin on feeding using licking microstructure analysis in mice. *Behav. Pharmacol.* **2016**, *27*, 516–527. [CrossRef]
50. Rubio-Martín, E.; García-Escobar, E.; Ruiz de Adana, M.S.; Lima-Rubio, F.; Peláez, L.; Caracuel, A.M.; Bermúdez-Silva, F.J.; Soriguer, F.; Rojo-Martínez, G.; Olveira, G. Comparison of the Effects of Goat Dairy and Cow Dairy Based Breakfasts on Satiety, Appetite Hormones, and Metabolic Profile. *Nutrients* **2017**, *9*, 877. [CrossRef]
51. Park, Y.W.; Juarez, M.; Ramos, M.; Haenlein, G.F.W. Physico-chemical characteristics of goat and sheep milk. *Small Rumin. Res.* **2007**, *68*, 88–113. [CrossRef]
52. Klockars, A.; Levine, A.S.; Olszewski, P.K. Hypothalamic Integration of the Endocrine Signaling Related to Food Intake. *Curr. Top. Behav. Neurosci.* **2018**. [CrossRef]
53. Levine, A.S.; Jewett, D.C.; Cleary, J.P.; Kotz, C.M.; Billington, C.J. Our journey with neuropeptide Y: Effects on ingestive behaviors and energy expenditure. *Peptides* **2004**, *25*, 505–510. [CrossRef]
54. Nixon, J.P.; Kotz, C.M.; Novak, C.M.; Billington, C.J.; Teske, J.A. Neuropeptides controlling energy balance: Orexins and neuromedins. *Handb. Exp. Pharmacol.* **2012**, *209*, 77–109.
55. Wirth, M.M.; Olszewski, P.K.; Yu, C.; Levine, A.S.; Giraudo, S.Q. Paraventricular hypothalamic alpha-melanocyte-stimulating hormone and MTII reduce feeding without causing aversive effects. *Peptides* **2001**, *22*, 129–134. [CrossRef]
56. Girardet, C.; Butler, A.A. Neural melanocortin receptors in obesity and related metabolic disorders. *Biochim. Biophys. Acta* **2014**, *1842*, 482–494. [CrossRef] [PubMed]
57. Olszewski, P.K.; Klockars, A.; Levine, A.S. Oxytocin: A Conditional Anorexigen whose Effects on Appetite Depend on the Physiological, Behavioural and Social Contexts. *J. Neuroendocrinol.* **2016**, *28*. [CrossRef] [PubMed]
58. Gosnell, B.A.; Levine, A.S.; Morley, J.E. The stimulation of food intake by selective agonists of mu, kappa and delta opioid receptors. *Life Sci.* **1986**, *38*, 1081–1088. [CrossRef]
59. Giraudo, S.Q.; Grace, M.K.; Welch, C.C.; Billington, C.J.; Levine, A.S. Naloxone's anorectic effect is dependent upon the relative palatability of food. *Pharmacol. Biochem. Behav.* **1993**, *46*, 917–921. [CrossRef]
60. Steffensen, S.C.; Bradley, K.D.; Hansen, D.M.; Wilcox, J.D.; Wilcox, R.S.; Allison, D.W.; Merrill, C.B.; Edwards, J.G. The role of connexin-36 gap junctions in alcohol intoxication and consumption. *Synapse* **2011**, *65*, 695–707. [CrossRef] [PubMed]
61. Skibicka, K.P.; Shirazi, R.H.; Rabasa-Papio, C.; Alvarez-Crespo, M.; Neuber, C.; Vogel, H.; Dickson, S.L. Divergent circuitry underlying food reward and intake effects of ghrelin: Dopaminergic VTA-accumbens projection mediates ghrelin's effect on food reward but not food intake. *Neuropharmacology* **2013**, *73*, 274–283. [CrossRef] [PubMed]
62. Kanoski, S.E.; Hayes, M.R.; Skibicka, K.P. GLP-1 and weight loss: Unraveling the diverse neural circuitry. *Am. J. Physiol. Regul. Integr. Comp. Physiol.* **2016**, *310*, R885–R895. [CrossRef] [PubMed]

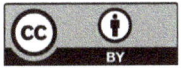 © 2019 by the authors. Licensee MDPI, Basel, Switzerland. This article is an open access article distributed under the terms and conditions of the Creative Commons Attribution (CC BY) license (http://creativecommons.org/licenses/by/4.0/).

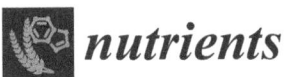

Article

Tryptophan-Tyrosine Dipeptide, the Core Sequence of β-Lactolin, Improves Memory by Modulating the Dopamine System

Yasuhisa Ano [1,*], Tatsuhiro Ayabe [1], Rena Ohya [1], Keiji Kondo [1], Shiho Kitaoka [2,3] and Tomoyuki Furuyashiki [2,3]

1. Research Laboratories for Health Science & Food Technologies, Kirin Company Ltd, Kanazawa-ku, Yokohama-shi, Kanagawa 236-0004, Japan; Tatsuhiro_Ayabe@kirin.co.jp (T.A.); Rena_Ohya@kirin.co.jp (R.O.); kondok@kirin.co.jp (K.K.)
2. Division of Pharmacology, Kobe University Graduate School of Medicine, Kobe 650-0017, Japan; skitaoka@med.kobe-u.ac.jp (S.K.); tfuruya@med.kobe-u.ac.jp (T.F.)
3. AMED-CREST, Chiyoda-ku 100-0004, Tokyo, Japan
* Correspondence: Yasuhisa_Ano@kirin.co.jp; Tel.: +81-45-330-9007

Received: 10 January 2019; Accepted: 3 February 2019; Published: 6 February 2019

Abstract: Tryptophan-tyrosine (WY)-related peptides including the β-lactopeptide of the glycine-threonine-tryptophan-tyrosine peptide, β-lactolin, improve spatial memory. However, whether and how the WY dipeptide as the core sequence in WY-related peptides improves memory functions has not been investigated. This study assessed the pharmacological effects of the WY dipeptide on memory impairment to elucidate the mechanisms. Here, we showed that oral administration of dipeptides of WY, tryptophan-methionine (WM), tryptophan-valine, tryptophan-leucine, and tryptophan-phenylalanine improved spontaneous alternation of the Y-maze test in scopolamine-induced amnesic mice. In contrast, tyrosine-tryptophan, methionine-tryptophan, tryptophan, tyrosine, and methionine had no effect. These results indicated that the conformation of dipeptides with N-terminal tryptophan is required for their memory improving effects. WY dipeptide inhibited the monoamine oxidase B activity in vitro and increased dopamine levels in the hippocampus and frontal cortex, whereas tryptophan did not cause these effects. In addition, the treatment with SCH-23390, a dopamine D1-like receptor antagonist, and the knockdown of the hippocampal dopamine D1 receptor partially attenuated the memory improvement induced by the WY dipeptide. Importantly, WY dipeptide improved the spontaneous alternations of the Y-maze test in aged mice. These results suggest that the WY dipeptide restores memory impairments by augmenting dopaminergic activity. The development of supplements rich in these peptides might help to prevent age-related cognitive decline.

Keywords: dipeptide; dopamine; hippocampus; memory; monoamine oxidase B

1. Introduction

The rapid growth of aging populations worldwide is associated with an increased incidence of cognitive decline and dementia that become a growing burden not only on patients and their families but also on national healthcare systems. Due to the lack of effective dementia therapies, increasing attention is given to preventive approaches. Recent epidemiological studies suggest that the consumption of certain dairy products reduces the risk of cognitive decline in the elderly and may prevent Alzheimer's disease [1].

Crichton et al. [2] reported that individuals who consumed low-fat dairy products, including yogurt and cheese, once a week had a higher cognitive function than those who did not. A survey-based study of self-reported health information showed that the consumption of low-fat dairy products was associated with increased memory recall, increased social functioning, and decreased stress [3,4]. Ozawa et al. [3,4] surveyed more than 1000 Japanese subjects who were living in the community, aged 60–79 years, and free from dementia to investigate their dietary patterns and any potential association with a reduced risk of dementia symptoms. The authors concluded that including milk or fermented dairy products in the diet reduces the risk of dementia in the general Japanese population. In a clinical trial, Ogata et al. [5] investigated the association between the intake of dairy products and short-term memory and found that the intake of dairy products is highly associated with improved short-term memory. It has also been demonstrated that the intake of dairy products fermented with *Penicillium candidum*, i.e., Camembert cheese, had preventive effects on Alzheimer's disease pathology in a mouse model [6].

We have previously identified tryptophan-tyrosine (WY)-related peptides, including the β-lactopeptide of glycine-threonine-tryptophan-tyrosine (GTWY) peptide, β-lactolin, derived from β-lactoglobulin in an enzymatic whey protein digest [7]. The β-lactolin was smoothly absorbed into the body and delivered to the brain where it was associated with a dopamine level increase, resulting in improved spatial and object memory [7]. In addition, we demonstrated that whey peptides rich in WY-related peptides improved memory and attention in a clinical trial [8]. These reports suggested that WY-related peptides improve cognitive function. However, whether and how the WY dipeptide, the core sequence of WY-related peptides, improves cognitive function has not been investigated. The gap in our knowledge about the pharmacological effects of the WY dipeptide on memory impairment hinders the assessment of the underlying mechanism of the effect of whey peptide preparations rich in WY-related peptides on cognitive performance in clinical trials.

In the present study, we examined the effects of tryptophan-containing dipeptides, including the WY dipeptide, on memory impairment and their mechanisms.

2. Materials and Methods

2.1. Materials

The dipeptides WY, tyrosine-tryptophan (YW), tryptophan-methionine (WM), methionine-tryptophan (MW), tryptophan-valine (WV), tryptophan-leucine (WL), and tryptophan-phenylalanine (WF) (purity > 98%) were purchased from NARD Chemicals, Ltd. (Amagasaki, Japan). Tryptophan, tyrosine, (−)-scopolamine hydrobromide trihydrate, and R(+)-SCH-23390 hydrochloride were purchased from Sigma Aldrich Co. (St. Louis, MO, USA).

2.2. Animals

Crl:CD1 (ICR) male mice, 6 weeks old, and C57BL/6J male mice, 7 months and 22 months old (Charles River Japan, Tokyo, Japan), were maintained at Kirin Company Ltd. Mice were maintained at room temperature (23 ± 1 °C) under a constant 12-h light/dark cycle (light period from 8:00 am to 8:00 pm) and were fed a standard rodent diet (CE-2 (Clea Japan, Tokyo, Japan)). Behavioral pharmacological tests were performed in a sound-isolated room with the same temperature and light/dark cycles. All efforts were made to minimize suffering. For euthanasia, mice were placed into a chamber filled with vapor of isoflurane (Wako, Osaka, Japan). All experiments were approved by the Animal Experiment Committee of Kirin Company Ltd and conducted in strict accordance with their guidelines in 2016.

2.3. Spontaneous Alteration Test

A spontaneous alternation test was conducted in accordance with our previous report [7]. The Y-maze is a three-arm maze with equal angles between all arms (25 cm long × 5 cm wide × 20 cm high). The maze walls were constructed from dark black, polyvinyl plastic. Each mouse was initially placed in one arm, and the sequence and number of arm entries were counted for 8 minutes. The alternation score (%) for each mouse was defined as the ratio of the actual number of alternations to the possible number (defined as the total number of arm entries minus two) multiplied by 100 as follows: % Alternation = ((Number of alternations) / (Total arm entries − 2)) × 100.

To evaluate the effects of the samples on scopolamine-induced memory impairment, 6-week-old Crl:CD1 male mice were orally administered distilled water with or without peptides to be tested 1 h before evaluation. Forty minutes after the oral administration, memory impairment was induced by the intraperitoneal administration of 0.85 mg/kg scopolamine dissolved in saline. One hour after the oral administration, mice were subjected to the Y-maze test. In some experiments, mice were administered 0.85 mg/kg scopolamine and 0.05 mg/kg SCH-23390 (dopamine D1 antagonist) intraperitoneally at 40 min after the oral administration of 0 or 1 mg/kg WY peptide and subjected to the Y-maze test at 1 h after the oral administration. There were 10 mice per group.

In other experiments, C57BL/6J mice were orally administered a daily dose of 0 or 1 mg/kg WY peptide for 14 days. One hour after the last administration, mice were subjected to a Y-maze trial.

2.4. Monoamine Analysis

To evaluate the levels of dopamine and its metabolites (DOPAC and HVA) in the brain, tissue was homogenized in 0.2 M perchloric acid (PCA, Wako, Tokyo, Japan) containing 100 µM EDTA·2Na (Sigma-Aldrich, St. Louis, MO, USA). After centrifugation, the supernatant was analyzed by high-performance liquid chromatography (HPLC) using an EICOMPAK SC-5ODS column and PREPAK column (Eicom, Kyoto, Japan) with an electrochemical detection (ECD) unit. The mobile phase consisted of 83% 0.1 M acetic acid in citric acid buffer (pH 3.5), 17% methanol (Wako), 190 mg/ml of sodium 1-octanesulfonate sodium (Wako), and 5 mg/mL EDTA·2Na. For ECD, the applied voltage was 750 mV vs. an Ag/AgCl reference electrode.

2.5. Monoamine Oxidase (MAO) Activity Assay

MAO-B activity was measured using the MAO assay kit (Cell Biolabs, San Diego, CA, USA) according to the manufacturer's instructions. Human MAO-B (50 µg/mL; Sigma-Aldrich) was incubated with 1 mM WY dipeptide or 1 mM tryptophan for 30 min. The substrates for MAO-B were added and the amount of hydrogen peroxide in the reaction was measured.

2.6. Injection of Adeno-Associated Viruses (AAV) to the Hippocampus

The adeno-associated virus (AAV) injection method used to knock down the dopamine D1 receptor and the following behavioral evaluation were performed as described in our previous study [9,10]. The AAV construct that expresses artificial microRNA (miRNA) targeting the dopamine D1 receptor with an emerald green fluorescent protein (EmGFP) under the control of the elongation factor (EF)1α promoter only in the presence of Cre recombinase (AAV10-EF1α-double-floxed inverted (DIO)-EmGFP-D1miRNA), an AAV construct that expresses control miRNA in the same arrangement (AAV10-EF1α-DIO-EmGFP-control), and an AAV construct that expresses Cre recombinase under the CMV promoter (AAV10-CMV-Cre) were produced as previously described [9]. After anesthetized with sodium pentobarbital, 8-week-old Crl:CD1 male mice were injected with 0.5 µL of the AAV solution (1.0×10^{12} genomics copies/mL) per site, applied at two sites in the hippocampal regions of both hemispheres (four sites per mouse; from bregma: posterior, −3.5 mm; lateral, ± 3 mm; ventral, −3.8 mm and −1.8 mm) according to the atlas of Paxinos and Franklin [11] and using a PV-830 Pneumatic PicoPump (World Precision Instruments, Sarasota, FL, USA). Mice were allowed to recover for 4 weeks and then used for the Y-maze test.

2.7. Statistical Analysis

All values are expressed as means ± standard error of the mean (SEM). Data was analyzed by one-way analysis of variance (ANOVA), followed by Tukey–Kramer test, Dunnett's test, or Student's t-test as described in the figure legends. All statistical analyses were performed using the Ekuseru–Toukei 2012 software program (Social Survey Research Information, Tokyo, Japan). A p-value < 0.05 was considered statistically significant.

3. Results

3.1. Tryptophan-Containing Dipeptides Improved Memory Impairment in Amnesic Mice

To evaluate the effects of the WY, WM, WV, WL, and WF dipeptides, which are known to be derived from milk proteins, on spatial memory, amnesia was induced by treatment with scopolamine, a muscarinic antagonist, according to a previous study [7]. The spontaneous alternation test using the Y-maze is well-established as a behavioral evaluation method for examining short-term spatial memory performance. A single dose of 1 mg/kg WY, WM, WV, WL, or WF dipeptide significantly increased the spontaneous alternation (Figure 1A–E, respectively). Further, the administration of 0.3 mg/kg WY or WM dipeptide already increased the alternation, which showed higher improvement than that of WV, WL, or WF (Figure 1A and B). The number of arm entries was not changed among the groups (data not shown). These results indicated that the administration of certain dipeptides with N-terminal tryptophan improved short-term spatial memory in amnestic mice.

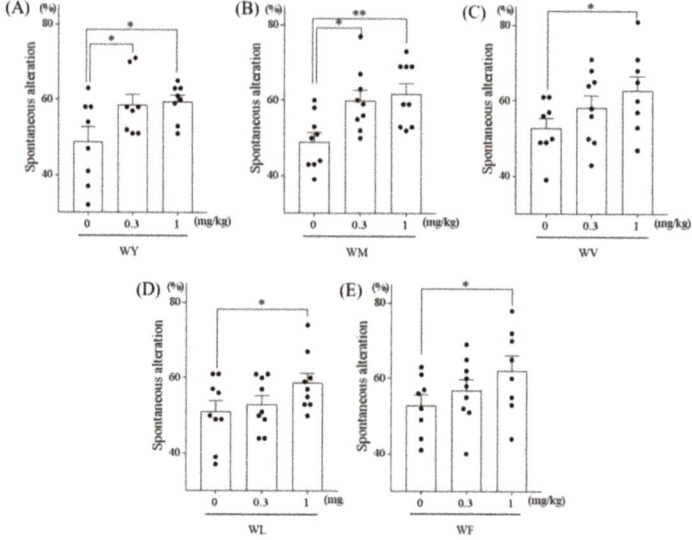

Figure 1. The effects of dipeptides (**A**) WY, (**B**) WM, (**C**) WV, (**D**) WL, and (**E**) WF on spatial memory in amnesic mice. Six-week-old Crl:CD1 male mice were orally administered 0, 0.3, or 1 mg/kg of dipeptide (WV, WM, WV, WL, and WF) and, 40 min later, injected intraperitoneally with 0.85 mg/kg of scopolamine. At 1 h after oral administration, each mouse was allowed to explore the Y-maze for 8 min. Spontaneous alternations were also measured. Data represent the mean ± SEM of 10 mice per group. The p values shown were calculated using the Dunnett's test. *$p < 0.05$ and **$p < 0.01$.

3.2. Dipeptides Containing Tryptophan at the N-Terminus But Not at the C-Terminus Improved Memory Impairment

Next, to evaluate the effect of the tryptophan position within the dipeptides, we assessed the effect of tryptophan, tyrosine, and the dipeptides WY and YW on spatial memory in the spontaneous alternation test. A single administration of 1 mg/kg WY dipeptide, but not tryptophan, tyrosine, or YW dipeptide, increased the spontaneous alternation (Figure 2A). We also tested the effect of tryptophan, methionine, and the dipeptides WM and MW on spatial memory. A single administration of 1 mg/kg WM peptide, but not tryptophan, methionine, or MW dipeptide, also increased the alternation (Figure 2B). These results suggested that the conformation of dipeptides with an N-terminal tryptophan is required to improve the spatial memory in amnestic mice.

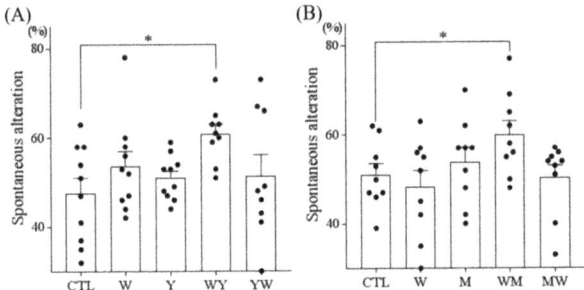

Figure 2. The effects of the dipeptides and single amino acids of (**A**) WY and (**B**) WM on spatial memory in amnesic mice. Six-week-old Crl:CD1 male mice were orally administered 0 or 1 mg/kg of dipeptide or single amino acid (WY, YW, WM, MW, tryptophan (W), tyrosine (Y), and methionine (M)) and, 40 min later, injected intraperitoneally with 0.85 mg/kg of scopolamine. At 1 h after oral administration, each mouse was allowed to explore the Y-maze for 8 min. Spontaneous alternations were also measured. Data represent the mean ± SEM of 10 mice per group. The p values shown were calculated using the Dunnett's test. * $p < 0.05$.

3.3. WY Peptide Increased Dopamine Levels in the Hippocampus and Frontal Cortex

Because we previously reported that the GTWY peptide inhibits MAO-B activity in vitro and in vivo and increases dopamine contents in the frontal cortex and hippocampus, we further evaluated the effect of the WY dipeptide on the catecholamine levels in the hippocampus and frontal cortex. In both the hippocampus and frontal cortex, a single administration of the WY dipeptide significantly increased the level of dopamine (Figure 3A–F). The levels of DOPAC and HVA appear to be slightly increased, though not statistically significant. Thus, the administration of WY dipeptide increased the level of dopamine in the brain without affecting the levels of its metabolites.

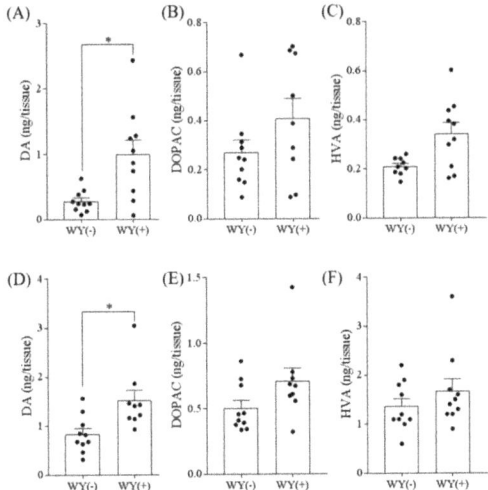

Figure 3. The levels of dopamine and its metabolites in the hippocampus and frontal cortex. Six-week-old Crl:CD1 male mice were orally administered 0 or 1 mg/kg of WY dipeptide. At 1 h after oral administration, the following monoamine levels were measured in the hippocampus (**A**–**C**) and frontal cortex (**D**–**F**) by HPLC: dopamine (DA) (**A**, **D**), 3,4-dihydroxyphenylacetic acid (DOPAC) (**B**, **E**), and homovanillic acid (HVA) (**C**, **F**). Data represent the mean ± SEM of 10 mice per group. The p values shown were calculated using the Student's t-test. * $p < 0.05$.

3.4. WY Peptide Inhibited the Activity of MAO

We evaluated the effect of WY dipeptide and tryptophan on MAO-B activity. Tyrosine and YW dipeptide were not tested in this assay because the compounds could not be dissolved in the assay buffer. Treatment with 1 mM WY dipeptide decreased MAO-B activity by $48 \pm 1.95\%$ compared to that of the control treatment. By contrast, treatment with 1 mM tryptophan did not inhibit MAO-B activity (Figure 4A). These results suggested that the WY dipeptide increased the dopamine content in the hippocampus by inhibiting MAO-B activity and that its chemical structure (Figure 4B) was important to inhibit the MAO-B activity.

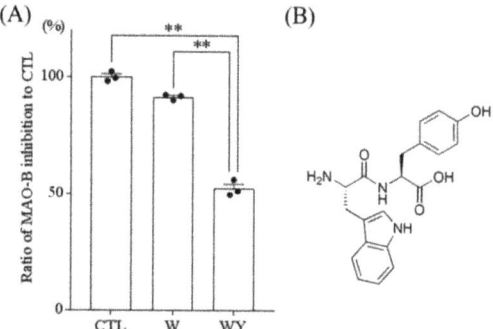

Figure 4. The inhibition of monoamine oxidase by the WY dipeptide and tryptophan and the chemical structure of the WY dipeptide. (**A**) The activity of monoamine oxidase B (MAO-B) was tested in the presence of 1 mM WY dipeptide or tryptophan (W). Data represent the mean $\pm$ SEM of triplicate per sample. The p values shown were calculated using the Dunnett's test. ** $p < 0.01$. (**B**) The chemical structure of the WY dipeptide.

3.5. Inhibition of the Dopamine D1 Receptor Attenuated the WY-Induced Memory Improvement

To investigate the link between dopamine and the memory-improving effect of the WY dipeptide, we examined the effect of SCH-23390, a dopamine D1-like receptor antagonist on the WY-dipeptide-induced memory improvement. Whereas WY-dipeptide increased spontaneous alteration in scopolamine-induced amnestic mice with prior treatment with saline (control group), SCH-23390 treatment abolished the memory improvement induced by the WY dipeptide (Figure 5A). These results indicated that the dopamine D1-like receptor was involved in the improvement of spatial memory induced by the WY dipeptide.

To further determine the involvement of the dopamine D1 receptor in the memory-improving effect of the WY dipeptide, the mRNA expression of the dopamine D1 receptor was knocked down in hippocampal neurons using the AAV system expressing artificial miRNA targeting this receptor according to our previous study [10]. While the WY dipeptide administration increased the spontaneous alternation in amnestic mice expressing control miRNA, this memory improvement was not significant with the dopamine D1 receptor knockdown in hippocampal neurons (Figure 5B). These results suggested that the dopamine D1 receptor in the hippocampus is involved in the memory improvement caused by the WY dipeptide at least in part.

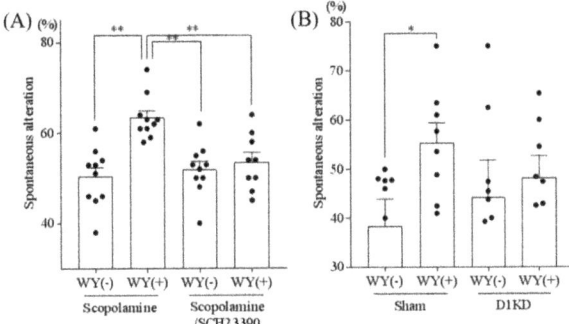

Figure 5. The dopamine receptor is involved in memory improvement linked to the WY dipeptide. (**A**) Six-week-old Crl:CD1 male mice were orally administered 0 or 1 mg/kg of WY dipeptide and, 40 min later, intraperitoneally injected with 0.85 mg/kg of scopolamine alone or scopolamine plus 0.05 mg/kg of SCH-23390. At 1 h after oral administration of the peptide, mice were allowed to explore the Y-maze for 8 min. Data represent the mean ± SEM of 10 mice per group. (**B**) Eight-week-old Crl:CD1 male mice were administered either a control microRNA or dopamine D_1 receptor microRNA containing AAV, which suppresses the dopamine D_1 receptor, to the hippocampus. Mice were orally administered 0 or 1 mg/kg of WY dipeptide and, 40 min later, intraperitoneally injected with 0.85 mg/kg of scopolamine. At 1 h after oral administration of the peptide, mice were allowed to explore the Y-maze for 8 min. Data represent the mean ± SEM of 7–8 mice per group. The p values were calculated using one-way ANOVA followed by the Tukey–Kramer test. ** $p < 0.01$ and * $p < 0.05$.

3.6. WY Peptide Improved Age-Related Memory Impairment

Our results showed that the WY dipeptide restored pharmacologically-induced memory impairment in mice. Therefore, we further examined whether the WY dipeptide would have a similar effect on memory impairment in aged mice. Aged (22 months) and young (7 months) C57BL/6J mice were orally administered WY dipeptide, and their performance in the spontaneous alternation test was evaluated. The proportion of spontaneous alternation was reduced in aged mice, compared with young mice, indicating age-related memory impairment. The administration of the WY dipeptide increased the proportion of spontaneous alteration in aged mice (Figure 6), indicating that WY dipeptide also restored memory impairment in aged mice.

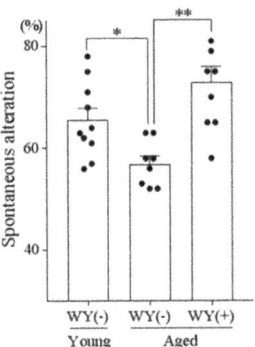

Figure 6. The effects of the WY peptide on aged mice: 7- and 22-month-old C57BL/6 mice were orally administered a daily dose 1 mg/kg of WY dipeptide for 14 days. At 1 h after oral administration of the peptide, mice were allowed to explore the Y-maze for 8 min. Data represent the mean ± SEM of 8–10 mice per group. The p values were calculated using one-way ANOVA followed by the Tukey–Kramer test. * $p < 0.05$ and ** $p < 0.01$.

4. Discussion

Epidemiological studies have reported that the consumption of fermented dairy products is beneficial for the prevention of cognitive decline in the elderly [1]. Our previous study demonstrated that WY-related peptides derived from enzymatic whey protein digests, such as the GTWY peptide β-lactolin, improve memory impairment in mice with pharmacologically-induced amnesia [7]. However, the underlying mechanism of the effects of the WY dipeptide core included in WY-related peptides on memory improvement is not well-understood. In the present study, we demonstrated that dipeptides with an N-terminal tryptophan, such as WY, WM, WV, WL, and WF improved memory impairment in scopolamine-induced amnesic mice. Especially, the WY dipeptide increased the dopamine levels in the hippocampus and frontal cortex, and the WY-induced memory improvement was attenuated by the blockade of the dopamine D1 receptor. Moreover, the WY dipeptide improved spatial memory impairment in aged mice. These results suggested that orally administered WY dipeptide improved spatial memory impairments in pharmacologically-induced amnestic mice and aged mice via modulating the dopamine system.

We showed that the WY dipeptide inhibited MAO-B activity and increased dopamine levels in the hippocampus and frontal cortex and improved spatial memory impairment in pharmacologically-induced amnestic mice and aged mice. Previous reports have indicated that dopamine is involved in hippocampus-dependent memory functions [12,13]. The dopamine neuronal network is related to an age-related decline in cognitive performance and executive function, and the dopamine precursor levodopa has been shown to improve the task-based learning rate and task performance in the elderly [14]. It has also been reported that MAO-B inhibitors improve cognitive function in rodents [15–17]. MAO-B is an enzyme for dopamine metabolism and thus decreases dopamine levels in the brain [18]. Therefore, MAO-B inhibitors have been used as drugs to induce dopamine levels [19]. It is suggested that some MAO-B inhibitors have a potential as therapeutic or preventive treatment for dementia including Alzheimer's disease [20,21]. We also showed that the administration of WY dipeptide increased total dopamine levels in the hippocampus and frontal cortex. These results suggest that WY dipeptide increase dopamine levels in the brain by inhibiting MAO-B activity. Those findings suggest that the WY dipeptide exerts its beneficial effect on the prevention of age-related cognitive decline by increasing dopaminergic activity in the brain.

In addition, we showed that dopamine D1 receptor is involved in the spatial memory improvement induced by the WY dipeptide. Dopamine exerts its functions via multiple receptor subtypes, D1-like (D1 and D5) and D2-like (D2, D3, and D4) receptors. In the present study, the treatment with D1-like receptor antagonist, SCH-23390 attenuated the improvement caused by the WY dipeptide in scopolamine-induced amnesic mice. It has been reported that activation of dopamine D1-like receptors enhances hippocampus-dependent memory functions [22–25]. Because the hippocampus is crucial for spatial memory as measured by the Y-maze test [26], we examined the involvement of the dopamine D1 receptor in the hippocampus in WY-dipeptide-induced memory improvement. Dopamine D1-like receptors are expressed in many brain areas including the hippocampus, but due to the lack of selective pharmacological drugs, most studies failed to discriminate dopamine receptor subtypes. Recently, the brain-region-specific knockdown of the dopamine D1 receptor subtype was achieved by injecting AAV vectors that express recombinant miRNA targeting this dopamine receptor subtype [9]. This technique made it possible to further examine a potential link between the spatial memory improvement by the WY dipeptide and the dopamine D1 receptors in the hippocampus. Dopamine D1 receptor knockdown in the hippocampus attenuated the improvement by the WY peptide, but it was a partial reduction. These data suggested that the dopamine D1 receptor in the hippocampus is involved in the WY-dipeptide-induced memory improvement for spatial information measured in the Y-maze test at least in part. The reason why the effect of the D1 receptor knockdown was partial remains unclear. It could be due to the partial knockdown of the dopamine D1 receptor in the hippocampus. This finding is consistent with previous reports suggesting that D1 receptor stimulation in the hippocampus augments spatial memory.

Alternatively, dopamine in the frontal cortex could be involved in the WY-dipeptide-induced memory improvement, since the WY dipeptide increased the dopamine levels in frontal cortex as well.

In the present study, we compared the effects of several dipeptides containing tryptophan and tryptophan as a single amino acid. We found that the administration of a single dose of dipeptides with an N-terminal tryptophan, WY, WM, WV, WL, and WF improved spatial memory in mice, whereas YW and MW dipeptides did not have this effect. These findings suggest that the dipeptide conformation with an N-terminal tryptophan is crucial for effectively improving the memory impairment after oral administration. It has been shown that dipeptides with an N-terminal tryptophan have a high affinity to peptide transporters, and among the dipeptide library, the WY dipeptide is one of the dipeptides with the highest affinities [27]. Thus, the conformation of dipeptides with an N-terminal tryptophan could be necessary for transporter-mediated absorption from the gut and delivery to the brain. On the other hand, based on our finding that the WY dipeptide, but not tryptophan as a single amino acid, inhibited MAO-B activity in vitro, the dipeptide conformation with an N-terminal tryptophan could be crucial for enhancing dopaminergic activity. Note that these two possibilities are not mutually exclusive but rather synergetic for the memory improving effect of the WY dipeptide.

5. Conclusions

In summary, the present study showed that the WY dipeptide improves pharmacologically-induced and age-related memory impairment in mice. Effective intake of the WY dipeptide and other dipeptides with N-terminal tryptophan via supplements or nutraceutical foods including certain whey peptide preparations might be beneficial for improving cognitive function in older age.

Author Contributions: Y.A., T.A., and R.O. conducted the experiments and analyzed the results. Y.A., S.K., and T.F. wrote the paper, and K.K. supervised this research.

Funding: This study was supported by Kirin Company, Ltd. and in part by a CREST grant from AMED (JP18gm0910012 to T.F.); Grants-in-Aids for Scientific Research (16H05132 and 17K19457 to T.F. and 17K08593 to S.K.) from the Japan Society for the Promotion of Science; and Grants-in-Aids for Scientific Research from the Ministry of Education, Culture, Sports, Science and Technology in Japan (18H05429 to T.F.)

Conflicts of Interest: Ano, Y., Ayabe, T., Ohya, R., and Kondo, K. are employed by Kirin Co. Ltd. All other authors declare no competing interests.

References

1. Ano, Y.; Nakayama, H. Preventive effects of dairy products on dementia and the underlying mechanisms. *Int. J. Mol. Sci.* **2018**, *19*, 1927. [CrossRef] [PubMed]
2. Crichton, G.E.; Bryan, J.; Murphy, K.J.; Buckley, J. Review of dairy consumption and cognitive performance in adults: Findings and methodological issues. *Dement. Geriatr. Cogn. Disord.* **2010**, *30*, 352–361. [CrossRef] [PubMed]
3. Ozawa, M.; Ninomiya, T.; Ohara, T.; Doi, Y.; Uchida, K.; Shirota, T.; Yonemoto, K.; Kitazono, T.; Kiyohara, Y. Dietary patterns and risk of dementia in an elderly Japanese population: The Hisayama Study. *Am. J. Clin. Nutr.* **2013**, *97*, 1076–1082. [CrossRef] [PubMed]
4. Ozawa, M.; Ohara, T.; Ninomiya, T.; Hata, J.; Yoshida, D.; Mukai, N.; Nagata, M.; Uchida, K.; Shirota, T.; Kitazono, T.; et al. Milk and dairy consumption and risk of dementia in an elderly Japanese population: The Hisayama Study. *J. Am. Geriatr. Soc.* **2014**, *62*, 1224–1230. [CrossRef] [PubMed]
5. Ogata, S.; Tanaka, H.; Omura, K.; Honda, C.; Hayakawa, K. Association between intake of dairy products and short-term memory with and without adjustment for genetic and family environmental factors: A twin study. *Clin. Nutr. (Edinburgh, Scotland)* **2016**, *35*, 507–513. [CrossRef] [PubMed]
6. Ano, Y.; Ozawa, M.; Kutsukake, T.; Sugiyama, S.; Uchida, K.; Yoshida, A.; Nakayama, H. Preventive effects of a fermented dairy product against Alzheimer's disease and identification of a novel oleamide with enhanced microglial phagocytosis and anti-inflammatory activity. *PloS ONE* **2015**, *10*, e0118512. [CrossRef] [PubMed]
7. Ano, Y.; Ayabe, T.; Kutsukake, T.; Ohya, R.; Takaichi, Y.; Uchida, S.; Yamada, K.; Uchida, K.; Takashima, A.; Nakayama, H. Novel lactopeptides in fermented dairy products improve memory function and cognitive decline. *Neurobiol. Aging* **2018**, *72*, 23–31. [CrossRef]

8. Kita, M.; Obara, K.; Kondo, S.; Umeda, S.; Ano, Y. Effect of supplementation of a whey peptide rich in tryptophan-tyrosine-related peptides on cognitive performance in healthy adults: A randomized, double-blind, placebo-controlled study. *Nutrients* **2018**, *10*, 899. [CrossRef]
9. Shinohara, R.; Taniguchi, M.; Ehrlich, A.T.; Yokogawa, K.; Deguchi, Y.; Cherasse, Y.; Lazarus, M.; Urade, Y.; Ogawa, A.; Kitaoka, S.; et al. Dopamine D1 receptor subtype mediates acute stress-induced dendritic growth in excitatory neurons of the medial prefrontal cortex and contributes to suppression of stress susceptibility in mice. *Mol. Psychiatr.* **2017**, *23*, 1717. [CrossRef]
10. Ano, Y.; Hoshi, A.; Ayabe, T.; Ohya, R.; Uchida, S.; Yamada, K.; Kondo, K.; Kitaoka, S.; Furuyashiki, T. Iso-alpha-acids, the bitter components of beer, improve hippocampus-dependent memory through vagus nerve activation. *FASEB J. Off. Publ. Fed. Am. Soc. Exp. Biol.* **2019**. [CrossRef]
11. Franklin, K.; Paxinos, G. *The Mouse Brain in Stereotaxic Coordinates, Compact*; Academic Press: San Diego, CA, USA, 2008.
12. McNamara, C.G.; Dupret, D. Two sources of dopamine for the hippocampus. *Trends Neurosci.* **2017**, *40*, 383–384. [CrossRef] [PubMed]
13. Takeuchi, T.; Duszkiewicz, A.J.; Sonneborn, A.; Spooner, P.A.; Yamasaki, M.; Watanabe, M.; Smith, C.C.; Fernandez, G.; Deisseroth, K.; Greene, R.W.; et al. Locus coeruleus and dopaminergic consolidation of everyday memory. *Nature* **2016**, *537*, 357–362. [CrossRef] [PubMed]
14. Chowdhury, R.; Guitart-Masip, M.; Lambert, C.; Dayan, P.; Huys, Q.; Duzel, E.; Dolan, R.J. Dopamine restores reward prediction errors in old age. *Nat. Neurosci.* **2013**, *16*, 648–653. [CrossRef] [PubMed]
15. Bar-Am, O.; Amit, T.; Kupershmidt, L.; Aluf, Y.; Mechlovich, D.; Kabha, H.; Danovitch, L.; Zurawski, V.R.; Youdim, M.B.; Weinreb, O. Neuroprotective and neurorestorative activities of a novel iron chelator-brain selective monoamine oxidase-A/monoamine oxidase-B inhibitor in animal models of Parkinson's disease and aging. *Neurobiol. Aging* **2015**, *36*, 1529–1542. [CrossRef] [PubMed]
16. Justo, L.A.; Duran, R.; Alfonso, M.; Fajardo, D.; Faro, L.R.F. Effects and mechanism of action of isatin, a MAO inhibitor, on in vivo striatal dopamine release. *Neurochem. Int.* **2016**, *99*, 147–157. [CrossRef] [PubMed]
17. Schulz, D.; Mirrione, M.M.; Henn, F.A. Cognitive aspects of congenital learned helplessness and its reversal by the monoamine oxidase (MAO)-B inhibitor deprenyl. *Neurobiol. Learn. Mem.* **2010**, *93*, 291–301. [CrossRef] [PubMed]
18. Gaweska, H.; Fitzpatrick, P.F. Structures and mechanism of the monoamine oxidase family. *Biomol. Concepts* **2011**, *2*, 365–377. [CrossRef]
19. Cai, Z. Monoamine oxidase inhibitors: Promising therapeutic agents for Alzheimer's disease (Review). *Mol. Med. Rep.* **2014**, *9*, 1533–1541. [CrossRef]
20. Wang, Y.; Sun, Y.; Guo, Y.; Wang, Z.; Huang, L.; Li, X. Dual functional cholinesterase and MAO inhibitors for the treatment of Alzheimer's disease: Synthesis, pharmacological analysis and molecular modeling of homoisoflavonoid derivatives. *J. Enzyme Inhib. Med. Chem.* **2016**, *31*, 389–397. [CrossRef]
21. Borroni, E.; Bohrmann, B.; Grueninger, F.; Prinssen, E.; Nave, S.; Loetscher, H.; Chinta, S.J.; Rajagopalan, S.; Rane, A.; Siddiqui, A.; et al. Sembragiline: A novel, selective monoamine oxidase type B inhibitor for the treatment of Alzheimer's disease. *J. Pharmacol. Exp. Ther.* **2017**, *362*, 413–423. [CrossRef]
22. Da Silva, W.C.; Kohler, C.C.; Radiske, A.; Cammarota, M. D1/D5 dopamine receptors modulate spatial memory formation. *Neurobiol. Learn. Mem.* **2012**, *97*, 271–275. [CrossRef] [PubMed]
23. De Bundel, D.; Femenia, T.; DuPont, C.M.; Konradsson-Geuken, A.; Feltmann, K.; Schilstrom, B.; Lindskog, M. Hippocampal and prefrontal dopamine D1/5 receptor involvement in the memory-enhancing effect of reboxetine. *Int. J. Neuropsychopharmacol.* **2013**, *16*, 2041–2051. [CrossRef] [PubMed]
24. Yuan Xiang, P.; Janc, O.; Grochowska, K.M.; Kreutz, M.R.; Reymann, K.G. Dopamine agonists rescue Abeta-induced LTP impairment by Src-family tyrosine kinases. *Neurobiol. Aging* **2016**, *40*, 98–102. [CrossRef] [PubMed]
25. Hao, J.R.; Sun, N.; Lei, L.; Li, X.Y.; Yao, B.; Sun, K.; Hu, R.; Zhang, X.; Shi, X.D.; Gao, C. L-Stepholidine rescues memory deficit and synaptic plasticity in models of Alzheimer's disease via activating dopamine D1 receptor/PKA signaling pathway. *Cell Death Dis.* **2015**, *6*, e1965. [CrossRef] [PubMed]

26. Pioli, E.Y.; Gaskill, B.N.; Gilmour, G.; Tricklebank, M.D.; Dix, S.L.; Bannerman, D.; Garner, J.P. An automated maze task for assessing hippocampus-sensitive memory in mice. *Behav. Brain Res.* **2014**, *261*, 249–257. [CrossRef] [PubMed]
27. Ito, K.; Hikida, A.; Kawai, S.; Lan, V.T.; Motoyama, T.; Kitagawa, S.; Yoshikawa, Y.; Kato, R.; Kawarasaki, Y. Analysing the substrate multispecificity of a proton-coupled oligopeptide transporter using a dipeptide library. *Nat. Commun.* **2013**, *4*, 2502. [CrossRef] [PubMed]

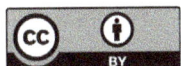
© 2019 by the authors. Licensee MDPI, Basel, Switzerland. This article is an open access article distributed under the terms and conditions of the Creative Commons Attribution (CC BY) license (http://creativecommons.org/licenses/by/4.0/).

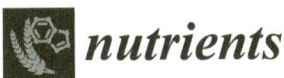

Review

The Potential Influence of the Bacterial Microbiome on the Development and Progression of ADHD

Stephanie Bull-Larsen and M. Hasan Mohajeri *

Institute of Anatomy, Department of medicine, University of Zurich, Winterthurerstrasse 190, 8057 Zürich, Switzerland; stephanie.bull-larsen@uzh.ch
* Correspondence: mhasan.mohajeri@uzh.ch; Tel.: +41-79-938-1203

Received: 15 October 2019; Accepted: 13 November 2019; Published: 17 November 2019

Abstract: The latest research cumulates staggering information about the correlation between the microbiota-gut-brain axis and neurodevelopmental disorders. This review aims to shed light on the potential influence of the microbiome on the development of the most prevalent neurodevelopmental disease, attention-deficit-hyperactive disorder (ADHD). As the etiology and pathophysiology of ADHD are still unclear, finding viable biomarkers and effective treatment still represent a challenge. Therefore, we focused on factors that have been associated with a higher risk of developing ADHD, while simultaneously influencing the microbial composition. We reviewed the effect of a differing microbial makeup on neurotransmitter concentrations important in the pathophysiology of ADHD. Additionally, we deduced factors that correlate with a high prevalence of ADHD, while simultaneously affecting the gut microbiome, such as emergency c-sections, and premature birth as the former leads to a decrease of the gut microbial diversity and the latter causes neuroprotective *Lactobacillus* levels to be reduced. Also, we assessed nutritional influences, such as breastfeeding, ingestion of short-chain fatty acids (SCFAs) and polyunsaturated fatty acids (PUFAs) on the host's microbiome and development of ADHD. Finally, we discussed the potential significance of *Bifidobacterium* as a biomarker for ADHD, the importance of preventing premature birth as prophylaxis and nutrition as a prospective therapeutic measurement against ADHD.

Keywords: microbiome; microbiota-gut-brain axis; ADHD; attention-deficit-hyperactive-disorder

---

1. Introduction

The microbiota-gut-brain axis is a bidirectional communication pathway between the microbiota, gut and central nervous system (CNS). It has been estimated that over 10^{14} microorganisms, which include bacteria, archaea, and eukaryota, reside in the gastrointestinal tract (GI-tract) [1]. According to the latest study, this results in an approximately equal number of microbial compared to human cells in an individual [2]. The microorganisms residing in the GI-tract play an important role in protecting humans from potential GI pathogens [3], and also exert neuroactive properties which explains why this ecosystem does not only influence the gut, but also the brain. Research shows the great importance of a healthy microbial composition in the gut at an early stage in life (2–3 years of age), a period also characterized by intense neurodevelopment in humans. Several reports conclude that early gut dysbiosis can influence the neurodevelopment in the short run and may also lead to mental health issues later in life [4,5].

Research highlights this risk, as gut dysbiosis in child or adulthood has not only been associated with various diseases, such as irritable bowel syndrome [6] or obesity [7], but also with psychiatric disorders as, for example, depression [8], Parkinson's disease (PD) [9], schizophrenia [10], autism spectrum disorder (AS) [11], and lastly, attention-deficite-hyperactive-disorder (ADHD) [12].

ADHD is an early onset neurodevelopmental disease that, according to the fifth edition of Diagnostic and Statistical Manual (DSM-V), can be characterized into different representations:

Hyperactivity and/or impulsivity, inattentiveness or all combined [13]. The worldwide prevalence of ADHD in children under the age of 18 ranges from 5.3% [14] to 7.2% [15], making it the most frequent neurobehavioral diagnosis in children. Interestingly, varying prevalence levels are reported in different geographies, which are primarily due to different characteristics of methods employed for ADHD diagnosis rather than geographic variations [14]. Nonetheless, 30–60% of the children continue to show symptoms into adulthood and thus, 1–6% of the population develop adult ADHD [16]. This is predominantly represented by the inattentive type [17].

This literature review attempts to identify and discuss factors that may influence the microbiome, and thus, could be associated with the development or progression of ADHD. Thereby we concentrate solely on the influence of bacteria rather than archaea and eukaryota. Furthermore, we evaluate the biochemical changes in ADHD patients and to what extent these can be related to microbial alterations in the gut. Finally, we reconfirm known biomarkers and deduce possible new ones for the diagnosis of ADHD and conclude what factors worsen or alleviate the development and progression of ADHD as this might lead to potential intervention methods of the neurodevelopmental disorder.

2. Materials and Methods

The key research question of this literature review is: What factors may influence the microbiome and could be associated with the development and/or progression of ADHD? The databases Pubmed and Scopus were searched until the 1 July 2019 with the following MeSH and search terms: "Microbiome", "microbiota", "gut-brain axis", "microbiota-gut-brain-axis", "ADHD". Most of the research papers included in this review were published between 2010 and 2019.

As our primary focus was on bacteria, we excluded studies that concentrated on archaea and eukaryota. The incorporated studies had to fulfill all of the following inclusion criteria:

- Articles were directly related to the topic;
- ADHD patients were diagnosed by a medical expert;
- Publication in a peer-reviewed journal;
- Availability of the full-text publication;
- Studies were written in English.

A total of 208 citations were included in this article.

3. Evidence Linking Microbiota to ADHD

3.1. Microbiome

The influence of the microbiome on the ADHD pathophysiology is being intensively researched. The microbiota consists of the different microorganisms [18], and the microbiome describes the entire genome of the microbiota [18]. The primary functions of the microbiota include: (i) Protecting the host organism against pathogens by increasing the mucine production, and thus, stabilizing the gut-blood barrier; (ii) support of the immune system [19]; (iii) the production of vitamins [20]; and (iv) short-chain fatty acids (SCFAs), whereby the latter are products of microbial catabolism of indigestible carbohydrates [21]. Throughout the GI-tract, the composition and density of microbes changes, increasing from 10^2 cells per gram of content in the stomach to 10^8 cells per gram in the cecum [22]. Additionally, up to 1000 different bacterial species have been found to inhabit the GI-tract of humans [23]. Thereby the composition in species of the microbiome can be influenced by genetics [24], geography [25], disease, medication [26], and age [27].

The GI-microbiota goes through a physiological change from its prenatal period until the age of three [27]. For a long time, it has been thought that the intrauterine environment is sterile and that the first bacterial colonization of the newborn happens during delivery [28]. However, numerous studies have shown that bacteria exist in the placenta, amniotic fluid [29–31], and meconium [32] indicating that the unique microbial composition in utero may already influence the development of the microbiome of the fetus before birth. Research demonstrates that the microbiome of the placenta is low in richness and diversity and is predominantly colonized by the phyla Proteobacteria and Bacteroidetes. The former is mostly represented by the spp. *Escherichia coli* and *Neisseria lactamica*, while Bacteroidetes is dominated by *Bacteroides* spp. [31]. Other important phyla include Firmicutes, Fusobacteria and Tenericutes [31], whereby the latter includes genera, such as *Mycoplasma* and *Ureaplasma* [33].

The colonization of the gut in the postnatal period is sensitive to environmental factors. Nonetheless, the normal composition of the microbiome in a newborn is low in diversity and shows dominance in Proteobacteria and Actinobacteria [34]. More specifically, Proteobacteria shows its peak at birth, whereas Actinobacteria increases and dominates at the age of four months [35]. At this point, Proteobacteria is still mostly represented by *Escherichia coli* and Actinobacteria by the genus *Bifidobacterium longum* [35]. As seen in Figure 1, at the age of three and onwards, the microbiome stabilizes to four major phyla: Firmicutes, Bacteroidetes, Actinobacteria, and Proteobacteria, which normally cover more than 90% of the total bacterial population in a human body [36].

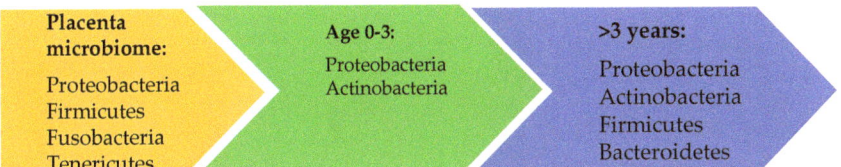

Figure 1. The most prevalent bacterial phyla in utero and in the GI-tract of humans. This figure represents the dynamic and development of the composition of the microbiome from fetuses in utero until the age of three years, at which point the microbiome gains its stability and consists of mostly four phyla: Proteobacteria, Actinobacteria, Firmicutes, and Bacteroides.

3.2. Gut-Brain Axis

The gut-brain axis describes the bidirectional communication between the microbes, enteric nervous system and the CNS [37]. So far, there are three known means of communication between these compartments: Neural, immune, and endocrine [4,38].

The neural pathway describes the hypothalamic-pituitary-adrenal axis (HPA axis), which is the most important efferent stress pathway. It is of great importance to understand to what extent the HPA axis plays a role in the pathogenesis of ADHD, as it influences pathways in the body that are often deviating in ADHD patients [39,40] as for example: Circadian rhythm [41], sleep [42], and emotions [43]. The stimulation of the HPA axis by stress or pro-inflammatory cytokines results in a release of corticotropin-releasing factor (CRF) from the hypothalamus, as well as adrenocorticotropic hormone (ACTH) from the pituitary gland, finally resulting in the secretion of cortisol from the suprarenal (adrenal) glands [38].

One study using 69 healthy children and 123 children with ADHD observed an increase in salivatory cortisol in ADHD patients after waking up in the morning [44]. The effect of stressors was studied in one paper showing that after being exposed to stress children with ADHD of combined type (high levels of hyperactivity and impulsivity) have decreased salivary cortisol levels in comparison to other ADHD patients [45]. In contrast, adult ADHD patients with an inattentive type showed higher levels of cortisol in comparison to the combined types, which showed normal levels of cortisol [46]. Finally, Lackschewitz et al. discovered that adults with ADHD who undergo a stress-inducing exam show a trend towards reduced cortisol levels [47]. These reports portray the association between altered cortisol levels and different types of ADHD. However, the heterogeneity of the results can be explained by various stressors on a differing target group all acting as confounders. Thus, only future studies using the same stressor, examining similar and large patient groups will allow drawing further reliable conclusions.

The neuroimmune communication pathway describes how intestinal microbes influence the function and maturation of immune cells in the CNS, whereby microglia cells play an important role [48]. These cells are activated, as well as produced, by pro-inflammatory cytokines, and are important regulators for autoimmunity, neuroinflammation, and neurogenesis [49]. Germ-free (GF) mice showed defects in microglia activation, which in turn lead to a deficient innate immune response when exposed to pathogenic bacteria [50]. The same study showed the immense effect the microbiome has on microglial cells, as introducing microbiota into GF mice resulted in restored microglial functions. Reversely, eradicating various bacteria in specific pathogen-free (SPF) mice resulted in microglial cells maturing less rapidly [50]. As neuroinflammation plays an important part in the pathophysiology of ADHD, the proper activation and maturation of microglia in ADHD patients have to be thoroughly investigated in order to determine if it has a pathogenic influence.

The enteric nervous system communicates with the brain mainly through the parasympathetic vagus nerve [51], and partially though the sympathetic spinal cord pathway [52]. Furthermore, the vagus nerve predominantly consists of afferent nerve fibers with a ratio of 9:1 to efferent fibers [53]. Even though a definite conclusion cannot be made, various studies have demonstrated that the autonomic nervous system of ADHD patients shows alterations. A study testing 19 children with ADHD showed that the patients had an underactive parasympathetic and an overactive sympathetic nervous system [54]. Another study comparing 32 ADHD patients to 34 healthy controls registered under-aroused parasympathetic nervous systems, while the sympathetic part did not show any difference between the groups [55].

It has become clear that all three ways of communication between the microbiome, gut, and CNS could play an important role in the pathophysiology of ADHD. The neural communication over the HPA axis shows abnormalities in ADHD patients. Additionally, studies detected that microbes influence the function of pro-inflammatory microglia, a key finding, as neuroinflammation in ADHD patients is commonly found. Finally, the autonomic nervous system shows aberrations as the main research results show an under-arousal of the parasympathetic nervous system.

3.3. Etiology of ADHD and the Genetic and Environmental Influences

As the exact pathophysiology of ADHD is still unclear, its causes are still being researched. Nevertheless, it has been established that there is an interplay between genes and the environment resulting in a complex etiology. Genetic predisposition plays an important part in the pathophysiology of ADHD as children from parents that have been diagnosed with ADHD have a 50% higher chance to be diagnosed with the same disorder [56]. Similarly, twin studies have shown a high heritability, as especially for inattentive and combined types an inheritance of 71–90% could be discovered [56,57]. On the other hand, one study showed, that 20–30% of the risk of developing ADHD is due to environmental factors [58]. These include perinatal maternal smoking, stress, mineral and micronutrient deficiencies and premature birth [59]. Additionally, research showed that 10–40% of the variance inheritance of ADHD could be caused due to the environment highlighting the interplay of genetic and environmental risk factors [60]. Due to these complex interactions, it is believed that ADHD can be manifested with highly heterogenous symptoms depending on the exact pathway and etiology involved [61].

Research shows that the dysfunction of monoaminergic neurotransmitters, including noradrenaline (NE), serotonin (5-HT) and dopamine (DA), plays an important role in the pathophysiology of ADHD [62].

3.3.1. Dopamine

DA is a catecholamine that acts both as a hormone and neurotransmitter (NT). It is a product of the essential amino acid L-phenylalanine, which must be provided in our diet. As seen in Figure 2, this is then turned into L-tyrosine, and finally into DA and NE [63].

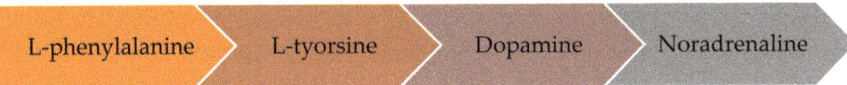

Figure 2. The synthesis pathway from L-phenylalanine to noradrenaline including all its intermediary products. Dopamine acts as an important metabolite for the emotional response and reward system [64].

The dopamine hypothesis links ADHD to alterations in dopamine metabolism. The hypothesis describes the increased expression of presynaptic dopamine transports (DAT) in ADHD patients leading to an increased dopamine transporter density (DTD), and finally results in a decreased level of the bioavailable NT [65]. The dopamine hypothesis gained attention due to the way methylphenidate (MPH) and amphetamines (AMP), the most commonly used pharmacotherapies to treat ADHD, interact with the DA and NE metabolism. MPH and AMP exert a stimulatory effect in ADHD as they inhibit the reuptake of NE and DA by blocking the metabolizing enzyme, monoamine oxidase (MAO), thereby increasing the concentration of the two monoamines in the synaptic cleft. One differentiates between MAO-A and MAO-B as the former is mostly expressed in the liver and GI-tract and the latter in blood platelets [66]. Nevertheless, both are manifested in the CNS and are able to break down DA [66]. Furthermore, amphetamines have the ability to release NTs from the presynaptic neuron, which additionally increases the monoaminergic concentration in the synapse [67].

Moreover, recent research shows that not only the metabolization, but also the production of DA plays an important role in the pathophysiology of ADHD. One of the influencers on the production of NTs seems to be the microbiome in the GI-tract [68]. Bacteria, such as the genus Bifidobacterium belonging to the phylum Actinobacteria potentially influence the levels of available DA in the body by encoding cyclohexadienyl dehydratase (CDT) [69]. This enzyme is important for the synthesis of the essential amino acid phenylalanine [69], which acts as a precursor of the amino acid tyrosine, which in turn is metabolized into DA and lastly to NE [70]. Aarts et al. found an increase in Bifidobacterium in ADHD patients, and thus, higher levels of CDT. By analyzing BOLD responses of the ventral striatal using fMRI measurements they deduced a negative correlation between the abundance of CDT and reward anticipation [69], a key symptom in ADHD [71], and target of DA [72]. Finally, this study concluded that high levels of phenylalanine might be a risk factor for abnormal dopamine signaling and could lead to a reduced reward response [69]. Although another study supports the findings by Aarts et al. [73], the correlation still appears to be inconsistent as two older studies found a decreased level of phenylalanine in ADHD patients [74,75], even if data of source [74] are not statistically significant. Finally, a more recent study found no correlation between phenylalanine levels and ADHD [76]. A summary of these finfings is given in Table 1.

Table 1. Various studies that tested phenylalanine levels in ADHD patients. ↑ represent the increase of phenylalanine found in ADHD patients and ↓ the decrease of the amino acid in comparison to healthy controls (HC). The symbol — describes that the study found no correlation between ADHD and phenylalanine levels. The accumulative data to date do not allow a definite correlation between a change in phenylalanine levels and ADHD. p levels less than 0.05 were considered statistically different.

Source	Levels of Phenylalanine in ADHD Patients	Sample Size (n)	Statistical Significance (p)
[69]	↑	96	$p < 0.001$
[73]	↑	79	$p < 0.001$
[74]	↓	44	$p < 0.1$
[75]	↓	48	$p < 0.05$
[76]	—	155	$p < 0.01$

3.3.2. Tryptophan and Serotonin

Upon intestinal absorption into the bloodstream, the essential amino acid tryptophan can cross the blood-brain barrier (BBB). Thereby tryptophan can act as the precursor of the neurotransmitter 5-HT, which plays an important part in the microbiome-gut-brain axis [77]. Although it is still unclear to what extent the microbiome influences the synthesis of 5-HT, it has been established that certain strains of bacteria, such as *Streptococcus* spp., *Enterococcus* spp., and *Escheria* spp. are capable of producing this NT [78]. Most of the 5-HT is produced and stored in gastrointestinal cells and affects peristalsis, nausea, satiety and abdominal pain [79]. Meanwhile, in the brain, it influences other NTs, such as DA, Cholin (CH) and GABA, which influence memory and mood [80].

Banerjee et al. showed that 5-HT may have an influence on hyperactive and impulsive symptoms in ADHD [81]. Another study implied lower levels of 5-HT in the CNS of ADHD patients due to a decreased transport capacity of its precursor, tryptophan, into the brain [82]. Finally, one study showed that inflammation in the intestine affects 5-HT signaling pathways due to a decreased function and expression of the serotonin selective reuptake transporter (SERT) resulting in an increased level of 5-HT in the body [79]. However, it is important to remember that serotonin is not able to cross the BBB, and thus, the 5-HT pools in the CNS and the periphery do not directly interact with each other.

To demonstrate the importance of microbes on the 5-HT system, one study concluded that GF male mice have a 1.3 fold increased level of 5-HT in their hippocampus. This is an important finding as certain therapeutic medications of ADHD, such as escitalopram and lithium increase serotonin levels in a similar amount [83]. Thus, the composition and the modulation of the gut microbiota might become an interesting, future therapeutic intervention strategy.

Although the studies do not allow us to make a precise conclusion in what way bacterial-produced 5-HT influences ADHD, they do make it clear that it is one of the several catecholamines that play an important role in the pathophysiology of ADHD.

3.3.3. Kynurenine Pathway

Although tryptophan is the key amino acid for the production of 5-HT, 90% of tryptophan is catabolized by the kynurenine pathway [84]. This process produces nicotinamide adenine dinucleotide (NAD) through the stimulation of inflammatory and glucocorticoid metabolites. The kynurenine pathway has received attention in regards to psychiatric diseases, such as depression and schizophrenia [80,85,86] as it uses most of the tryptophan, and thus, leaves a limiting amount of substrate for the synthesis of serotonin.

Intermediate products, such as kynurenine, kynurenic acid (KA), xanthurenic acid (XA) and quilonoic acid (QA) can influence the immune system and neurotransmission [87]. The three former metabolites have anti-inflammatory properties as KA inhibits the NMDA-gated ion channels [88], and XA interferes with the glutamatergic neurotransmission [89]. Also, these products decrease the amount of pro-inflammatory IFN gamma in comparison to the anti-inflammatory IL-10 [87]. In contrast, QA stimulates microglial cells and increases the ratio of IFN gamma/IL-10 [87], resulting in pro-inflammatory effects [90]. Although KA shows neuroprotective properties, human and animal studies show that high levels of KA are associated with cognitive abnormalities, such as attention and memory issues typically associated with psychiatric disease [91,92].

Studies regarding levels of tryptophan and metabolites of the kynurenine pathway show inconclusive results. A Norwegian study, using 133 adult ADHD patients and 133, did not find that the ADHD group had lower levels of tryptophan and neuroprotective KA and XA [86]. These data were confirmed by another study testing ADHD children, which exhibited lower KA and XA levels [93]. These researchers, however, recorded higher levels of tryptophan in ADHD subjects [93]. These data do suggest an association between low levels of KA and XA in ADHD, but as there are still too few studies on this topic, it is difficult to deduce a definitive connection between tryptophan, its metabolites, and ADHD.

The various steps of the kynurenine pathway are dependent on coenzymes, such as the activated form of vitamin B6, pyridoxal 5′-phosphate (PLP). One study found an inverse correlation between serum levels of vitamin B6 and ADHD including its symptom severity [94]. Similarly, Aarsland et al. also observed a decrease in vitamin B6 in their patient group. Other data suggested that vitamin B6 metabolism plays a key part in the pathophysiology of ADHD, as vitamin B6 dependent enzymes show severe abnormalities in the ADHD test group [95]. Thus, lower levels of intermediate metabolites could be related to a deficiency of enzyme substrate. This data supports the importance of optimal coverage of ADHD patients with vitamin B6. The microbiome could play a potentially important role, as bacteria in the large intestine produce this vitamin [96]. As the correlation between levels of vitamin B6 and ADHD are relatively new, future studies are warranted to asses to what extent the microbiome can influence vitamin B6 levels on a therapeutic level.

3.3.4. Gut Dysbiosis and Immunology

High variability in gut flora prevents the growth of pathogenic bacteria, and thus, stops gut dysbiosis [97]. The term dysbiosis describes a microbial imbalance in which there is a shift from protective to pathogenic microbes in the GI-tract [98]. This can lead to a growing GI-permeability which leads to an increase in migration of pathogenic microbes and translocation of their metabolites into the systemic circulation potentially resulting in systemic inflammation [99]. This can, in turn, decrease the permeability of the BBB, which can lead to inflammation of brain parenchyma [100]. Severe dysbiosis has been associated with chronic inflammatory intestinal disorders and psychiatric illnesses, such as schizophrenia, anxiety, depression [98], and ADHD [90,101]. A systematic review supports the latter findings concluding that patients with ADHD have increased levels of inflammatory cytokines [102]. Similarly, Verlaet et al. also detected increased levels of pro-inflammatory cytokines (IFN gamma and IL-6) in the serum of ADHD patients [101].

An imbalance of pro-inflammatory cytokines can also lead to allergic disease [103], and a positive correlation between ADHD and allergies has been shown in different cohorts [104–106]. Additionally, research has shown an association between an altered gut microbial composition and the tendency to suffer from the allergic disease [107].

An important pro-inflammatory cytokine is interleukin (IL-6). This has been inversely associated with the bacterium *Dialister* spp. [108]. *Dialister* spp. is shown to correlate with an altered temperament and impulsiveness in toddlers positively. These commonly found ADHD symptoms were measured using the Early Childhood Behavior Questionnaire (ECBQ), which measures extroversion, activity levels and feelings of high-intensity pleasure [109]. Furthermore, a review evaluating multiple studies concluded an increase in pro-inflammatory metabolites, such as IL-6 and IL-1 in patients with ADHD [110]. Nonetheless, one study showed that ADHD patients had significantly lower levels of *Dialister* spp. in comparison to healthy controls (HC), hinting towards decreased feelings of activity and lower levels of intense pleasure, and finally higher levels of IL-6 [111].

Although the association between *Dialister* spp. and feelings of pleasure are new findings; and it is important to note that pro-inflammatory interleukin levels are increased in ADHD patients. As high levels of pro-inflammatory interleukins can be linked to neurological inflammation that can lead to a decrease of cortical volume and altered behavior [110,112], reducing the activity of these pro-inflammatory cytokines could represent a vital prophylaxis strategy in ADHD management.

Patients with th2-mediated atopic disorders, such as eczema, asthma and allergic rhinitis have a 30–50% higher chance of developing ADHD [113]. Eczema is an inflammatory skin disease and is the most prevalent chronic condition in early childhood [114]. Children suffering from atopic dermatitis (eczema) have a 50% likelihood of developing asthma and allergic rhinitis, exhibiting airway inflammation and clear nasal discharge, respectively [115]. Th2-cytokines are important for eosinophilic recruitment and the production of IgE by B-lymphocytes. All of these processes are associated with allergies and inflammation of the skin (e.g., eczema) [116,117] as they activate the production of pro-inflammatory cytokines, such as IL-6, IL-1beta, TNF-alpha and IL-8 [103]. Studies have shown that these atopic diseases are associated with a low level of *Faecalbacteria* spp. In the gut [118]. This species is known to have anti-inflammatory effects on the organisms [119,120]. As explained above, patients with ADHD seem to exhibit higher levels of inflammatory markers which could potentially support the hypothesis that low levels of *Feacalbacteria* spp. Cause an increase of inflammation which affects the development of the brain, and finally the pathogenesis of ADHD.

4. Results

4.1. Obstetric Mode of Delivery: Vaginal Birth vs. Caesarean Section (C-Section)

As infants delivered by vaginal birth move through the birth canal, they get colonized by their mother's vaginal microbiota, and thus, adopted a resembling gut microbiome. In contrast, infants born via c-section are colonized by the microbiota of their mother's skin. Therefore, the delivery mode affects the composition of the gut microbiota in infants [121].

Results of various studies showed that in comparison to vaginally born infants, babies delivered by c-section had a decreased gut microbiota diversity including lower levels of *Bifidobacterium* spp. and Bacteroidetes, but increased levels *Clostridium difficile* [122] up until the age of two years [123].

Several research groups studied the correlation between c-section delivery and ADHD (see Table 2). An animal study showed a correlation between offspring born via c-section and altered dopamine metabolism throughout development [124]. It is important to note that these results might have been confounded by indication, which means that the altered dopamine response might be due to triggers that lead to a c-section [125]. In contrast to the above findings, two previous case-control studies found no significant correlation between c-sections and ADHD [126,127] in humans. A systematic review by Curran et al. initially showed a slight increase in the prevalence of ADHD in children born via c-section [128]. This correlation was challenged in their later study due to confounders, such as not differentiating between elective and emergency c-sections [129]. The only correlation that still seemed to be consistent was an increased prevalence of ADHD in children born via emergency c-sections. Confirmative data were obtained in a prospective cohort study using 671,592 Danish children. They found a significantly increased chance of children developing ADHD (Hazard Ratio 1.21) for intrapartum c-sections, but no effect when born by an elective c-section [130]. In contrast, the Millenium UK cohort study testing 13,141 children found no correlation between ADHD and mode of delivery despite differentiating between emergency, planned and induced c-sections [131].

Table 2. List of seven studies that tested the effects of c-section delivery on the development of ADHD. The table describes if the studies differentiated between the types of c-sections and their effects, and finally shows the sample size and statistical significance level of the individual studies. The symbol - represents that for these studies, this information could not be found as the studies were systematic reviews. The data shows that elective vs. emergency c-sections seem to have different effects on ADHD. p levels less than 0.05 were considered statistically different.

Source	Type of C-Section	Effect	Sample Size (n)	Statistical Significance (p)
[124]	No differentiation	Altered dopamine response	-	-
[126]	No differentiation	No effect	248	$p = 0.005$
[127]	No differentiation	No effect	12,991	$p < 0.05$
[128]	No differentiation	Positive correlation to ADHD	-	-
[129]	Elective vs. intrapartum	Only intrapartum c-sections showed a positive correlation to ADHD	1,722,548	$p < 0.05$
[130]	Elective vs. intrapartum	Only intrapartum c-sections showed a positive correlation to ADHD	671,592	$p < 0.05$
[131]	Elective vs. intrapartum	No effect	13,141	$p < 0.05$

The reasons for finding a positive correlation between intrapartum c-sections and ADHD development cannot unequivocally be explained as multiple confounders, such as unobserved familial factors, birth weight or gestational age also directly influence the mode of delivery and ADHD. However, there is a strong indication that the microbiota plays a subordinate role in this correlation as Axelsson et al. discovered that exposure of the newborn to ruptured vs. non-ruptured membranes prior to c-section did not influence the correlation between c-section and ADHD development [130].

To conclude, the accumulative data show that the mode of delivery affects the composition of the gut microbiota. However, a clear correlation between c-section delivery and a higher chance of developing ADHD cannot be found as results depend on various confounders and the type of c-section, whereby intrapartum c-sections show a positive correlation with the development of ADHD in comparison to elective c-sections.

4.2. Stress of the Mother

A prospective follow up study, and a Dutch population-based cohort study concluded a correlation between prenatal maternal stress exposure and an increase in ADHD in their offspring [132,133]. This data was confirmed by a Canadian study enrolling 203 pregnant women exposed to stress. Sixty-two of them were exposed to severe prenatal stress (experienced physical or sexual abuse, or death of a close relative) and delivered children with more severe ADHD symptoms in comparison to the 48 mothers who experienced moderate stress (financial or marital troubles) [134].

An animal study using quantitative PCR determined that maternal stress significantly decreased one of the most abundant taxa in the maternal vaginal flora, *Lactobacillus* spp. [135]. Consequently, *Lactobacillus* spp. was also significantly decreased in the distal colon of the offspring of stress exposed mothers. Additionally, a review focusing on the immunomodulatory effects of *Lactobacillus* spp. shows that stress reduces the abundance of this species independent of the host being pregnant or not [136]. *Lactobacillus* spp. is important for the synthesis of acetylcholine, while together with *Bifidobacteria* spp. it is contributing to the production of the main inhibitory neurotransmitter GABA [137]. Alterations in the GABAergic system have been associated with neurodevelopmental diseases, such as autism spectrum disorder and ADHD. This system is especially susceptible to alterations during development as GABAergic neurons originate from a different part of the neural tube than GABA's most important counterpart, the glutamatergic system. ADHD symptoms may be explained by the hypothesis that inhibitory functions of the cerebral cortex are reduced, leading to a reduction of filtering sensory influences, and finally having difficulties choosing the right behavioral reaction [138].

As described above, several studies have associated low levels of cerebral GABA concentrations with symptoms of ADHD [139–141]. Furthermore, a randomized controlled study showed that *Lactobacillus rhamnosus* also has a preventive effect as the administration of this bacterium in the first six months of life reduced the risk of ADHD and Asperger Syndrome (AS) [142]. The positive effects of this species may be due to the fact that *Lactobacillus rhamnosus* is, on the one hand, implicated in the development of tight junctions responsible for a strong gut barrier, and on the other hand, important for the immunoglobulin A and mucin production [143].

Various factors influence the development of ADHD, among which the neuroinhibitory neurotransmitter GABA seems to play a crucial role. However, to what extent low levels of *Lactobacillus* spp. and decreased concentrations of GABA are associated and how they precisely affect the development of ADHD remains unclear and has to be thoroughly investigated.

4.3. Preterm

Preterm babies that, thus, have gone through stressful situations similarly show lower levels of *Lactobacillus* spp. [144], and simultaneously have a significant increase in the prevalence of ADHD [58,145,146]. More specifically, Barrett et al. showed an increased abundance of *Proteobacteria* spp., while discovering undetectable levels of *Lactobacillus* spp. and *Bifidobacteria* spp. [144,147]. Chou et al. discovered that certain strains of *Lactobacillus* spp. show a protective trait towards the CNS. Preterm babies received strains of *Lactobacillus reuteri* and *Lactobacillus rhamnous* as probiotics for six weeks. This treatment resulted in a significantly reduced number of babies with neurological aberrations at one year of age in comparison to the group fed with *Lactobacillus acidophilus* and *Bifidobacterium infantis* [148].

It is widely known that preterm infants own an immature immune system as the innate and adaptive immune system has not developed fully. Due to their immature immune response and their usual extended hospital stay, infants are highly susceptible to nosocomial spread infections [149]. The increased number of infections may impair the neurodevelopment, and thus, might influence the development of the most common neurodevelopmental disorder ADHD. In addition to this, the weeks before term delivery (between 37 0/7 and 41 6/7) [150] represent an important stage in the neurodevelopment of the brain usually occurring in the protective womb of the mother [151,152]. Thus, preterm babies suffer from underdeveloped brain structures that in combination with postnatal complications, such as infections can lead to cell death of neurons, and finally lead to a decrease in the volume of specific areas of the brain [153].

As the prevalence of infection in premature newborns is high, the use of therapeutic antibiotics is similarly increased. Antibiotics have been associated with altering functions in the host's brain [154], while simultaneously, they are notoriously known for reducing the diversity of the microbiota [155]. Nevertheless, the direct effects of a lower microbiota diversity on the neurodevelopment have still not been thoroughly researched on, and thus, a concrete correlation cannot be made.

To summarize, a preterm baby is exposed to increased levels of stress, may have underdeveloped brain structures and owns an immature immune system. All of these result in a higher susceptibility to infections, and finally may lead to increased exposure to therapeutic antibiotics. These factors influence the neurodevelopment either directly through inflammatory processes during infections or indirectly by changing the composition of the gut microbiome.

4.4. Breastfeeding vs. Formula Feeding

Studies have associated breastfeeding with a lower prevalence of ADHD [156]. In contrast, formula-fed newborns showed a strong correlation with ADHD diagnosis [157–159]. The nutritious breast milk not only contains human milk oligosaccharides acting as prebiotics important for establishing a healthy gut microbiome, but also consists of vitamins and antibodies [160]. The latter being important in the first couple of months for the maturation of the innate immune system of the newborn [161]. Additionally, breast milk is marked to have a rich fat content due to its high levels of long-chain fatty acids, which are said to have protective effects on the CNS and the development of ADHD [162,163]. The gut microbiota of breastfed infants is less diverse in comparison to formula-fed infants [164]. Importantly, various groups utilizing differing methods for microbiome analysis, such as 16S sequencing or cytogenic FISH technique discovered that in both groups, the most prevalent genus is *Bifidobacterium* [122,164,165].

A systematic review by Guaraldi et al. showed that bottle-fed infants have a higher number of *Escherichia coli, Clostridium difficile, Bacteroides* spp. and *Lactobacilli* [166]. As seen in Table 3, research papers demonstrated that increased levels of *Lactobacillus acidophilus* [122], *Streptococcus, Veillonella parvula* [164], and *Clostridium coccoides* [165], were found in formula-fed infants. Although *Bifidobacterium* is the most prevalent genus found in both groups, breastfed infants show more than double of *Bifidobacteria* cells in comparison to formula-fed infants [164]. *Bifidobacterium infantis* has protective properties against pathogens as it supports the barrier function of the mucosa and concurrently has anti-inflammatory properties, thus, promotes a healthy immunological response [167,168].

Although the effect on the microbial composition could be the main cause of developing ADHD when being formula-fed, one has to consider the fact that other ingredients in the formula may also act as important influences. One study found that there were more cases of ADHD in formula-fed infants in 2007, than in December 2011. During the latter, the neurotoxic chemical Bisphenol A (BPA) was significantly reduced in formula cans and baby bottles in comparison to the former, suggesting that BPA might be the actual trigger of the correlation [169].

Table 3. Listing the different genera, predominantly found in formula-fed vs. breastfed infants. The arrow ↑ describes that this genus is increased in variously fed infants, while '-' represents that there is no significant change in this genus. One can clearly see that microbial diversity is increased in formula-fed in comparison to breastfed infants. p levels less than 0.05 were considered statistically different.

Genus	Formula-Fed	Sample Size (n)	Statistical Significance (p)	Breastfed	Sample Size (n)	Statistical Significance (p)
Bifidobacterium	↑ [122]	232	$p < 0.01$	↑ [122]	700	$p < 0.01$
	↑ [164]	6	$p < 0.05$	↑ [164]	6	$p < 0.05$
	↑ [165]	182	$p < 0.001$	↑ [165]	312	$p < 0.001$
Escherichia coli	↑ [122]	232	$p < 0.01$	-	700	$p < 0.01$
Bacteroides	↑ [122]	232	$p < 0.01$	-	700	$p < 0.01$
Lactobacillus	↑ [122]	232	$p < 0.01$	-	700	$p < 0.01$
Veillonella parvula	↑ [164]	6	$p < 0.05$	-	6	$p < 0.05$
Streptococcus	↑ [164]	6	$p < 0.05$	-	6	$p < 0.05$
Clostridium coccoides	↑ [165]	182	$p < 0.014$	-	312	$p < 0.014$

In summary, studies show that breastfeeding correlates negatively with the risk of developing ADHD, whereas formula-feeding increases this risk. Nevertheless, despite the highly nutritious content of breast milk, the gut microbiota of breastfed infants seems less diverse, but still contains the same or higher amount of protective components than formula-fed infants. Thus, alteration of the microbiome composition could potentially be a reason for the positive correlation between formula-feeding and the risk of developing ADHD.

4.5. Short Chain Fatty Acids

SCFAs are products of polysaccharides which could not be properly digested by the human digestive system, and thus, are broken down by microbial fermentation. Bacteria, such as *Bacteroides* spp. and *Clostridiae* spp., are two of the most important microbes for the production of SCFAs [21]. SCFAs represent not only a major energy source for microorganisms, but also show neuroactive and anti-inflammatory effects on the host [170,171]. A study by MacFabe et al. demonstrated that when SCFAs, such as propionic acid are intracebreoventriculary (ICV), administered to rodents, they show biochemical alterations similar to individuals who from autism [172]. Besides, the same authors found that high levels of the SCFA worsened symptoms of autistic individuals [172].

As ADHD, similar to autism, is a neurodevelopmental disease, it seems likely that SCFAs may affect the development of ADHD. Research shows that SCFAs influence the immune system, and as discussed earlier, this can influence the CNS [50]. An animal study using mice showed that the microbiome could influence the levels of the brain-derived neurotrophic factor (BDNF) via SCFA production [173]. The neurotrophin BDNF is important for neurogenesis and has a positive effect on the survival of neurons meaning that the microbiome can indirectly influence neural functions via SCFA's modulating effect on the BDNF production. The same study showed that GF mice whose BDNF levels had been decreased displayed problems with their working memory [173]. Confirmatory data were generated by Corominas-Roso et al. who showed in a human study that adults with ADHD have lower levels of BDNF compared to healthy controls [174]. Similarly, Akay et al. tested the effects of methylphenidate on BDNF levels on 50 drug-naïve ADHD boys and detected significantly increased BDNF levels in the serum and improved ADHD symptoms after eight weeks of methylphenidate treatment [175]. The same findings were found by an older study by Amiri et al. [176]. This is a direct confirmation of a potential link between the dopaminergic system, BDNF function, and ADHD. In contrast, another study enrolling 41 untreated ADHD and 107 control patients concluded that drug-naïve ADHD children had higher levels of BDNF in their plasma and that these levels are positively associated with the severity of inattentiveness [177].

Besides hypothesizing a compensatory mechanism in ADHD children, a potential reason for these differing results could be varying methodology as Akay et al. measured BDNF levels in the serum, known to have a higher BDNF concertation in comparison to the plasma [178].

In conclusion, SCFAs most probably affect the development of ADHD indirectly by influencing the production of BDNF.

4.6. Polyunsaturated Fatty Acids

Another regulator of BDNF seems to be omega-3 polyunsaturated fatty acids (PUFAs). PUFAs are long chains of carbon atoms characterized by a carboxyl group at one end and a methyl group at the other end. As they are unsaturated, they own one or more double bonds between the carbon atoms. Naturally, plant and fish oils, such as flaxseed or salmon have a high content of omega-3 PUFAs [179]. PUFAs play an important role in membrane fluidity, neuronal membranes, neurotransmission, and receptor function [180]. Furthermore, the omega-3 fatty acid, docosahexaenoic acid (DHA), is indispensable for cognition function throughout the lifespan [181]. Indeed, already intrauterine PUFA deficiencies lead to altered cognitive and attentive skills [182].

An animal study showed that omega-3 PUFAs did not only affect the levels of BDNF, but also of glial cell-derived neurotrophic factor (GDNF). The latter is especially important for the recovery of dopaminergic neurons in Parkinson's disease (PD) as it promotes the survival of the dopamine system in the nigrostriatum. Hence, GDNF is shown to be neuroprotective and supporting dopaminergic neurons in PD models, and thus, could potentially be utilized as a therapy against neurodegenerative diseases, especially PD [183,184]. Furthermore, another study found that lower levels of omega-3 fatty acids were associated with lower levels of BDNF in the frontal cortex of rats [185], a part of the brain where various psychiatric illnesses, such as bipolar disease can be manifested [186]. Additionally, omega-3 PUFAs show antimicrobial effects as they increase levels of *Enterobacteria* and *Bifidobacteria*, which both strengthen intestinal permeability, reducing the risk of inflammation [187]. Finally, omega-3 PUFAs have the ability to stimulate macrophages that inhibit the activation of the NLRP3 inflammasome, and thus, decrease levels of the previously mentioned pro-inflammatory IL-1beta [188]. Nevertheless, it is important to note that an excess of omega-6 PUFAs benefits the development of endotoxemia leading to low-grade systematic inflammation, explaining why a low ratio of omega-6/omega-3 PUFAs should be targeted [189,190].

Human studies have discovered a negative correlation between patients with ADHD and levels of PUFAs. An Italian study examined the levels of PUFAs in the blood of 51 ADHD and 22 non-ADHD patients. PUFA levels in the blood of ADHD patients were significantly lower and correlated with behavioral symptoms, but were not associated with cognitive skills [191]. Similarly, a systematic review concluded that in all randomized control trials (RCT) analyzed (7 RCTs, n = 534), omega-3 PUFA supplementation led to an improvement in clinical ADHD symptoms. Furthermore, in three out of the seven RCT's (n = 396), the omega-3 PUFA supplementation was associated with improvements in cognitive skills [192]. Due to these findings, questions of PUFAs being a potential therapeutic medication for ADHD patients seem to be warranted.

Moreover, a double-blind trial [193] assessed the effects of inducing the noradrenaline reuptake inhibitor (Atomoxetine) conventionally used to treat ADHD, to the patient and control group and PUFAs, such as eicosapentanoic acid (EPA) and DHA solely to the ADHD patients. The medication was given on a daily basis for four months to a total of 50 children. Although PUFAs improved ADHD symptoms, this experiment showed no clinically significant difference in the ADHD Conners Parent rating scale, questioning the overall therapeutic effect of PUFAs against ADHD, even if some beneficial effects are evident [193]. Supporting these results, a systematic review discussing results of 14 meta-analyses inducing PUFAs to ADHD children showed a very small effect size when parents and teachers rated children's behavior using the Conners scale [194].

Lastly, on a microbial level, an RCT showed that the intake of PUFAs does not seem to affect the alpha or beta diversity of the microbiota of the participants. Nevertheless, it did show a reversible increase in genera, such as *Bifidobacterium roseburia* and *Lactobaccilus* spp., all of which are important for the production of SCFAs and maintain an anti-inflammatory environment [195]. Similarly, a commentary discussing the importance of long-chain PUFAs as a mean to restore a healthy gut microbiome, deduced that PUFA ingestion may act as a protector from developing systemic inflammation and in the long term, chronic disease. It is, therefore, hypothesized that PUFA supplementation would not only be of therapeutic importance for ADHD, but also a prophylactic measurement against cancer as inflammation leads to immunosuppression and activates immune checkpoints resulting in an optimal tumor microenvironment [196].

Although the collected data show inconclusive results concerning the effect of PUFA supplementation as a therapeutic measurement for ADHD, the indirect effects of ingesting PUFAs and its impact on the microbiome may as well be crucial determinants that could modify the metabolism and consequently the behavioral and cognitive symptoms of ADHD.

4.7. Antibiotics

Although the development of antibiotics has made it possible to treat life-threatening infections, the use of antibiotics reduces the microbiota diversity in the GI-tract [197]. Consequently, the use of antibiotics may elevate the number of pathogenic bacteria, such as *Enterobacter, Klebsiella, Citrobacter, and Pseudomonas* and decrease anaerobic bacteria [197]. For example, a human study analyzing the short term parenteral-neonatal antibiotic usage showed that it reduced the number of protective *Bifidobacteria* in the first couple of months of life [198]. Supporting these results, Penders et al. not only found a decrease of *Bifidobacteria*, but also of *Bacteroides* when infants administered antibiotics [122].

Results concerning the correlation of early antibiotic use and later risk of developing ADHD seem to be incoherent. A Danish population-based cohort study did not find an association in sibling-stratified Cox model between antibiotic use in the first two years of life and the risk of developing ADHD [130]. Another study, however, using 871 European newborns examined the effects of early antibiotic treatment on cognitive functions with the help of IQ and reading tests, and on symptoms of ADHD using the mentioned Conners Rating Scale-Revised (CRS-R). Thereby they discovered that children who consumed antibiotics in the first year of life showed a reduced reading ability score, higher scores on the CRS-R, rated by parents, and increased symptoms of ADHD at the ages of 7–11 years. Nonetheless, this association was not made for babies and children that used antibiotics between the ages of 12 months and 3.5 years. This indicates that one of the vital factors for developing ADHD is the age in which the newborn consumes the antibiotics. It seems that during the first 12 months of life, important developments of the gut-brain axis take place, which when disrupted influence the neurodevelopment, and thus, the CNS in the long run [12]. These data, however, must be interpreted with caution, as this was not an RCT. Accordingly, direct causation between the antibiotic use and later seen ADHD cannot be correctly made [199].

4.8. Probiotics

By definition of the FAO/WHO probiotics are "live microorganisms which when administered in adequate amounts confer a health benefit on the host" [200]. Benefits of probiotics include reinforcing a more desirable environment in the gut, a healthy digestive system, and finally an adequate immune system [201]. Thereby probiotics help to sustain and produce healthy enzymes while eradicating potentially harmful pathogens [202,203]. Naturally occurring probiotic sources include lactic acid fermented vegetables, such as kimchi or fermented dairy products as, for example, yogurt [204].

The influence of probiotic strains on psychiatric diseases has been examined by multiple studies, concluding a positive effect on such illnesses and are, thus, described as "psychobiotics" [90]. An animal study using mice showed that probiotic ingestion of *Bifidobacterium longum* and *breve* led to a reduction of depression and anxiety symptoms [205].

The seminal study by Pärtty et al. researched the effects of probiotic use on the development of ADHD in children by randomly administering strains of *Lactobacillus rhamnosus* into 75 infants.

The infants were monitored at three weeks, 3, 6, 12, 18 and 24 months, and finally, at 13 years of age. The authors concluded that at the age of 13 years, ADHD was diagnosed in 6/35 (17.1%) children using the placebo, whereas no children had this disorder in the probiotic group. These results, even if encouraging, do not identify any specific composition of the microbiota to the neurodevelopmental disease, and thus, might mean that probiotics decrease ADHD in a different way rather than influencing the composition of the microbiome [142]. However, it is important to conclude that these findings potentially represent a method to reduce the risk of developing ADHD.

5. Discussion

This literature review demonstrates that the ADHD population has a different gut microbial composition in comparison to healthy controls as the phylum Actinobacteria is more and Firmicutes less abundant in ADHD patients. The genus *Bifidobacterium*, belonging to the phylum Actinobacteria, seems to play a significant role in the pathogenesis of ADHD and is recurrently influenced by several factors. *Bifidobacteria* do not only protect the barrier function in the gut and support a healthy immune response [168], but also influence the dopamine system by elevating the production of CDT which increases phenylalanine levels, and finally, results in higher levels of dopamine. This review showed that *Bifidobacterium* was decreased in offspring that were born (i) via c-section delivery ([122,123], (ii) as preterms [144,206], (iii) were breastfed [164] or (iv) were given antibiotics in the first months of life [122,198]. All of these factors are simultaneously associated with an increased risk of developing ADHD. Nevertheless, using *Bifidobacterium* as a potential biomarker for diagnosis of ADHD seems uncertain due to varying results regarding *Bifidobacterium* levels in ADHD patients. Although Pärtty et al. observed decreased levels of *Bifidobacterium* in 3 and 6-month-old ADHD patients [142], Aarts et al. detected slightly increased levels of the genus using a larger sample size and a more sensitive methodology [69]. Thus, for future research, well-designed studies, using a larger sample size, are needed to deduce a definite correlation between levels of *Bifidobacterium* and ADHD and the importance of this genus as a biomarker.

Additionally, this article concludes that the concertation of neuroprotective BDNF, indirectly influenced by the microbiome [173], plays a vital role in the pathogenesis of ADHD. The majority of reports showed a negative correlation between levels of BDNF and ADHD [173,174,207]. As the levels of SCFAs [173], and PUFAs [185] are positively correlated with BDNF, omega-3 fatty acids may prove to be of therapeutic importance. So far, various studies have shown that adding PUFAs to the diet only marginally decreases the symptoms of ADHD [193,194,208]. Future studies could assess the effects of various concentrations of PUFAs and age at which these were ingested on the symptom development of ADHD. BDNF shows properties important for neurogenesis in the critical stages of neurodevelopment. The production of SCFAs by the microbiome has been positively associated with levels of BDNF [173]. Therefore, increasing SCFAs through fiber-rich nutrition in combination with the appropriate gut microbial composition could also be a beneficial means for the treatment of ADHD symptoms.

It is widely known that c-section delivery causes the offspring's microbiome to be more similar to the mother's skin rather than her vaginal flora. However, it is still under debate to what extent this change impacts the development of ADHD. We decided to concentrate on the more recent papers, that used a large sample size and a precise methodology by differentiating between elective and emergency c-sections. These studies show that not every c-section increases the risk of developing ADHD, but only those that were done intrapartum [129,130]. Although this correlation is most probably not due to a differing microbial composition and rather due to various confounders, such as gestational age and birth weight [130], it is still important to note that emergency c-sections bear an intrinsic risk for the offspring developing ADHD.

Additionally, it has become increasingly clear to what extent prematurity plays a role in the development of ADHD. As the GI-tract and its colonization with bacteria are still underdeveloped, the microbiome shows lower levels of neuroprotective *Lactobacillus* [144]. Nonetheless, this decrease of the genus has not yet been directly associated with the development of ADHD. Much more important seems to be the combination of premature infants having underdeveloped brain structures and an immature immune system resulting in being more prone to neuronal cell death and infections that promote neuroinflammation, and finally influence the neurodevelopment. It is difficult to deduce the exact impact of microbial changes in preterms on the development of ADHD, as there are numerous confounders [153]. Thus, future studies should elucidate and concentrate on levels of pro-inflammatory cytokines in neonates and determine the extent to which underdeveloped brain structures influence the development of ADHD. Once these have been thoroughly understood, one can assess in what way the microbiome plays a role in the pathophysiology of prenates having a higher prevalence of ADHD. As the topic of this literature review is relatively new, only a limited number of studies examining the link between ADHD and the microbiota could be found. Hence, it was challenging to draw concrete conclusions from the scarce available data. A solid conclusion will require future investigations enrolling larger populations with defined pathologies to be able to analyze the study outcomes using robust statistical analysis. Finally, it is important that future trials use standardized methodologies for an unambiguous comparison of the outcomes and results. This literature review has made it clear that certain factors are associated with ADHD, while simultaneously changing the guts microbiome. Nevertheless, it remains yet to be determined to what extent the composition of the microbiome in the gut influences the development of ADHD.

6. Conclusions

To determine to what extent the microbiome plays a role in the pathophysiology of ADHD, further studies are needed. We discussed several triggers that have been associated with ADHD, how these correlate with an altered microbial composition, and thus, how various microbes might act as possible biomarkers for ADHD. Further research, on the microbial composition of ADHD patients using large, well-diagnosed cohorts is needed in order to find future conclusive biomarkers and therapeutic methods to treat ADHD.

Author Contributions: Conceptualization, S.B.-L. and M.H.M.; Methodology, S.B.-L. and M.H.M.; Validation, M.H.M.; Formal Analysis, S.B.-L., and M.H.M.; Investigation, S.B.-L., and M.H.M., Resources, S.B.-L. and M.H.M.; Data curation, S.B.-L.; Writing—Original Draft Preparation, S.B.-L.; Writing—Review and Editing, S.B.-L. and M.H.M.; Visualization, S.B.-L.; Supervision, M.H.M.; Project Administration, M.H.M. and S.B.-L.

Funding: This research received no external funding.

Acknowledgments: We thank David Wolfer for helpful discussions and for critically reading this manuscript.

Conflicts of Interest: The authors declare no conflict of interest.

References

1. Thursby, E.; Juge, N. Introduction to the human gut microbiota. *Biochem. J.* **2017**, *474*, 1823–1836. [CrossRef] [PubMed]
2. Sender, R.; Fuchs, S.; Milo, R. Revised Estimates for the Number of Human and Bacteria Cells in the Body. *PLoS Biol.* **2016**, *14*, 1002533. [CrossRef] [PubMed]
3. Bäumler, A.J.; Sperandio, V. Interactions between the microbiota and pathogenic bacteria in the gut. *Nature* **2016**, *535*, 85–93. [CrossRef] [PubMed]
4. Mohajeri, M.H.; La Fata, G.; Steinert, R.E.; Weber, P. Relationship between the gut microbiome and brain function. *Nutr. Rev.* **2018**, *76*, 481–496. [CrossRef]
5. Mohajeri, M.H.; Brummer, R.J.M.; Rastall, R.A.; Weersma, R.K.; Harmsen, H.J.M.; Faas, M.; Eggersdorfer, M. The role of the microbiome for human health: From basic science to clinical applications. *Eur. J. Nutr.* **2018**, *57*, 1–14. [CrossRef]
6. Dinan, T.G.; Cryan, J.F. The Microbiome-Gut-Brain Axis in Health and Disease. *Gastroenterol. Clin. N. Am.* **2017**, *46*, 77–89. [CrossRef]

7. Cotillard, A.; ANR MicroObes consortium; Kennedy, S.P.; Kong, L.C.; Prifti, E.; Pons, N.; Le Chatelier, E.; Almeida, M.; Quinquis, B.; Levenez, F.; et al. Dietary intervention impact on gut microbial gene richness. *Nature* **2013**, *500*, 585–588. [CrossRef]
8. Stower, H. Depression linked to the microbiome. *Nat. Med.* **2019**, *25*, 358. [CrossRef]
9. Gerhardt, S.; Mohajeri, M.H. Changes of Colonic Bacterial Composition in Parkinson's Disease and Other Neurodegenerative Diseases. *Nutrients* **2018**, *10*, 708. [CrossRef]
10. Dickerson, F.; Severance, E.; Yolken, R. The microbiome, immunity, and schizophrenia and bipolar disorder. *Brain Behav. Immun.* **2017**, *62*, 46–52. [CrossRef]
11. Srikantha, P.; Mohajeri, M.H. The Possible Role of the Microbiota-Gut-Brain-Axis in Autism Spectrum Disorder. *Int. J. Mol. Sci.* **2019**, *20*, 2115. [CrossRef] [PubMed]
12. Borre, Y.E.; O'Keeffe, G.W.; Clarke, G.; Stanton, C.; Dinan, T.G.; Cryan, J.F. Microbiota and neurodevelopmental windows: Implications for brain disorders. *Trends Mol. Med.* **2014**, *20*, 509–518. [CrossRef] [PubMed]
13. Association, A.P. *Diagnostic and Statistical Manual of Mental Disorders*; American Psychiatric Pub: Washington, DC, USA, 2013.
14. Polanczyk, G.; De Lima, M.S.; Horta, B.L.; Biederman, J.; Rohde, L.A. The Worldwide Prevalence of ADHD: A Systematic Review and Metaregression Analysis. *Am. J. Psychiatry* **2007**, *164*, 942–948. [CrossRef] [PubMed]
15. Thomas, R.; Sanders, S.; Doust, J.; Beller, E.; Glasziou, P. Prevalence of Attention-Deficit/Hyperactivity Disorder: A Systematic Review and Meta-analysis. *Pediatrics* **2015**, *135*, e994–e1001. [CrossRef]
16. Wender, P.H.; Wolf, L.E.; Wasserstein, J. Adults with ADHD. An overview. *Ann. N. Y. Acad. Sci.* **2001**, *931*, 1–16. [CrossRef]
17. Wilens, T.E.; Biederman, J.; Faraone, S.V.; Martelon, M.; Westerberg, D.; Spencer, T.J. Presenting ADHD symptoms, subtypes, and comorbid disorders in clinically referred adults with ADHD. *J. Clin. Psychiatry* **2009**, *70*, 1557–1562. [CrossRef]
18. Ding, H.T.; Taur, Y.; Walkup, J.T. Gut Microbiota and Autism: Key Concepts and Findings. *J. Autism. Dev. Disord.* **2017**, *47*, 480–489. [CrossRef]
19. Rescigno, M. Intestinal microbiota and its effects on the immune system. *Cell. Microbiol.* **2014**, *16*, 1004–1013. [CrossRef]
20. Bora, S.A.; Kennett, M.J.; Smith, P.B.; Patterson, A.D.; Cantorna, M.T. The Gut Microbiota Regulates Endocrine Vitamin D Metabolism through Fibroblast Growth Factor. *Front. Immunol.* **2018**, *9*, 408. [CrossRef]
21. Macfarlane, S.; Macfarlane, G.T. Regulation of short-chain fatty acid production. *Proc. Nutr. Soc.* **2003**, *62*, 67–72. [CrossRef]
22. Dethlefsen, L.; Eckburg, P.B.; Bik, E.M.; Relman, D.A. Assembly of the human intestinal microbiota. *Trends Ecol. Evol.* **2006**, *21*, 517–523. [CrossRef] [PubMed]
23. Douglas-Escobar, M.; Elliott, E.; Neu, J. Effect of Intestinal Microbial Ecology on the Developing Brain. *JAMA Pediatr.* **2013**, *167*, 374. [CrossRef] [PubMed]
24. Goodrich, J.K.; Davenport, E.R.; Waters, J.L.; Clark, A.G.; Ley, R.E. Cross-species comparisons of host genetic associations with the microbiome. *Science* **2016**, *352*, 532–535. [CrossRef] [PubMed]
25. Carmody, R.N.; Gerber, G.K.; Luevano, J.M.; Gatti, D.M.; Somes, L.; Svenson, K.L.; Turnbaugh, P.J. Diet dominates host genotype in shaping the murine gut microbiota. *Cell Host Microbe* **2015**, *17*, 72–84. [CrossRef]
26. Bik, E.M. The Hoops, Hopes, and Hypes of Human Microbiome Research. *Yale J. Boil. Med.* **2016**, *89*, 363–373.
27. Buie, T. Potential Etiologic Factors of Microbiome Disruption in Autism. *Clin. Ther.* **2015**, *37*, 976–983. [CrossRef]
28. Koenig, J.E.; Spor, A.; Scalfone, N.; Fricker, A.D.; Stombaugh, J.; Knight, R.; Angenent, L.T.; Ley, R.E. Succession of microbial consortia in the developing infant gut microbiome. *Proc. Natl. Acad. Sci. USA* **2011**, *108*, 4578–4585. [CrossRef]
29. Collado, M.C.; Rautava, S.; Aakko, J.; Isolauri, E.; Salminen, S. Human gut colonisation may be initiated in utero by distinct microbial communities in the placenta and amniotic fluid. *Sci. Rep.* **2016**, *6*, 23129. [CrossRef]
30. MacIntyre, D.A.; Chandiramani, M.; Lee, Y.S.; Kindinger, L.; Smith, A.; Angelopoulos, N.; Lehne, B.; Arulkumaran, S.; Brown, R.; Teoh, T.G.; et al. The vaginal microbiome during pregnancy and the postpartum period in a European population. *Sci. Rep.* **2015**, *5*, 8988. [CrossRef]
31. Aagaard, K.; Ma, J.; Antony, K.M.; Ganu, R.; Petrosino, J.; Versalovic, J. The Placenta Harbors a Unique Microbiome. *Sci. Transl. Med.* **2014**, *6*, 237ra65. [CrossRef]

32. Human Microbiome Jumpstart Reference Strains Consortium; Nelson, K.E.; Weinstock, G.M.; Highlander, S.K.; Worley, K.C.; Creasy, H.H.; Wortman, J.R.; Rusch, D.B.; Mitreva, M.; Sodergren, E.; et al. A catalog of reference genomes from the human microbiome. *Science* **2010**, *328*, 994–999. [CrossRef] [PubMed]
33. Brotman, R.M. Vaginal microbiome and sexually transmitted infections: An epidemiologic perspective. *J. Clin. Investig.* **2011**, *121*, 4610–4617. [CrossRef] [PubMed]
34. Dogra, S.; Sakwinska, O.; Soh, S.-E.; Ngom-Bru, C.; Brück, W.M.; Berger, B.; Brüssow, H.; Karnani, N.; Lee, Y.S.; Yap, F.; et al. Rate of establishing the gut microbiota in infancy has consequences for future health. *Gut Microbes* **2015**, *6*, 321–325. [CrossRef] [PubMed]
35. Bäckhed, F.; Roswall, J.; Peng, Y.; Feng, Q.; Jia, H.; Kovatcheva-Datchary, P.; Li, Y.; Xia, Y.; Xie, H.; Zhong, H.; et al. Dynamics and Stabilization of the Human Gut Microbiome during the First Year of Life. *Cell Host Microbe* **2015**, *17*, 852. [CrossRef]
36. Latorre, R.; Sternini, C.; De Giorgio, R.; Greenwood-Van Meerveld, B. Enteroendocrine cells: A review of their role in brain-gut communication. *Neurogastroenterol. Motil.* **2016**, *28*, 620–630. [CrossRef]
37. Mayer, E.A.; Knight, R.; Mazmanian, S.K.; Cryan, J.F.; Tillisch, K. Gut microbes and the brain: Paradigm shift in neuroscience. *J. Neurosci.* **2014**, *34*, 15490–15496. [CrossRef]
38. Cryan, J.F.; Dinan, T.G. Mind-altering microorganisms: The impact of the gut microbiota on brain and behaviour. *Nat. Rev. Neurosci.* **2012**, *13*, 701–712. [CrossRef]
39. Shaw, P.; Stringaris, A.; Nigg, J.; Leibenluft, E. Emotion dysregulation in attention deficit hyperactivity disorder. *Am. J. Psychiatry* **2014**, *171*, 276–293. [CrossRef]
40. Cortese, S.; Brown, T.E.; Corkum, P.; Gruber, R.; O'Brien, L.M.; Stein, M.; Weiss, M.; Owens, J. Assessment and Management of Sleep Problems in Youths With Attention-Deficit/Hyperactivity Disorder. *J. Am. Acad. Child. Adolesc. Psychiatry* **2013**, *52*, 784–796. [CrossRef]
41. Baird, A.L.; Coogan, A.N.; Siddiqui, A.; Donev, R.M.; Thome, J. Adult attention-deficit hyperactivity disorder is associated with alterations in circadian rhythms at the behavioural, endocrine and molecular levels. *Mol. Psychiatry* **2012**, *17*, 988–995. [CrossRef]
42. Van Lenten, S.A.; Doane, L.D. Examining multiple sleep behaviors and diurnal salivary cortisol and alpha-amylase: Within- and between-person associations. *Psychoneuroendocrinology* **2016**, *68*, 100–110. [CrossRef] [PubMed]
43. Tsigos, C.; Chrousos, G.P. Hypothalamic–pituitary–adrenal axis, neuroendocrine factors and stress. *J. Psychosom. Res.* **2002**, *53*, 865–871. [CrossRef]
44. Freitag, C.M.; Hänig, S.; Palmason, H.; Meyer, J.; Wüst, S.; Seitz, C. Cortisol awakening response in healthy children and children with ADHD: Impact of comorbid disorders and psychosocial risk factors. *Psychoneuroendocrinology* **2009**, *34*, 1019–1028. [CrossRef] [PubMed]
45. Blomqvist, M.; Holmberg, K.; Lindblad, F.; Fernell, E.; Ek, U.; Dahllöf, G. Salivary cortisol levels and dental anxiety in children with attention deficit hyperactivity disorder. *Eur. J. Oral Sci.* **2007**, *115*, 1–6. [CrossRef]
46. Corominas-Roso, M.; Palomar, G.; Ferrer, R.; Real, A.; Nogueira, M.; Corrales, M.; Casas, M.; Ramos-Quiroga, J.A. Cortisol Response to Stress in Adults with Attention Deficit Hyperactivity Disorder. *Int. J. Neuropsychopharmacol.* **2015**, *18*, 18. [CrossRef]
47. Lackschewitz, H.; Hüther, G.; Kröner-Herwig, B. Physiological and psychological stress responses in adults with attention-deficit/hyperactivity disorder (ADHD). *Psychoneuroendocrinology* **2008**, *33*, 612–624. [CrossRef]
48. Principi, N.; Esposito, S. Gut microbiota and central nervous system development. *J. Infect.* **2016**, *73*, 536–546. [CrossRef]
49. Sato, K. Effects of Microglia on Neurogenesis. *Glia* **2015**, *63*, 1394–1405. [CrossRef]
50. Erny, D.; De Angelis, A.L.H.; Jaitin, D.; Wieghofer, P.; Staszewski, O.; David, E.; Keren-Shaul, H.; Mahlakoiv, T.; Jakobshagen, K.; Buch, T.; et al. Host microbiota constantly control maturation and function of microglia in the CNS. *Nat. Neurosci.* **2015**, *18*, 965–977. [CrossRef]
51. Critchley, H.D.; Eccles, J.; Garfinkel, S.N. Interaction between cognition, emotion, and the autonomic nervous system. *Stroke* **2013**, *117*, 59–77.
52. Koopman, F.A.; Stoof, S.P.; Straub, R.H.; Van Maanen, M.A.; Vervoordeldonk, M.J.; Tak, P.P. Restoring the Balance of the Autonomic Nervous System as an Innovative Approach to the Treatment of Rheumatoid Arthritis. *Mol. Med.* **2011**, *17*, 937–948. [CrossRef] [PubMed]
53. Lyte, M. Microbial Endocrinology and the Microbiota-Gut-Brain Axis. *Adv. Exp. Med. Biol.* **2014**, *817*, 3–24. [PubMed]

54. Negrao, B.L.; Bipath, P.; Van Der Westhuizen, D.; Viljoen, M. Autonomic Correlates at Rest and during Evoked Attention in Children with Attention-Deficit/Hyperactivity Disorder and Effects of Methylphenidate. *Neuropsychobiology* **2011**, *63*, 82–91. [CrossRef] [PubMed]
55. Musser, E.D.; Backs, R.W.; Schmitt, C.F.; Ablow, J.C.; Measelle, J.R.; Nigg, J.T. Emotion regulation via the autonomic nervous system in children with attention-deficit/hyperactivity disorder (ADHD). *J. Abnorm. Child. Psychol.* **2011**, *39*, 841–852. [CrossRef] [PubMed]
56. Tandon, M.; Pergjika, A. Attention Deficit Hyperactivity Disorder in Preschool-Age Children. *Child Adolesc. Psychiatr Clin. N. Am.* **2017**, *26*, 523–538. [CrossRef] [PubMed]
57. Willcutt, E.G.; Nigg, J.T.; Pennington, B.F.; Solanto, M.V.; Rohde, L.A.; Tannock, R.; Loo, S.K.; Carlson, C.L.; McBurnett, K.; Lahey, B.B. Validity of DSM-IV attention deficit/hyperactivity disorder symptom dimensions and subtypes. *J. Abnorm. Psychol.* **2012**, *121*, 991–1010. [CrossRef]
58. Thapar, A.; Cooper, M.; Eyre, O.; Langley, K. What have we learnt about the causes of ADHD? *J. Child. Psychol. Psychiatry* **2013**, *54*, 3–16. [CrossRef]
59. Starobrat-Hermelin, B. The effect of deficiency of selected bioelements on hyperactivity in children with certain specified mental disorders. *Ann. Acad. Med. Stetin.* **1998**, *44*, 297–314.
60. Sciberras, E.; Mulraney, M.; Silva, D.; Coghill, D. Prenatal Risk Factors and the Etiology of ADHD—Review of Existing Evidence. *Curr. Psychiatry Rep.* **2017**, *19*, 1. [CrossRef]
61. Dias, T.G.C.; Kieling, C.; Graeff-Martins, A.S.; Moriyama, T.S.; Rohde, L.A.; Polanczyk, G.V. Developments and challenges in the diagnosis and treatment of ADHD. *Braz. J. Psychiatry* **2013**, *35*, S40–S50. [CrossRef]
62. Sharma, A.; Couture, J. A review of the pathophysiology, etiology, and treatment of attention-deficit hyperactivity disorder (ADHD). *Ann. Pharmacother.* **2014**, *48*, 209–225. [CrossRef] [PubMed]
63. Daubner, S.C.; Le, T.; Wang, S. Tyrosine hydroxylase and regulation of dopamine synthesis. *Arch. Biochem. Biophys.* **2011**, *508*, 1–12. [CrossRef] [PubMed]
64. Arias-Carrión, O.; Stamelou, M.; Murillo-Rodriguez, E.; Menéndez-González, M.; Pöppel, E. Dopaminergic reward system: A short integrative review. *Int. Arch. Med.* **2010**, *3*, 24. [CrossRef] [PubMed]
65. Dougherty, D.D.; Bonab, A.A.; Spencer, T.J.; Rauch, S.L.; Madras, B.K.; Fischman, A.J. Dopamine transporter density in patients with attention deficit hyperactivity disorder. *Lancet* **1999**, *354*, 2132–2133. [CrossRef]
66. Tong, J.; Meyer, J.H.; Furukawa, Y.; Boileau, I.; Chang, L.-J.; Wilson, A.A.; Houle, S.; Kish, S.J. Distribution of monoamine oxidase proteins in human brain: Implications for brain imaging studies. *Br. J. Pharmacol.* **2013**, *33*, 863–871. [CrossRef]
67. Seiden, L.S.; Sabol, K.E.; Ricaurte, G.A. Amphetamine: Effects on catecholamine systems and behavior. *Annu. Rev. Pharmacol. Toxicol.* **1993**, *33*, 639–677. [CrossRef]
68. Strandwitz, P. Neurotransmitter modulation by the gut microbiota. *Brain Res.* **2018**, *1693*, 128–133. [CrossRef]
69. Aarts, E.; Ederveen, T.H.A.; Naaijen, J.; Zwiers, M.P.; Boekhorst, J.; Timmerman, H.M.; Smeekens, S.P.; Netea, M.G.; Buitelaar, J.K.; Franke, B.; et al. Gut microbiome in ADHD and its relation to neural reward anticipation. *PLoS ONE* **2017**, *12*, e0183509. [CrossRef]
70. Lou, H. Dopamine precursors and brain function in phenylalanine hydroxylase deficiency. *Acta Paediatr.* **1994**, *83*, 86–88. [CrossRef]
71. Scheres, A.; Milham, M.P.; Knutson, B.; Castellanos, F.X. Ventral Striatal Hyporesponsiveness During Reward Anticipation in Attention-Deficit/Hyperactivity Disorder. *Boil. Psychiatry* **2007**, *61*, 720–724. [CrossRef]
72. Ming, X.; Chen, N.; Ray, C.; Brewer, G.; Kornitzer, J.; Steer, R.A. A Gut Feeling: A Hypothesis of the Role of the Microbiome in Attention-Deficit/Hyperactivity Disorders. *Child Neurol. Open* **2018**, *5*, 2329048X18786799. [CrossRef] [PubMed]
73. Antshel, K.M.; Waisbren, S.E. Developmental timing of exposure to elevated levels of phenylalanine is associated with ADHD symptom expression. *J. Abnorm. Child Psychol.* **2003**, *31*, 565–574. [CrossRef] [PubMed]
74. Baker, G.; Bornstein, R.; Rouget, A.; Ashton, S.; Van Muyden, J.; Coutts, R. Phenylethylaminergic mechanisms in attention-deficit disorder. *Boil. Psychiatry* **1991**, *29*, 15–22. [CrossRef]
75. Bornstein, R.; Baker, G.B.; Carroll, A.; King, G.; Wong, J.T.; Douglass, A.B. Plasma amino acids in attention deficit disorder. *Psychiatry Res.* **1990**, *33*, 301–306. [CrossRef]
76. Bergwerff, C.E.; Luman, M.; Blom, H.J.; Oosterlaan, J. No Tryptophan, Tyrosine and Phenylalanine Abnormalities in Children with Attention-Deficit/Hyperactivity Disorder. *PLoS ONE* **2016**, *11*, e0151100. [CrossRef]

77. O'Mahony, S.; Clarke, G.; Borre, Y.; Dinan, T.; Cryan, J.; Dinan, T. Serotonin, tryptophan metabolism and the brain-gut-microbiome axis. *Behav. Brain Res.* **2015**, *277*, 32–48. [CrossRef]
78. Dinan, T.G.; Stanton, C.; Cryan, J.F. Psychobiotics: A Novel Class of Psychotropic. *Boil. Psychiatry* **2013**, *74*, 720–726. [CrossRef]
79. Mawe, G.M.; Hoffman, J.M. Serotonin signalling in the gut—Functions, dysfunctions and therapeutic targets. *Nat. Rev. Gastroenterol. Hepatol.* **2013**, *10*, 473–486. [CrossRef]
80. Mechan, A.O.; Fowler, A.; Seifert, N.; Rieger, H.; Wöhrle, T.; Etheve, S.; Wyss, A.; Schüler, G.; Colletto, B.; Kilpert, C.; et al. Monoamine reuptake inhibition and mood-enhancing potential of a specified oregano extract. *Br. J. Nutr.* **2011**, *105*, 1150–1163. [CrossRef]
81. Banerjee, E.; Nandagopal, K. Does serotonin deficit mediate susceptibility to ADHD? *Neurochem. Int.* **2015**, *82*, 52–68. [CrossRef]
82. Johansson, J.; Landgren, M.; Fernell, E.; Vumma, R.; Åhlin, A.; Bjerkenstedt, L.; Venizelos, N. Altered tryptophan and alanine transport in fibroblasts from boys with attention-deficit/hyperactivity disorder (ADHD): An in vitro study. *Behav. Brain Funct.* **2011**, *7*, 40. [CrossRef] [PubMed]
83. Clarke, G.; Grenham, S.; Scully, P.; Fitzgerald, P.; Moloney, R.D.; Shanahan, F.; Dinan, T.G.; Cryan, J.F. The microbiome-gut-brain axis during early life regulates the hippocampal serotonergic system in a sex-dependent manner. *Mol. Psychiatry* **2013**, *18*, 666–673. [CrossRef] [PubMed]
84. Badawy, A.A. Tryptophan metabolism, disposition and utilization in pregnancy. *Biosci. Rep.* **2015**, *35*, e00261. [CrossRef] [PubMed]
85. Wu, H.Q.; Okuyama, M.; Kajii, Y.; Pocivavsek, A.; Bruno, J.P.; Schwarcz, R. Targeting kynurenine aminotransferase II in psychiatric diseases: Promising effects of an orally active enzyme inhibitor. *Schizophr. Bull.* **2014**, *40*, S152–S158. [CrossRef] [PubMed]
86. Aarsland, T.I.M.; Landaas, E.T.; Hegvik, T.-A.; Ulvik, A.; Halmøy, A.; Ueland, P.M.; Haavik, J. Serum concentrations of kynurenines in adult patients with attention-deficit hyperactivity disorder (ADHD): A case-control study. *Behav. Brain Funct.* **2015**, *11*, 36. [CrossRef] [PubMed]
87. Maes, M.; Mihaylova, I.; De Ruyter, M.; Kubera, M.; Bosmans, E. The immune effects of TRYCATs (tryptophan catabolites along the IDO pathway): Relevance for depression- and other conditions characterized by tryptophan depletion induced by inflammation. *Neuro Endocrinol. Lett.* **2007**, *28*, 826–831. [PubMed]
88. Moroni, F.; Cozzi, A.; Sili, M.; Mannaioni, G. Kynurenic acid: A metabolite with multiple actions and multiple targets in brain and periphery. *J. Neural Transm.* **2012**, *119*, 133–139. [CrossRef]
89. Neale, S.A.; Copeland, C.S.; Uebele, V.N.; Thomson, F.J.; Salt, T.E. Modulation of Hippocampal Synaptic Transmission by the Kynurenine Pathway Member Xanthurenic Acid and Other VGLUT Inhibitors. *Neuropsychopharmacology* **2013**, *38*, 1060–1067. [CrossRef]
90. Cenit, M.C.; Nuevo, I.C.; Codoñer-Franch, P.; Sanz, Y.; Dinan, T.G. Gut microbiota and attention deficit hyperactivity disorder: New perspectives for a challenging condition. *Eur. Child. Adolesc. Psychiatry* **2017**, *8*, 429–1092. [CrossRef]
91. Kozak, R.; Campbell, B.M.; Strick, C.A.; Horner, W.; Hoffmann, W.E.; Kiss, T.; Chapin, D.S.; McGinnis, D.; Abbott, A.L.; Roberts, B.M.; et al. Reduction of Brain Kynurenic Acid Improves Cognitive Function. *J. Neurosci.* **2014**, *34*, 10592–10602. [CrossRef]
92. Vécsei, L.; Szalárdy, L.; Fülöp, F.; Toldi, J. Kynurenines in the CNS: Recent advances and new questions. *Nat. Rev. Drug Discov.* **2013**, *12*, 64–82. [CrossRef] [PubMed]
93. Evangelisti, M.; De Rossi, P.; Rabasco, J.; Donfrancesco, R.; Lionetto, L.; Capi, M.; Sani, G.; Simmaco, M.; Nicoletti, F.; Villa, M.P. Changes in serum levels of kynurenine metabolites in paediatric patients affected by ADHD. *Eur. Child. Adolesc. Psychiatry* **2017**, *26*, 1433–1441. [CrossRef] [PubMed]
94. Landaas, E.T.; Aarsland, T.I.; Ulvik, A.; Halmøy, A.; Ueland, P.M.; Haavik, J. Vitamin levels in adults with ADHD. *BJPsych Open* **2016**, *2*, 377–384. [CrossRef] [PubMed]
95. Dolina, S.; Margalit, D.; Malitsky, S.; Rabinkov, A. Attention-deficit hyperactivity disorder (ADHD) as a pyridoxine-dependent condition: Urinary diagnostic biomarkers. *Med. Hypotheses* **2014**, *82*, 111–116. [CrossRef]
96. Said, Z.M.; Subramanian, V.S.; Vaziri, N.D.; Said, H.M. T1881 Pyridoxine Uptake By Colonocytes: A Specific and Regulated Carrier-Mediated Process. *Am. J. Physiol. Cell Physiol.* **2008**, *294*, C1192–C1197. [CrossRef]

97. Gagliardi, A.; Totino, V.; Cacciotti, F.; Iebba, V.; Neroni, B.; Bonfiglio, G.; Trancassini, M.; Passariello, C.; Pantanella, F.; Schippa, S. Rebuilding the Gut Microbiota Ecosystem. *Int. J. Environ. Res. Public Health* **2018**, *15*, 1679. [CrossRef]
98. Fond, G.; Boukouaci, W.; Chevalier, G.; Regnault, A.; Eberl, G.; Hamdani, N.; Dickerson, F.; MacGregor, A.; Boyer, L.; Dargel, A.; et al. The "psychomicrobiotic": Targeting microbiota in major psychiatric disorders: A systematic review. *Pathol. Boil.* **2015**, *63*, 35–42. [CrossRef]
99. Saltzman, E.T.; Palacios, T.; Thomsen, M.; Vitetta, L. Intestinal Microbiome Shifts, Dysbiosis, Inflammation, and Non-alcoholic Fatty Liver Disease. *Front. Microbiol.* **2018**, *9*, 61. [CrossRef]
100. Varatharaj, A.; Galea, I. The blood-brain barrier in systemic inflammation. *Brain Behav. Immun.* **2017**, *60*, 1–12. [CrossRef]
101. Verlaet, A.A.J.; Noriega, D.B.; Hermans, N.; Savelkoul, H.F.J. Nutrition, immunological mechanisms and dietary immunomodulation in ADHD. *Eur. Child. Adolesc. Psychiatry* **2014**, *23*, 519–529. [CrossRef]
102. Mitchell, R.H.; Goldstein, B.I. Inflammation in children and adolescents with neuropsychiatric disorders: A systematic review. *J. Am. Acad. Child Adolesc. Psychiatry* **2014**, *53*, 274–296. [CrossRef] [PubMed]
103. Di Cesare, A.; Di Meglio, P.; Nestle, F.O. A role for Th17 cells in the immunopathogenesis of atopic dermatitis? *J. Investig. Dermatol.* **2008**, *128*, 2569–2571. [CrossRef] [PubMed]
104. Chen, M.H.; Su, T.P.; Chen, Y.S.; Hsu, J.W.; Huang, K.L.; Chang, W.H.; Bai, Y.M. Attention deficit hyperactivity disorder, tic disorder, and allergy: Is there a link? A nationwide population-based study. *J. Child. Psychol. Psychiatry* **2013**, *54*, 545–551. [CrossRef] [PubMed]
105. Tsai, M.C.; Lin, H.K.; Lin, C.H.; Fu, L.S. Prevalence of attention deficit/hyperactivity disorder in pediatric allergic rhinitis: A nationwide population-based study. *Allergy Asthma Proc.* **2011**, *32*, 41–46. [CrossRef] [PubMed]
106. Genuneit, J.; Braig, S.; Brandt, S.; Wabitsch, M.; Florath, I.; Brenner, H.; Rothenbacher, D. Infant atopic eczema and subsequent attention-deficit/hyperactivity disorder–a prospective birth cohort study. *Pediatr. Allergy Immunol.* **2014**, *25*, 51–56. [CrossRef] [PubMed]
107. Lynch, S.V. Gut Microbiota and Allergic Disease. New Insights. *Ann. Am. Thorac. Soc.* **2016**, *13*, S51–S54.
108. Martínez, I.; Lattimer, J.M.; Hubach, K.L.; Case, J.A.; Yang, J.; Weber, C.G.; Louk, J.A.; Rose, D.J.; Kyureghian, G.; Peterson, D.A.; et al. Gut microbiome composition is linked to whole grain-induced immunological improvements. *ISME J.* **2013**, *7*, 269–280. [CrossRef]
109. Christian, L.M.; Galley, J.D.; Hade, E.M.; Schoppe-Sullivan, S.; Kamp Dush, C.; Bailey, M.T. Gut microbiome composition is associated with temperament during early childhood. *Brain Behav. Immun.* **2015**, *45*, 118–127. [CrossRef]
110. Buske-Kirschbaum, A.; Schmitt, J.; Plessow, F.; Romanos, M.; Weidinger, S.; Roessner, V. Psychoendocrine and psychoneuroimmunological mechanisms in the comorbidity of atopic eczema and attention deficit/hyperactivity disorder. *Psychoneuroendocrinology* **2013**, *38*, 12–23. [CrossRef]
111. Jiang, H.-Y.; Zhou, Y.-Y.; Zhou, G.-L.; Li, Y.-C.; Yuan, J.; Li, X.-H.; Ruan, B. Gut microbiota profiles in treatment-naïve children with attention deficit hyperactivity disorder. *Behav. Brain Res.* **2018**, *347*, 408–413. [CrossRef]
112. Marshall, P. Attention deficit disorder and allergy: A neurochemical model of the relation between the illnesses. *Psychol. Bull.* **1989**, *106*, 434–446. [CrossRef]
113. Van Der Schans, J.; De Vries, T.W.; Hak, E.; Hoekstra, P.J.; Çiçek, R. Association of atopic diseases and attention-deficit/hyperactivity disorder: A systematic review and meta-analyses. *Neurosci. Biobehav. Rev.* **2017**, *74*, 139–148. [CrossRef] [PubMed]
114. Schmitt, J.; Romanos, M.; Meurer, M.; Kirch, W. Atopic Eczema and Attention-Deficit/Hyperactivity Disorder in a Population-Based Sample of Children and Adolescents. *JAMA* **2009**, *301*, 724. [CrossRef] [PubMed]
115. Strachan, D.; Sibbald, B.; Weiland, S.; Aït-Khaled, N.; Anabwani, G.; Anderson, H.R.; Asher, M.I.; Beasley, R.; Björkstén, B.; Burr, M.; et al. Worldwide variations in prevalence of symptoms of allergic rhinoconjunctivitis in children: The International Study of Asthma and Allergies in Childhood (ISAAC). *Pediatr. Allergy Immunol.* **1997**, *8*, 161–176. [CrossRef] [PubMed]
116. Leung, D.Y.; Bieber, T. Atopic dermatitis. *Lancet* **2003**, *361*, 151–160. [CrossRef]
117. Novak, N. Immune mechanisms leading to atopic dermatitis. *J. Allergy Clin. Immunol.* **2003**, *112*, S128–S139. [CrossRef]

118. Penders, J.; Thijs, C.; van den Brandt, P.A.; Kummeling, I.; Snijders, B.; Stelma, F.; Adams, H.; van Ree, R.; Stobberingh, E.E. Gut microbiota composition and development of atopic manifestations in infancy: The KOALA Birth Cohort Study. *Gut* **2007**, *56*, 661–667. [CrossRef]
119. Qiu, X.; Zhang, M.; Yang, X.; Hong, N.; Yu, C. Faecalibacterium prausnitzii upregulates regulatory T cells and anti-inflammatory cytokines in treating TNBS-induced colitis. *J. Crohns Colitis* **2013**, *7*, e558–e568. [CrossRef]
120. Quévrain, E.; Maubert, M.A.; Michon, C.; Chain, F.; Marquant, R.; Tailhades, J.; Miquel, S.; Carlier, L.; Bermúdez-Humarán, L.G.; Pigneur, B.; et al. Identification of an anti-inflammatory protein from Faecalibacterium prausnitzii, a commensal bacterium deficient in Crohn's disease. *Gut* **2016**, *65*, 415–425.
121. Dominguez-Bello, M.G.; Costello, E.K.; Contreras, M.; Magris, M.; Hidalgo, G.; Fierer, N.; Knight, R. Delivery mode shapes the acquisition and structure of the initial microbiota across multiple body habitats in newborns. *Proc. Natl. Acad. Sci. USA* **2010**, *107*, 11971–11975. [CrossRef]
122. Penders, J.; Thijs, C.; Vink, C.; Stelma, F.F.; Snijders, B.; Kummeling, I.; Brandt, P.A.V.D.; Stobberingh, E.E. Factors Influencing the Composition of the Intestinal Microbiota in Early Infancy. *Pediatrics* **2006**, *118*, 511–521. [CrossRef] [PubMed]
123. Jakobsson, H.E.; Abrahamsson, T.R.; Jenmalm, M.C.; Harris, K.; Quince, C.; Jernberg, C.; Björkstén, B.; Engstrand, L.; Andersson, A.F. Decreased gut microbiota diversity, delayed Bacteroidetes colonisation and reduced Th1 responses in infants delivered by caesarean section. *Gut* **2014**, *63*, 559–566. [CrossRef] [PubMed]
124. Boksa, P.; El-Khodor, B.F. Birth insult interacts with stress at adulthood to alter dopaminergic function in animal models: Possible implications for schizophrenia and other disorders. *Neurosci. Biobehav. Rev.* **2003**, *27*, 91–101. [CrossRef]
125. Salas, M.; Hotman, A.; Stricker, B.H. Confounding by Indication: An Example of Variation in the Use of Epidemiologic Terminology. *Am. J. Epidemiol.* **1999**, *149*, 981–983. [CrossRef] [PubMed]
126. Ketzer, C.R.; Gallois, C.; Martinez, A.L.; Rohde, L.A.; Schmitz, M. Is there an association between perinatal complications and attention-deficit/hyperactivity disorder-inattentive type in children and adolescents? *Braz. J. Psychiatry* **2012**, *34*, 321–328. [CrossRef] [PubMed]
127. Silva, D.; Colvin, L.; Hagemann, E.; Bower, C. Environmental risk factors by gender associated with attention-deficit/hyperactivity disorder. *Pediatrics* **2014**, *133*, e14–e22. [CrossRef] [PubMed]
128. Curran, E.A.; O'Neill, S.M.; Cryan, J.F.; Kenny, L.C.; Dinan, T.G.; Khashan, A.S.; Kearney, P.M. Research review: Birth by caesarean section and development of autism spectrum disorder and attention-deficit/hyperactivity disorder: A systematic review and meta-analysis. *J. Child Psychol. Psychiatry* **2015**, *56*, 500–508. [CrossRef]
129. Curran, E.A.; Khashan, A.S.; Dalman, C.; Kenny, L.C.; Cryan, J.F.; Dinan, T.G.; Kearney, P.M. Obstetric mode of delivery and attention-deficit/hyperactivity disorder: A sibling-matched study. *Int. J. Epidemiol.* **2016**, *45*, 532–542. [CrossRef]
130. Axelsson, P.B.; Clausen, T.D.; Petersen, A.H.; Hageman, I.; Pinborg, A.; Kessing, L.V.; Bergholt, T.; Rasmussen, S.C.; Keiding, N.; Løkkegaard, E.C.L. Investigating the effects of cesarean delivery and antibiotic use in early childhood on risk of later attention deficit hyperactivity disorder. *J. Child Psychol. Psychiatry* **2019**, *60*, 151–159. [CrossRef]
131. Curran, E.A.; Cryan, J.F.; Kenny, L.C.; Dinan, T.G.; Kearney, P.M.; Khashan, A.S. Obstetrical Mode of Delivery and Childhood Behavior and Psychological Development in a British Cohort. *J. Autism Dev. Disord.* **2016**, *46*, 603–614. [CrossRef]
132. Li, J.; Olsen, J.; Vestergaard, M.; Obel, C. Attention-deficit/hyperactivity disorder in the offspring following prenatal maternal bereavement: A nationwide follow-up study in Denmark. *Eur. Child. Adolesc. Psychiatry* **2010**, *19*, 747–753. [CrossRef] [PubMed]
133. Van den Bergh, B.R.; Marcoen, A. High antenatal maternal anxiety is related to ADHD symptoms, externalizing problems, and anxiety in 8- and 9-year-olds. *Child Dev.* **2004**, *75*, 1085–1097. [CrossRef] [PubMed]
134. Grizenko, N.; Shayan, Y.R.; Polotskaia, A.; Ter-Stepanian, M.; Joober, R. Relation of maternal stress during pregnancy to symptom severity and response to treatment in children with ADHD. *J. Psychiatry Neurosci.* **2008**, *33*, 10–16. [PubMed]
135. Jašarević, E.; Howerton, C.L.; Howard, C.D.; Bale, T.L. Alterations in the Vaginal Microbiome by Maternal Stress Are Associated With Metabolic Reprogramming of the Offspring Gut and Brain. *Endocrinology* **2015**, *156*, 3265–3276. [CrossRef] [PubMed]
136. Galley, J.D.; Bailey, M.T. Impact of stressor exposure on the interplay between commensal microbiota and host inflammation. *Gut Microbes* **2014**, *5*, 390–396. [CrossRef] [PubMed]

137. Barrett, E.; Ross, R.P.; O'Toole, P.W.; Fitzgerald, G.F.; Stanton, C. γ-Aminobutyric acid production by culturable bacteria from the human intestine. *J. Appl. Microbiol.* **2012**, *113*, 411–417. [CrossRef]
138. Edden, R.A.E.; Crocetti, D.; Zhu, H.; Gilbert, D.L.; Mostofsky, S.H. Reduced GABA concentration in attention-deficit/hyperactivity disorder. *Arch. Gen. Psychiatry* **2012**, *69*, 750–753. [CrossRef]
139. Bollmann, S.; Ghisleni, C.; Poil, S.-S.; Martin, E.; Ball, J.; Eich-Höchli, D.; Edden, R.A.E.; Klaver, P.; Michels, L.; Brandeis, D.; et al. Developmental changes in gamma-aminobutyric acid levels in attention-deficit/hyperactivity disorder. *Transl. Psychiatry* **2015**, *5*, e589. [CrossRef]
140. Sumner, P.; Edden, R.A.E.; Bompas, A.; Evans, C.J.; Singh, K.D. More GABA, less distraction: A neurochemical predictor of motor decision speed. *Nat. Neurosci.* **2010**, *13*, 825–827. [CrossRef]
141. Wiebking, C.; Duncan, N.W.; Tiret, B.; Hayes, D.J.; Marjańska, M.; Doyon, J.; Bajbouj, M.; Northoff, G. GABA in the insula—A predictor of the neural response to interoceptive awareness. *Neuroimage* **2014**, *86*, 10–18. [CrossRef]
142. Pärtty, A.; Kalliomäki, M.; Wacklin, P.; Salminen, S.; Isolauri, E. A possible link between early probiotic intervention and the risk of neuropsychiatric disorders later in childhood: A randomized trial. *Pediatr. Res.* **2015**, *77*, 823–828. [CrossRef]
143. Kalliomäki, M.; Salminen, S.; Arvilommi, H.; Kero, P.; Koskinen, P.; Isolauri, E. Probiotics in primary prevention of atopic disease: A randomised placebo-controlled trial. *Lancet* **2001**, *357*, 1076–1079. [CrossRef]
144. Barrett, E.; Kerr, C.; Murphy, K.; O'Sullivan, O.; Ryan, C.A.; Dempsey, E.M.; Murphy, B.P.; O'Toole, P.W.; Cotter, P.D.; Fitzgerald, G.F.; et al. The individual-specific and diverse nature of the preterm infant microbiota. *Arch. Dis. Child Fetal Neonatal Ed.* **2013**, *98*, F334–F340. [CrossRef] [PubMed]
145. Bhutta, A.T.; Cleves, M.A.; Casey, P.H.; Cradock, M.M.; Anand, K.J.S. Cognitive and behavioral outcomes of school-aged children who were born preterm: A meta-analysis. *JAMA* **2002**, *288*, 728–737. [CrossRef] [PubMed]
146. Johnson, S.; Hollis, C.; Kochhar, P.; Hennessy, E.; Wolke, D.; Marlow, N. Psychiatric disorders in extremely preterm children: Longitudinal finding at age 11 years in the EPICure study. *J. Am. Acad. Child Adolesc. Psychiatry* **2010**, *49*, 453–463.e1. [CrossRef]
147. Ask, H.; Gustavson, K.; Ystrom, E.; Havdahl, K.A.; Tesli, M.; Askeland, R.B.; Reichborn-Kjennerud, T. Association of Gestational Age at Birth With Symptoms of Attention-Deficit/Hyperactivity Disorder in Children. *JAMA Pediatr.* **2018**, *172*, 749–756. [CrossRef]
148. Chou, I.-C.; Kuo, H.-T.; Chang, J.-S.; Wu, S.-F.; Chiu, H.-Y.; Su, B.-H.; Lin, H.-C. Lack of Effects of Oral Probiotics on Growth and Neurodevelopmental Outcomes in Preterm Very Low Birth Weight Infants. *J. Pediatr.* **2010**, *156*, 393–396. [CrossRef]
149. Melville, J.M.; Moss, T.J. The immune consequences of preterm birth. *Front. Neurosci.* **2013**, *7*, 79. [CrossRef]
150. Quinn, J.-A.; Munoz, F.M.; Gonik, B.; Frau, L.; Cutland, C.; Mallett-Moore, T.; Kissou, A.; Wittke, F.; Das, M.; Nunes, T.; et al. Preterm birth: Case definition & guidelines for data collection, analysis, and presentation of immunisation safety data. *Vaccine* **2016**, *34*, 6047–6056.
151. Lindström, K.; Lindblad, F.; Hjern, A. Preterm birth and attention-deficit/hyperactivity disorder in schoolchildren. *Pediatrics* **2011**, *127*, 858–865. [CrossRef]
152. D'Onofrio, B.M.; Class, Q.A.; Rickert, M.E.; Larsson, H.; Langström, N.; Lichtenstein, P. Preterm birth and mortality and morbidity: A population-based quasi-experimental study. *JAMA Psychiatry* **2013**, *70*, 1231–1240. [CrossRef] [PubMed]
153. Farooqi, A.; Hägglöf, B.; Sedin, G.; Gothefors, L.; Serenius, F. Mental Health and Social Competencies of 10- to 12-Year-Old Children Born at 23 to 25 Weeks of Gestation in the 1990s: A Swedish National Prospective Follow-up Study. *Pediatrics* **2007**, *120*, 118–133. [CrossRef] [PubMed]
154. Sternbach, H.; State, R. Antibiotics: Neuropsychiatric effects and psychotropic interactions. *Harv. Rev. Psychiatry* **1997**, *5*, 214–226. [CrossRef] [PubMed]
155. Becattini, S.; Taur, Y.; Pamer, E.G. Antibiotic-Induced Changes in the Intestinal Microbiota and Disease. *Trends Mol. Med.* **2016**, *22*, 458–478. [CrossRef] [PubMed]
156. Park, S.; Kim, B.N.; Kim, J.W.; Shin, M.S.; Yoo, H.J.; Cho, S.C. Protective effect of breastfeeding with regard to children's behavioral and cognitive problems. *Nutr. J.* **2014**, *13*, 111. [CrossRef] [PubMed]
157. Mimouni-Bloch, A.; Kachevanskaya, A.; Mimouni, F.B.; Shuper, A.; Raveh, E.; Linder, N. Breastfeeding may protect from developing attention-deficit/hyperactivity disorder. *Breastfeed Med.* **2013**, *8*, 363–367. [CrossRef] [PubMed]

158. Stadler, D.D.; Musser, E.D.; Holton, K.F.; Shannon, J.; Nigg, J.T. Recalled Initiation and Duration of Maternal Breastfeeding Among Children with and Without ADHD in a Well Characterized Case-Control Sample. *J. Abnorm. Child. Psychol.* **2016**, *44*, 347–355. [CrossRef]
159. Golmirzaei, J.; Namazi, S.; Amiri, S.; Zare, S.; Rastikerdar, N.; Hesam, A.A.; Rahami, Z.; Ghasemian, F.; Namazi, S.S.; Paknahad, A.; et al. Evaluation of Attention-Deficit Hyperactivity Disorder Risk Factors. *Int. J. Pediatr.* **2013**, *2013*, 1–6. [CrossRef]
160. Newburg, D.S.; Walker, W.A. Protection of the neonate by the innate immune system of developing gut and of human milk. *Pediatr. Res.* **2007**, *61*, 2–8. [CrossRef]
161. Cacho, N.T.; Lawrence, R.M. Innate Immunity and Breast Milk. *Front. Immunol.* **2017**, *8*, 584. [CrossRef]
162. Richardson, A.; Puri, B. The potential role of fatty acids in attention-deficit/hyperactivity disorder. *Prostaglandins Leukot. Essent. Fat. Acids* **2000**, *63*, 79–87. [CrossRef] [PubMed]
163. Richardson, A.J. Omega-3 fatty acids in ADHD and related neurodevelopmental disorders. *Int. Rev. Psychiatry* **2006**, *18*, 155–172. [CrossRef] [PubMed]
164. Bezirtzoglou, E.; Tsiotsias, A.; Welling, G.W. Microbiota profile in feces of breast- and formula-fed newborns by using fluorescence in situ hybridization (FISH). *Anaerobe* **2011**, *17*, 478–482. [CrossRef] [PubMed]
165. Fallani, M.; Young, D.; Scott, J.; Norin, E.; Amarri, S.; Adam, R.; Aguilera, M.; Khanna, S.; Gil, A.; Edwards, C.A.; et al. Intestinal Microbiota of 6-week-old Infants Across Europe: Geographic Influence Beyond Delivery Mode, Breast-feeding, and Antibiotics. *J. Pediatr. Gastroenterol. Nutr.* **2010**, *51*, 77–84. [CrossRef]
166. Guaraldi, F.; Salvatori, G. Effect of Breast and Formula Feeding on Gut Microbiota Shaping in Newborns. *Front. Microbiol.* **2012**, *2*, 94. [CrossRef]
167. Underwood, M.A.; Kalanetra, K.M.; Bokulich, N.A.; Lewis, Z.T.; Mirmiran, M.; Tancredi, D.J.; Mills, D.A. A comparison of two probiotic strains of bifidobacteria in premature infants. *J. Pediatr.* **2013**, *163*, 1585–1591.e9. [CrossRef]
168. Underwood, M.A.; German, J.B.; Lebrilla, C.B.; Mills, D.A. Bifidobacterium longum subspecies infantis: Champion colonizer of the infant gut. *Pediatr. Res.* **2015**, *77*, 229–235. [CrossRef]
169. Adesman, A.; Soled, D.; Rosen, L. Formula Feeding as a Risk Factor for Attention-Deficit/Hyperactivity Disorder: Is Bisphenol A Exposure a Smoking Gun? *J. Dev. Behav. Pediatr.* **2017**, *38*, 545–551.e9. [CrossRef]
170. Mariadason, J.M.; Corner, G.A.; Augenlicht, L.H. Genetic reprogramming in pathways of colonic cell maturation induced by short chain fatty acids: Comparison with trichostatin A, sulindac, and curcumin and implications for chemoprevention of colon cancer. *Cancer Res.* **2000**, *60*, 4561–4572.
171. Canani, R.B.; Di Costanzo, M.; Leone, L.; Pedata, M.; Meli, R.; Calignano, A. Potential beneficial effects of butyrate in intestinal and extraintestinal diseases. *World J. Gastroenterol.* **2011**, *17*, 1519–1528. [CrossRef]
172. Macfabe, D.F. Enteric short-chain fatty acids: Microbial messengers of metabolism, mitochondria, and mind: Implications in autism spectrum disorders. *Microb. Ecol. Heal. Dis.* **2015**, *26*, 28177. [CrossRef] [PubMed]
173. Bercik, P.; Denou, E.; Collins, J.; Jackson, W.; Lu, J.; Jury, J.; Deng, Y.; Blennerhassett, P.; Macri, J.; McCoy, K.D.; et al. The Intestinal Microbiota Affect Central Levels of Brain-Derived Neurotropic Factor and Behavior in Mice. *Gastroenterology* **2011**, *141*, 599–609.e3. [CrossRef] [PubMed]
174. Corominas-Roso, M.; Ramos-Quiroga, J.A.; Ribases, M.; Sanchez-Mora, C.; Palomar, G.; Valero, S.; Bosch, R.; Casas, M. Decreased serum levels of brain-derived neurotrophic factor in adults with attention-deficit hyperactivity disorder. *Int. J. Neuropsychopharmacol.* **2013**, *16*, 1267–1275. [CrossRef] [PubMed]
175. Akay, A.P.; Resmi, H.; Güney, S.A.; Erkuran, H.; Özyurt, G.; Sargin, E.; Topuzoglu, A.; Tufan, A.E. Serum brain-derived neurotrophic factor levels in treatment-naïve boys with attention-deficit/hyperactivity disorder treated with methylphenidate: An 8-week, observational pretest-posttest study. *Eur. Child Adolesc. Psychiatry* **2018**, *27*, 127–135. [CrossRef]
176. Amiri, A.; Torabi Parizi, G.; Kousha, M.; Saadat, F.; Modabbernia, M.J.; Najafi, K.; Atrkar Roushan, Z. Changes in plasma Brain-derived neurotrophic factor (BDNF) levels induced by methylphenidate in children with Attention deficit-hyperactivity disorder (ADHD). *Prog. Neuropsychopharmacol. Biol. Psychiatry* **2013**, *47*, 20–24. [CrossRef]
177. Shim, S.H.; Hwangbo, Y.; Kwon, Y.J.; Jeong, H.Y.; Lee, B.H.; Lee, H.J.; Kim, Y.K. Increased levels of plasma brain-derived neurotrophic factor (BDNF) in children with attention deficit-hyperactivity disorder (ADHD). *Prog. Neuropsychopharmacol. Biol. Psychiatry* **2008**, *32*, 1824–1828. [CrossRef]

178. Fujimura, H.; Chen, R.; Nakamura, T.; Nakahashi, T.; Kambayashi, J.-I.; Sun, B.; Altar, C.A.; Tandon, N.N. Brain-derived neurotrophic factor is stored in human platelets and released by agonist stimulation. *Thromb. Haemost.* **2002**, *87*, 728–734. [CrossRef]

179. Amjad Khan, W.; Chun-Mei, H.; Khan, N.; Iqbal, A.; Lyu, S.W.; Shah, F. Bioengineered Plants Can Be a Useful Source of Omega-3 Fatty Acids. *Biomed. Res. Int.* **2017**, *2017*, 7348919. [CrossRef]

180. Cryan, J.F.; O'Mahony, S.M. The microbiome-gut-brain axis: From bowel to behavior. *Neurogastroenterol. Motil.* **2011**, *23*, 187–192. [CrossRef]

181. Weiser, M.J.; Butt, C.M.; Mohajeri, M.H. Docosahexaenoic Acid and Cognition throughout the Lifespan. *Nutrients* **2016**, *8*, 99. [CrossRef]

182. Robertson, R.C.; Oriach, C.S.; Murphy, K.; Moloney, G.M.; Cryan, J.F.; Dinan, T.G.; Ross, R.P.; Stanton, C. Omega-3 polyunsaturated fatty acids critically regulate behaviour and gut microbiota development in adolescence and adulthood. *Brain Behav. Immun.* **2017**, *59*, 21–37. [CrossRef] [PubMed]

183. Choi-Lundberg, D.L.; Lin, Q.; Chang, Y.-N.; Chiang, Y.L.; Hay, C.M.; Mohajeri, H.; Davidson, B.L.; Bohn, M.C. Dopaminergic Neurons Protected from Degeneration by GDNF Gene Therapy. *Science* **1997**, *275*, 838–841. [CrossRef] [PubMed]

184. Bohn, M.C.; Connor, B.; Kozlowski, D.A.; Mohajeri, M.H. Gene transfer for neuroprotection in animal models of Parkinson's disease and amyotrophic lateral sclerosis. *Novartis Found Symp.* **2000**, *231*, 70–93. [PubMed]

185. Rao, J.S.; Ertley, R.N.; Lee, H.J.; DeMar, J.C.; Arnold, J.T.; Rapoport, S.I.; Bazinet, R.P. N-3 polyunsaturated fatty acid deprivation in rats decreases frontal cortex BDNF via a p38 MAPK-dependent mechanism. *Mol. Psychiatry* **2007**, *12*, 36–46. [CrossRef]

186. Soares, J.C.; Kochunov, P.; Monkul, E.S.; Nicoletti, M.A.; Brambilla, P.; Sassi, R.B.; Mallinger, A.G.; Frank, E.; Kupfer, D.J.; Lancaster, J.; et al. Structural brain changes in bipolar disorder using deformation field morphometry. *NeuroReport* **2005**, *16*, 541–544. [CrossRef]

187. Costantini, L.; Molinari, R.; Farinon, B.; Merendino, N. Impact of Omega-3 Fatty Acids on the Gut Microbiota. *Int. J. Mol. Sci.* **2017**, *18*, 2645. [CrossRef]

188. Yan, Y.; Jiang, W.; Spinetti, T.; Tardivel, A.; Castillo, R.; Bourquin, C.; Guarda, G.; Tian, Z.; Tschopp, J.; Zhou, R. Omega-3 Fatty Acids Prevent Inflammation and Metabolic Disorder through Inhibition of NLRP3 Inflammasome Activation. *Immunity* **2013**, *38*, 1154–1163. [CrossRef]

189. Kaliannan, K.; Li, X.-Y.; Wang, B.; Pan, Q.; Chen, C.-Y.; Hao, L.; Xie, S.; Kang, J.X. Multi-omic analysis in transgenic mice implicates omega-6/omega-3 fatty acid imbalance as a risk factor for chronic disease. *Commun. Boil.* **2019**, *2*, 276. [CrossRef]

190. Kaliannan, K.; Wang, B.; Li, X.Y.; Kim, K.J.; Kang, J.X. A host-microbiome interaction mediates the opposing effects of omega-6 and omega-3 fatty acids on metabolic endotoxemia. *Sci. Rep.* **2015**, *5*, 11276. [CrossRef]

191. Crippa, A.; Agostoni, C.; Mauri, M.; Molteni, M.; Nobile, M. Polyunsaturated Fatty Acids Are Associated With Behavior But Not With Cognition in Children With and Without ADHD: An Italian study. *J. Atten. Disord.* **2018**, *22*, 971–983. [CrossRef]

192. Chang, J.P.; Su, K.P.; Mondelli, V.; Pariante, C.M. Omega-3 Polyunsaturated Fatty Acids in Youths with Attention Deficit Hyperactivity Disorder: A Systematic Review and Meta-Analysis of Clinical Trials and Biological Studies. *Neuropsychopharmacology* **2018**, *43*, 534–545. [CrossRef] [PubMed]

193. Anand, P.; Sachdeva, A. Effect of Poly Unsaturated Fatty Acids Administration on Children with Attention Deficit Hyperactivity Disorder: A Randomized Controlled Trial. *J. Clin. Diagn. Res.* **2016**, *10*, OC01–OC05. [CrossRef] [PubMed]

194. Gillies, D.; Sinn, J.K.; Lad, S.S.; Leach, M.J.; Ross, M.J. Polyunsaturated fatty acids (PUFA) for attention deficit hyperactivity disorder (ADHD) in children and adolescents. *Cochrane Database Syst. Rev.* **2012**, *7*, CD007986. [CrossRef] [PubMed]

195. Watson, H.; Mitra, S.; Croden, F.C.; Taylor, M.; Wood, H.M.; Perry, S.L.; Spencer, J.A.; Quirke, P.; Toogood, G.J.; Lawton, C.L.; et al. A randomised trial of the effect of omega-3 polyunsaturated fatty acid supplements on the human intestinal microbiota. *Gut* **2018**, *67*, 1974–1983. [CrossRef] [PubMed]

196. Ilag, L.L. Are Long-Chain Polyunsaturated Fatty Acids the Link between the Immune System and the Microbiome towards Modulating Cancer? *Medicines* **2018**, *5*, 102. [CrossRef] [PubMed]

197. Bennet, R.; Eriksson, M.; Nord, C.E. The fecal microflora of 1-3-month-old infants during treatment with eight oral antibiotics. *Infection* **2002**, *30*, 158–160. [CrossRef] [PubMed]

198. Hussey, S.; Wall, R.; Gruffman, E.; O'Sullivan, L.; Ryan, C.A.; Murphy, B.; Fitzgerald, G.; Stanton, C.; Ross, R.P. Parenteral antibiotics reduce bifidobacteria colonization and diversity in neonates. *Int. J. Microbiol.* **2011**, *2011*, 130574. [CrossRef] [PubMed]
199. Slykerman, R.F.; Thompson, J.; Waldie, K.E.; Murphy, R.; Wall, C.; Mitchell, E.A. Antibiotics in the first year of life and subsequent neurocognitive outcomes. *Acta Paediatr.* **2017**, *106*, 87–94. [CrossRef]
200. Reid, G.; Hammond, J.A. Probiotics. Some evidence of their effectiveness. *Can. Fam. Physician* **2005**, *51*, 1487–1493.
201. Hill, C.; Guarner, F.; Reid, G.; Gibson, G.R.; Merenstein, D.J.; Pot, B.; Morelli, L.; Canani, R.B.; Flint, H.J.; Salminen, S.; et al. Expert consensus document. The International Scientific Association for Probiotics and Prebiotics consensus statement on the scope and appropriate use of the term probiotic. *Nat. Rev. Gastroenterol. Hepatol.* **2014**, *11*, 506–514. [CrossRef]
202. Kumar, M.; Nagpal, R.; Verma, V.; Kumar, A.; Kaur, N.; Hemalatha, R.; Gautam, S.K.; Singh, B. Probiotic metabolites as epigenetic targets in the prevention of colon cancer. *Nutr. Rev.* **2013**, *71*, 23–34. [CrossRef] [PubMed]
203. Reid, G.; Younes, J.A.; Van der Mei, H.C.; Gloor, G.B.; Knight, R.; Busscher, H.J. Microbiota restoration: Natural and supplemented recovery of human microbial communities. *Nat. Rev. Microbiol.* **2011**, *9*, 27–38. [CrossRef] [PubMed]
204. Rezac, S.; Kok, C.R.; Heermann, M.; Hutkins, R. Fermented Foods as a Dietary Source of Live Organisms. *Front. Microbiol.* **2018**, *9*, 1785. [CrossRef]
205. Savignac, H.M.; Kiely, B.; Dinan, T.G.; Cryan, J.F. Bifidobacteria exert strain-specific effects on stress-related behavior and physiology in BALB/c mice. *Neurogastroenterol. Motil.* **2014**, *26*, 1615–1627. [CrossRef] [PubMed]
206. Felice, V.D.; O'Mahony, S.M. The microbiome and disorders of the central nervous system. *Pharmacol. Biochem. Behav.* **2017**, *160*, 1–13. [CrossRef] [PubMed]
207. Tsai, S.J. Attention-deficit hyperactivity disorder may be associated with decreased central brain-derived neurotrophic factor activity: Clinical and therapeutic implications. *Med. Hypotheses* **2007**, *68*, 896–899. [CrossRef] [PubMed]
208. Pelsser, L.M.; Frankena, K.; Toorman, J.; Rodrigues Pereira, R. Diet and ADHD, Reviewing the Evidence: A Systematic Review of Meta-Analyses of Double-Blind Placebo-Controlled Trials Evaluating the Efficacy of Diet Interventions on the Behavior of Children with ADHD. *PLoS ONE* **2017**, *12*, e0169277. [CrossRef] [PubMed]

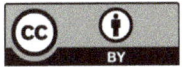

© 2019 by the authors. Licensee MDPI, Basel, Switzerland. This article is an open access article distributed under the terms and conditions of the Creative Commons Attribution (CC BY) license (http://creativecommons.org/licenses/by/4.0/).

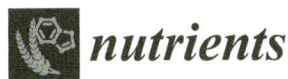

Review

From Probiotics to Psychobiotics: Live Beneficial Bacteria Which Act on the Brain-Gut Axis

Luis G. Bermúdez-Humarán [1],*, Eva Salinas [2], Genaro G. Ortiz [3], Luis J. Ramirez-Jirano [3], J. Alejandro Morales [4] and Oscar K. Bitzer-Quintero [3],*

- [1] INRA, Micalis Institute, INRA, AgroParisTech, Université Paris-Saclay, 78352 Jouy-en-Josas, France
- [2] Department of Microbiology, Center of Basic Science, Universidad Autónoma de Aguascalientes, Aguascalientes 20131, Mexico; emsalin@correo.uaa.mx
- [3] Neurosciences Division, Centro de Investigación Biomédica de Occidente, Instituto Mexicano del Seguro Social, Guadalajara 44340, Jalisco, Mexico; genarogabriel@yahoo.com (G.G.O.); ramirez_jirano@hotmail.com (L.J.R.-J.)
- [4] Department of Computer Sciences, Universidad de Guadalajara, Guadalajara 44430, Jalisco, Mexico; jalejandro.morales@academicos.udg.mx
- * Correspondence: luis.bermudez@inra.fr (L.G.B.-H.); neuronim26@yahoo.com (O.K.B.-Q.); Tel.: +33-1-34-652463 (L.G.B.-H.); +52-1-33-1605-6856 (O.K.B.-Q.)

Received: 21 March 2019; Accepted: 18 April 2019; Published: 20 April 2019

Abstract: There is an important relationship between probiotics, psychobiotics and cognitive and behavioral processes, which include neurological, metabolic, hormonal and immunological signaling pathways; the alteration in these systems may cause alterations in behavior (mood) and cognitive level (learning and memory). Psychobiotics have been considered key elements in affective disorders and the immune system, in addition to their effect encompassing the regulation of neuroimmune regulation and control axes (the hypothalamic-pituitary-adrenal axis or HPA, the sympathetic-adrenal-medullary axis or SAM and the inflammatory reflex) in diseases of the nervous system. The aim of this review is to summarize the recent findings about psychobiotics, the brain-gut axis and the immune system. The review focuses on a very new and interesting field that relates the microbiota of the intestine with diseases of the nervous system and its possible treatment, in neuroimmunomodulation area. Indeed, although probiotic bacteria will be concentrated after ingestion, mainly in the intestinal epithelium (where they provide the host with essential nutrients and modulation of the immune system), they may also produce neuroactive substances which act on the brain-gut axis.

Keywords: probiotics; microbiota; beneficial bacteria; psychobiotics; human health

1. Introduction

The skin and mucosal surfaces of vertebrates contain a wide collection of microorganisms (collectively named microbiota) which includes bacteria, fungi, parasites and viruses. The human gut harbors one of the most complex and abundant ecosystems composed of up to 10^{13}–10^{14} microorganisms which is between 1 to 10 times more than the number of eukaryotic cells in the body [1,2]. The collective adult human gut microbiota is composed of a maximum of 500–1000 bacterial species [1,3,4].

Hundreds of years of co-evolution have led to a mutual symbiosis between the host and gut microbiome. Indeed, the gut is rich in molecules that can be used as nutrients by the microorganisms, favoring microbiota colonization [1]. Gut colonization begins at birth and is established in the first 3 years of life. The initial interaction between gut microbiota and the host is indispensable for the maturation of the nervous system, the immune system and for the developmental regulation of intestinal physiology [1,5,6]. At this stage, gut microbiota is also able to modulate the process of angiogenesis [7]. Furthermore, microorganisms also display anti-microbial activities, thus maintaining a stable gut ecosystem. Alterations in the process of microbial colonization of the human gut in early life have been shown to influence the risk of disease [8].

Later in life, microbial colonization of the intestine has a significant impact on the host neurophysiology, behavior and function of the nervous system [9–11]. Given the immunomodulatory properties of gut microbiota, it has been shown that different immune pathways, inside and outside the central nervous system (CNS) are involved in important mechanisms like microbial mediation of brain functions and behavior. It has been discovered that neuroimmune modulation by the microbiota is able to contribute to etio-pathogenesis or to display important signs and symptoms in neurodegenerative and behavioral disorders such as autism spectrum disorders (ASD), anxiety, depression, Alzheimer's disease (AD) and Parkinson's disease (PD) [9].

Furthermore, different bacteria, which are commonly present in a large diversity of food products, transit through our gut every day, interacting with the food products themselves, the host microbiota, and our own cells in either a healthy or a pathological context. Many of the latter microorganisms are known as probiotics. Probiotics are defined as "live microorganisms which when administered in adequate amounts confer a health benefit on the host" [12]. This concept is based on the observations made by Élie Metchnikoff in 1907 in which the regular consumption of lactic acid bacteria (LAB) in fermented dairy products, such as yogurt, was associated with enhanced health and longevity in many people living in Bulgarian villages.

In association with probiotics, the concept of prebiotic was firstly introduced by Gibson and Roberfroid in 1995 as a "nondigestible food ingredient that beneficially affects the host by selectively stimulating the growth and/or activity of one or a limited number of bacteria already resident in the colon" [13]. This definition implies their ability to resist host digestion and their unique activity on microbiota intestinal. However, the progress in prebiotic study has forced the evolution of this definition, as they can also be directly administered to other sites of the body that are also colonized by commensal bacteria, such as skin or vagina. Recently, the International Scientific Association for Probiotics and Prebiotics (ISAPP) in a consensus panel proposed a new definition of prebiotics as "a substrate that is selectively utilized by host microorganisms conferring a health benefit", considering that dietary ones must not be degraded by host enzymes [14]. Substrates that fit with this definition include oligosaccharides (OS), polyunsaturated fatty acid, conjugated linoleic acid, plant polyphenols, and certain fermentable fibers. Among prebiotics highlight fructooligosaccharides (FOS), inulin, galactooligosaccharides (GOS), mannanoligosaccharides (MOS), xylooligosaccharides (XOS) and human milk oligosaccharides (HMO), being FOS and GOS the most studied as well as the classically accepted ones [14]. Prebiotics have been demonstrated to exert beneficial effects on the gastrointestinal tract, immune system, bones, lipid and sugar metabolism, and on mental health.

Dinan and coworkers [15] originally defined psychobiotics as probiotics that, upon ingestion in adequate amounts, yield positive influence on mental health. Because prebiotics have demonstrated benefit on mental health and they support the growing of specific commensal bacteria with psychophysiological effects, prebiotics can be included in the definition of psychobiotics [16]. In this sense, most prebiotic substrates analyzed for their neural effects are FOS and GOS, which favorably stimulate the growth of bifidobacteria and lactobacilli.

The effect of psychobiotics is not limited to the regulation of the neuroimmune axes (hypothalamic pituitary adrenal (HPA)-axis, sympatho-adrenal medullary (SAM)-axis and the inflammatory reflex) and in diseases that involve the nervous system, but they are also related to cognitive, memory, learning and behavior. Psychobiotics have thus opened a very broad and interesting panorama that changes the current paradigm of symbiosis between bacteria and humans. From this new point of view, this relationship seems to be more a commensalism, rather than a pure symbiosis.

2. Axes of Neuroimmune Control and Regulation

It has been shown that there is an important neural control of the immune system [17]. A well-known principle of the physiology in mammals is that the nervous system is responsible for achieving homeostasis by modulating of the function of other systems in the body through the HPA axis, the inflammatory reflex, the enteric nervous system (ENS) and finally the brain-gut axis.

Microglia is the resident immune cell in the CNS which represents 5 to 20% of glial cells. It is a myeloid cell, phagocytic, and has the activity of an antigen presenting cell (APC). In addition, it releases cytokines and can activate inflammatory-type responses [18,19]. During the early development stage, the microglia "brand" and "clean" synapses through a process called "synaptic pruning", promotes the "wiring" of neuronal circuits and releases cytokines and chemokines that assist and guide the process of neuronal differentiation [18,20]. The microbiota has a direct influence on the maturation and function of the microglia. In germ-free (GF)-animals, the microglia display a longer development process and with more derivations, with high levels in the expression of receptor-1 of the colony stimulating factor (CSF1R), F4/80 and CD31, factors that decrease in expression during development. This suggests that there is an important effect of the microbiota on the microglia, which depends on the stage of development and/or the time of microbial colonization.

The microglia of adult GF-mice can be functionally damaged when there are alterations caused by lipopolysaccharide (LPS) or by lymphocytic choriomeningitis virus, which in turn causes alterations in the correct activation of the immune system, including an increase in the release of proinflammatory cytokines such as tumor necrosis factor (TNF)-α, interleukin (IL)-1β and IL-6. These functional deficits are consistent with the concept that the naive microglia of adult GF-mice has a significant decrease in the expression of several genes important to interferon (IFN)-mediated responses, in genes for innate immune responses and genes for viral defense response and effector processes [9,21].

The mechanisms through which intestinal microbes exert their influence on microglia in the brain are not clear but it seems that there is a "microglial modulation" according to a specific type of bacteria [9]. This has raised the question of whether the effects of microbiota on microglia are not regulated by bacteria in general, by the microbiome, or if very specific microbial species are required [9]. The alterations in the morphology of the microglia in GF-animals and the alteration in the expression of genes can be normalized thanks to the post-natal supplementation with short-chain fatty acids (SCFAs), which are products of bacterial fermentation [22,23], suggesting that the bacterial species producing SCFAs are able to restore the alterations that occur in the microglia in GF-mice or treated with antibiotics [9].

The coordination of information between neurons, microglia and the responses at the central level with the periphery is carried out through the different axes of regulation and control; the HPA axis, and the inflammatory reflex (Figure 1). The coordination of these defense responses is mediated by signaling pathways related to the hypothalamus, the pituitary gland and the adrenal glands (e.g., HPA-axis), which causes the release of chemical molecules capable of altering behavior, including glucocorticoids, mineralocorticoids, and catecholamines. The activity of the HPA-axis is regulated by multiple sympathetic, parasympathetic and limbic circuits (amygdala, hippocampus and medial prefrontal cortex) that will directly or indirectly activate the hypothalamic paraventricular nucleus (PVN) [24]. Under normal conditions HPA-axis activity exhibits continuous oscillatory activity synchronized with circadian as well as ultradian rhythms [25,26].

The sympathic nervous system (SNS) and HPA-axis activation are the main components of neurotransmitter release and of neuroendocrine molecules of the stress response [27]. To respond to stress, the SNS is responsible for increasing catecholamine levels in the systemic circulation and tissues, with the concomitant release of corticotropin releasing factor (CRF) from hypothalamic paraventricular neurons, then the release of the adrenocorticotropic hormone (ACTH) from the anterior pituitary gland is stimulated, and ACTH travels through the circulation systemic and induces the synthesis and release of glucocorticoids from adrenals, cortisol in humans and corticosterone in animals. The primary function of the SNS and HPA-axis activation is to prepare the body to respond to damage by increasing the level of glucose in the blood through gluconeogenesis, the suppression of the immune system (suppression of cytokines) and increasing the metabolism of fats and proteins [27,28].

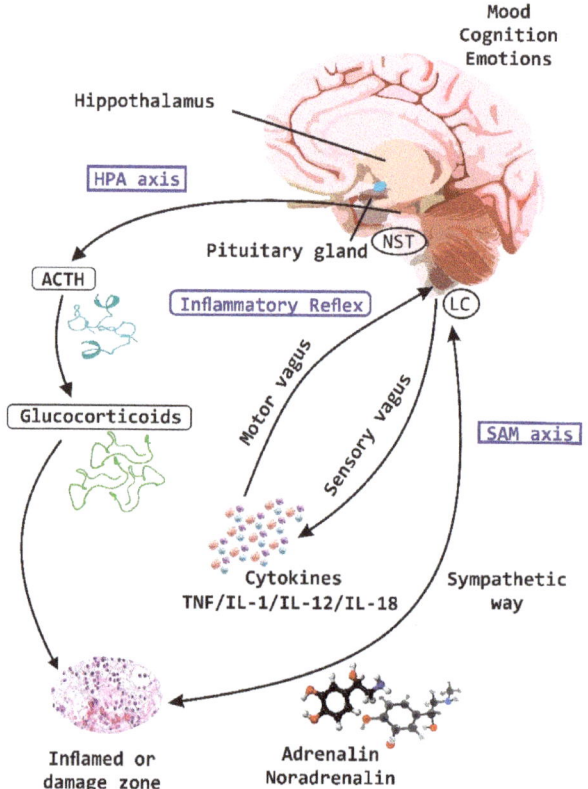

Figure 1. Regulation and control of neuroimmune axes. The three systems of regulation and control of information between the central nervous system (CNS) and the periphery are the hypothalamic pituitary adrenal (HPA)-axis, the sympatho-adrenal medullary (SAM)-axis and the inflammatory reflex. These systems are permanently sensing through nociceptive receptors and send information in real time to the CNS. ACTH, adrenocorticotropic hormone; NST Nucleus of the solitary tract; LC Locus coeruleus; TNF, tumor necrosis factor; IL, interleukin.

The responses of the HPA-axis as well as other variables of the stress response are regulated by exposure to psychological and physical stressors, such as infections [29]. The response of the HPA-axis and the SAM axis to psychological stress is mediated by neurotransmitter systems such as serotonin (5-HT), norepinepherine (NE) and endorphins, which play an important inhibitory role [29].

In addition, the HPA axis is strongly regulated to react efficiently to pathogens such as *Escherichia coli*. This response is mediated by the synthesis of prostanoids induced by the enzyme cyclo-oxygenase (COX). The elevation in corticosterone levels correlates with the increase in prostaglandin (PG) E2 in the circulation [29].

Interestingly, prebiotic intake in early life has been associated with beneficial neurological effects in adulthood. To demonstrate this effect, William and co-workers [30] fed neonatal rats (3 days old) with B-GOS during 19 or 53 days and showed that levels of the N-methyl-D-aspartate receptor (NMDAR) N2A subunit, synaptophysin and the brain-derived neurotrophic factor (BDNF) in the hippocampus of adult rats were elevated as compared with control fed animals. As the expression of the microtubule-associated-protein-2 (MAP2) was not affected, authors propose that neonatal B-GOS feeding impacts on neurotransmission, but not on synaptic architecture. Similar results were reported by Oliveros group [31] supplementing rat pups with 2'-fucosyllactose (FL) during the lactation period. When animals were evaluated just after weaning there was no change in behavior, although 2'-FL-feed rats evoked more intense long-term potentiation (LTP) than control ones. Same animals were evaluated at the age of 1 year and they performed significantly better in behavioral tests and still evoked more intense and longer TLP than the control group. Taken together, these results show that prebiotic administration early in life improves cognitive abilities both in childhood and in adulthood. However, in a randomized controlled trial, no significant improvement in neurodevelopmental outcomes was observed in preterm infants fed with breast milk or preterm formula supplemented with short-chain GOS/long-chain FOS/pectin-derived acidic OS between days 3 and 30 of life when they were evaluated at one or two years of age [32,33].

The basic organizational unit of the nervous system is the reflex arc, which is composed of sensory neurons (afferent) that report information to the CNS and motor neurons (efferent) that send "regulatory" signals to "target" tissues in the periphery. Recent advances in both neuroscience and immunology have revealed that there are neural reflexes that can regulate immune function in a wide range of species through evolution, from *Caenorhabditis elegans* to more complex mammals [17,34,35].

Inflammation is a key process of mammals in order to fight against pathogenic microorganisms and in the mechanism of wound healing. The molecular products of a bacterial invasion and of damaged tissue are rapidly detected by pattern recognition receptors (PRRs), which activate the cells of the innate immune system. The early response of these cells starts a cascade of events whose main function is the exclusion of pathogens and the subsequent restoration of homeostasis. This process includes the synthesis and release of proinflammatory cytokines and leukocyte recruitment [17].

It is crucial for the host to regulate and control an inflammatory response. Different mechanisms of regulation and control of inflammatory mediators have been described; for example, the release of inhibitory cytokines and soluble receptors to cytokines, as well as the activation of different subtypes of regulatory lymphocytes [36]. It is interesting to note that PRRs (Toll-like receptors, TLRs, and Nucleotide-binding and oligomerization domain (NOD)-like receptors, NLRs), in addition to the receptors for cytokines and PG are also expressed by sensory neurons [37]. This provides a molecular mechanism by which the CNS acquires information from a process of inflammation localized in the periphery. In addition, sensory nerves can react to the presence of microbial products independently of the activation of the immune system [17]. These nerves form a dense network along the external surfaces of the organism, and it has been suggested that this type of innervation provides the anatomical basis for a very precise "sensing" by the CNS against a potential infection with a pathogen, a tissue damage or an inflammatory process [17,37]. Reciprocally, many of the cells of the immune system express receptors for neurotransmitters such as dopamine (DA), acetylcholine (Ach) and norepinephrine (NE), all of which in turn regulate the differentiation and activity of leukocytes [17,38–40].

In this phenomenon, afferent signals are transmitted through the "vagus nerve", which are processed at the central level (CNS) and return to the periphery via the vagus efferent nerve, a process by which the release of cytokines is regulated by splenic macrophages [17,41]. Spleen is the major organ where TNF-α is synthesized and released systematically during an endotoxic process (endotoxemia). It has been shown that electrical stimulation of the vagus nerve significantly reduces the release of TNF-α in the spleen. However, the vagus nerve does not directly supply the spleen, the signal travels to the celiac ganglion, where the splenic adrenergic nerve also flows. The electrical stimulation of the latter also reduces the synthesis of TNF-α in the spleen. For this inhibition to occur, activation of the $\alpha 7$ subunit of the nicotinic acetylcholine receptor ($\alpha 7$nAchR) in splenic macrophages is necessary. The adrenergic nerve terminals are very close to a sub-type of T lymphocytes in the spleen that expresses the enzyme choline acetyltransferase (AchT), which has the ability to synthesize Ach, a neurotransmitter that is necessary to inhibit the synthesis and release of TNF-α in the spleen [42].

The vagus nerve, in addition to the splenic and splanchnic nerves, provide an important line of communication with the HPA-axis [29]. For instances, 2 h after vagal stimulation in rodents there is an increase in the expression of the mRNA of CRF in the hypothalamus and corticotropin-releasing hormone (CRH) which in turn increases the levels of ACTH and plasma corticosterone levels. The clinical relevance is the fact that vagal stimulation is associated with clinical benefits (signs and symptoms) antidepressants, together with the "normalization" of HPA-axis parameters in patients with refractory depression [43].

The impact of other prebiotics on brain physiology and biochemistry has also been experimentally studied. Rats that received a diet for 5 weeks supplemented with 2'-FL, the most abundant HMO, experienced increased BNDF levels in the striatum and hippocampus [44]. The expression of other two brain functional markers involved in the LTP process, the postsynaptic density protein (PSD)-95 and phosphorylated calcium/calmodulin-dependent kinase II (pCaMKII), was also augmented at frontal cortex and hippocampus, and at hippocampus, respectively. In accordance, authors reported an enhancement of synaptic plasticity in rats with that feeding regimen and in mice with a 2'-FL long-term feeding (12 weeks) protocol. Both species improved input/output curves and LPT experimentally evoked at hippocampal synapses, with a better performance of the animals in different applied tests of learning behavior.

Finally, some studies have addressed the impact of prebiotics in experimental models of neural dysfunctions. The first one was focused on analyzing the effect of GOS intake in a mouse model of amyotrophic lateral sclerosis (ALS) [45]. Animals started to receive the prebiotic at the age of 8 weeks on a daily basis until the end of the protocol. Mice orally fed with GOS experienced delayed onset of the disease, extended lifespan, improved muscle atrophy, attenuated oxidative stress of skeletal muscles, suppressed astrocyte and microglia activation, inflammatory response and apoptosis in spinal cord tissue. Authors attributed neuroprotective effects of GOS on ALS-sick mice to the amelioration on homocysteine serum levels, an amino acid related to neurotoxic effects in the pathogenesis of ALS, and to the increases in the amount of VitB12 and folato, both of which are involved in homocysteine metabolism [46]. Besides, beneficial effects of GOS have been also described in neuropsychiatric disorders where anxiety and neuroinflammation are clinically involved [47]. In this sense, the supplementation of 8 weeks-old mice standard diet with B-GOS incorporated to drink water during 3 weeks reduced LPS-induced anxiety. B-GOS intake also decreased elevated cortical IL-1β and 5-HT2A receptor expression mediated by LPS in the frontal cortex, in the absence of altered 5-HT metabolism. Thus, the anti-inflammatory effect of the prebiotic is probably modulating its anxiolytic activity. A similar link between anti-inflammation and neuroprotection was reported for chitosan oligosaccharides (CHO) [48] and FOS [49] in a rat model of AD. When CHO was orally administered to amyloid-β_{1-42}-induced rats during 2 weeks, the learning and memory deficits were reduced, and the hippocampal cell death decreased. At the same time, CHO treatment inhibited oxidative stress together with a reduction in proinflammatory cytokines expression at the hippocampus, particularly IL-1β and TNF-α [48]. In the case of a study done with FOS, it was orally and daily administered to amyloid-β_{1-42}-induced rats for 4 weeks or to D-Galactose-induced rats for 8 weeks, with similar outcomes. FOS intake improves inflammation and oxidative stress disorder, ameliorates learning and memory difficulties, and regulates the synthesis and secretion of neurotransmitters such as NE, DA, 5-HT, and 5-hydroxyindole acetic acid (5-HIAA) [49]. All these FOS-induced effects on AD are mediated by the regulation of the gut microbiota.

3. The Interaction of Microbiota with Enteric Nervous System and Brain-Gut Axes

In the last 10 years the importance of the brain-gut axis has been highlighted [50–52]. A connection has been established between the gut and the CNS, which is essential to achieve host homeostasis. It has been called the "brain-gut axis" or "GB axis" [53] (Figure 2). The brain-gut axis includes: the CNS, neuroendocrine and neuroimmune systems, the sympathetic and parasympathetic "arms" of the autonomic nervous system (ANS), the enteric nervous system (ENS) and noticeably the intestinal microbiota [29]. All these components interact and form a very complex network of reflexes, with afferent fibers (input) that project towards integrative structures of the CNS and efferent fibers (output) with projections towards the smooth muscle. This bi-directional communication network enables the sending of signals from the brain and influences the motor, sensory and secretory part of the gut, and conversely, visceral messages from the intestine can influence brain functions, especially in areas dedicated to the regulation of stress at the hypothalamic level [29].

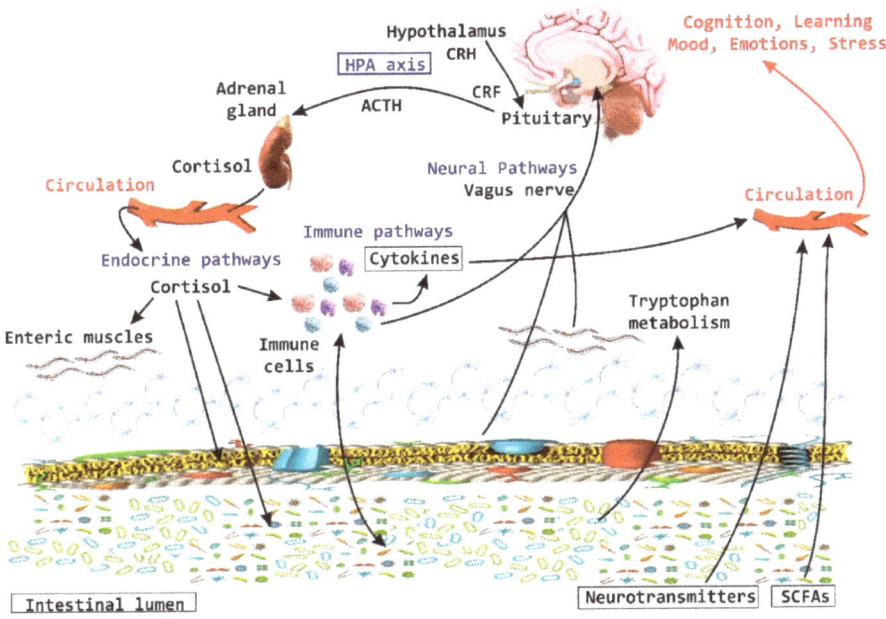

Figure 2. Brain-Gut Axis. The brain-gut axis is essential for the regulation established between the intestine and the brain. It includes the central nervous system and the endocrine and neuroimmune systems; as well as the enteric nervous system. CRH, corticotropin-releasing hormone; CRF, corticotropin releasing factor; SCFAs, short chain fatty acids; ACTH, adrenocorticitropic hormone; HPA, hypothalamic pituitary adrenal.

The sympathetic nervous system (SNP) enables the selective presentation of enteric bacteria to the mucosal immune system. Nerve fibers containing NE have been identified very close to the epithelium surrounding the lymphoid follicles in the jejunum of pigs; the administration of NE increases the reception of pathogenic bacteria inside the follicles [7]. In this sense, it has been suggested that the release of biogenic amines, such as NE, can influence the composition of the intestinal microbiota. For instance, it has been observed that this neurotransmitter stimulates the growth of both pathogenic and nonpathogenic *Escherichia coli in vitro*, in addition to influencing its adherence to the mucous membranes [48,54,55]. Changes in the physiology of the host that originated within the gut or from signals from the CNS, produce changes in the bacterial composition of the gut [7].

The ENS is a complex neuronal network that involves multiple neurotransmitters such as 5-HT, Ach and CRF, where a prominent role is given to the CRF that is mediating changes at the level of gastrointestinal function. At the ENS level, this CRF demonstrates that peripheral pathways also play a preponderant role in the local regulation of the intestine and its function in states of stress [56]. The activation of CRF-1 receptor (CRFR1) in the intestine induced by stress increases the motility of the colon, defecation, permeability of the intestine and the sensation of visceral pain [57]. The activation of CRFR2 inhibits gastric emptying, suppresses the motor function of stimulating the colon and prevents hypersensitivity generated by colorectal distension. It has been proposed that CRFR2 may have a key role in stress-induced patency dysfunction and in mucosal immune modulation and in inflammatory responses in the colon [58]. CRF can directly activate mesenteric neurons to increase motility, permeability and stimulate diarrhea in rodents [59].

The contrasting actions of CRFR1 and CRFR2 are associated with differential expression patterns. CRFR2 is present in anterior regions of the intestinal tract [60], whereas CRFR1 is mostly distributed in the colon, and is expressed in a very important way in the cells of the colon mucosa [56]. The presence of CRFR2 in the colonic mucus has been demonstrated and it has been proposed that in this area it may also have an important role in the stress-induced patency dysfunction in the modulation of immune and inflammatory responses within the colon mucosa [61]. The evidence shows that stress causes the recruitment and activation of CRF receptors in the colon, which induces changes related to the same stress in the intestinal function and in turn causes an increase in sensitivity to stress that results in an altered expression of receptors to CRF [29].

5-HT is recognized as the most important biological substrate in the pathogenesis of mood disorders [62]. There is evidence of the role of serotonergic signaling in the neurobiology of anxiety [63,64]. In GF-mice, altered levels of 5-HT have been reported in the striatum and in the hippocampus, which suggest an association between the microbiota and serotonergic signaling [62]. In addition to its role as a neurotransmitter in the brain, monoamine 5-HT is a potent regulator in the gut. More than 90% of all 5-HT in the body is synthesized in the intestine, where it activates 14 different types of receptors located in enterocytes [65,66], in enteric neurons [67] and in cells of the immune system [68]. In addition, circulating platelets sequester 5-HT from the gut and release it for the purpose of distributing it in different parts of the body [69]. 5-HT derived from the intestine regulates various functions including motor and secretory reflexes, platelet aggregation, regulation of immune responses, bone development, and cardiac function [69]. A dysregulation of peripheral 5-HT levels is implicated in the pathogenesis of diseases such as irritable bowel syndrome (IBS), cardiovascular diseases [70] and in osteoporosis processes. The molecular mechanisms that control the metabolism of 5-HT at the intestinal level are still unclear, but it has been shown to be synthesized by specialized endocrine cells called enterochromaffin cells (ECs), as well as by mast cells of the mucosa and by mesenteric neurons (Figure 3) [69].

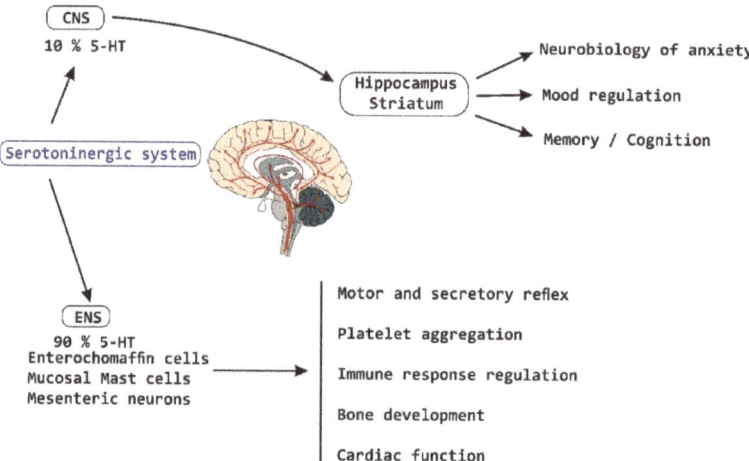

Figure 3. Serotoninergic system. The serotoninergic system is involved in the pathogenesis of diseases at the intestinal level, as well as in the regulation of different functions at a systemic level, which includes the regulation of memory processes, cognition and humor, among others. CNS, central nervous system; 5-HT, serotonin; ENS, enteric nervous system.

Exposure to chronic psychosocial stress decreases the levels of *Bacteroides* spp. and increases the levels of *Clostridium* spp. in the caecum, while increasing circulating levels of IL-6 and CCL2 chemokine (monocyte chemoattractant protein, MCP-1), which is indicative of an immune activation. The levels of IL-6 and CCL2 correlate with changes in the levels of *Coprococcus* spp., *Pseudobutyrivibrio* spp. and *Dorea* spp. induced by stressors directly in the intestine [53].

Some types of bacteria, such as lactobacilli, are able to convert nitrate to nitric oxide (NO), a potent regulator of responses to different levels of immune and nervous system. Lactobacilli also increase the activity of the enzyme indol-amine-2,3-dioxygenase (IDO), involved in the catabolism of tryptophan (TRP) and in formation of neuroactive compounds of kinuric and quinolinic acid [71]. Modification of the intestinal microbiota in adult mice causes changes in behavior, which may be related to immune, neural and hormonal mechanisms. In relation to immune mechanisms, it is known that TLR-2, 4 and 5 are over-regulated in the gut during colonization, which implies that there is interaction between these receptors and the microbiota [72,73]. The dendritic cells (DCs) of the gut break the epithelial layer and interact with commensal bacteria to induce the production of immunoglobulin-A (IgA) by B-lymphocytes and plasma cells. The secreted IgA confines penetration of the microbiota through the epithelium. This mechanism hampers an inflammatory response to commensal bacteria under normal conditions. The DCs are very close to nerve areas of the gut, the neuropeptide sensor calcitonin gene-related peptide (CGRP) modulates the function of these DCs [74] and can send signals about the presence of commensal bacteria to the brain via the vagus nerve [75]. The vagus nerve plays an important role in signaling the gut to the brain and can be stimulated by bacterial products such as endotoxins or inflammatory cytokines such as IL-1β and TNF-α [75]. The vagal response to stimulation by peripheral inflammatory events is the suppression in the release of pro-inflammatory cytokines from intestinal macrophages mediated by α7nAchR [76,77].

Dai, et al. [78] showed that certain probiotics are able to trigger IL-10 mediated anti-inflammatory responses by downregulating the proinflammatory cytokines TNF-α and IL-6. Both of these proinflammatory cytokines, along with IL-2 and IL-1β, are key participants in depressive states and other affective disorders (78). Several other microbe associated molecular patterns (MAMPs) are able to trigger or block inflammatory responses that are associated with different bacterial genera, e.g., bifidobacteria inhibits TLR activation, preventing the inflammatory response [79,80]. Other MAMPs-TLR interactions include OS and the intestinal epithelium. The inflammatory response is directly responsible for the intestinal barrier permeability, nutrient absorption, and microbiome translocation. That is the case in acute stress, that initiates inflammation and secondary dysbiosis, due to aberrant translocation, where the probiotic *Lactobacillus helveticus R0052* has been shown to be able to restore the intestinal barrier [16,79,81,82].

Colonization with *Bacteroides thetaiotaomicron* induces a 2- to 5-fold increase in the expression of mRNA that codes for the synaptic protein-33 associated with vesicles, which is involved in synaptic neurotransmission. This finding confirms that commensal bacteria can influence nervous system functions [7,50]. The intestinal microbiota is essential for the normal development of the immune and mucosal systems, which are intimately associated with the impact of the same microbiota on brain development and function [50].

4. Behavior, Cognition, and Emotion

It has been demonstrated that bi-directional communication exists between the intestine and the brain and that it involves neurological, metabolic, hormonal and immunological signaling pathways; and that disturbance or alteration in these systems can result in altered behavior [83]. A clear example is intestinal inflammation, which has been associated with changes in bowel-brain interactions, as well as a high morbidity between inflammatory bowel disorder and anxiety states (Figure 4) [84].

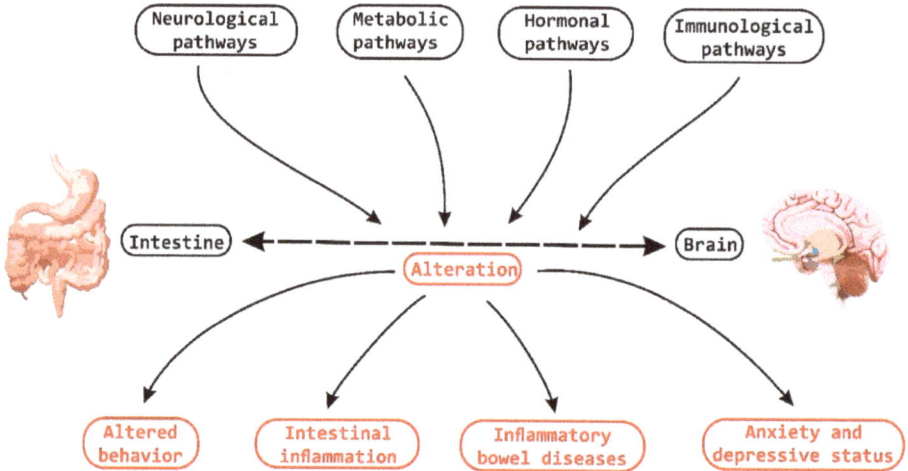

Figure 4. Brain-Gut Homeostasis. The relationship between the intestine and the brain involves signaling pathways at a neural, metabolic, hormonal and immune system levels. The alteration in these pathways is capable of causing changes in cognitive and behavioral processes, as well as inducing inflammatory processes at the periphery level.

The role of microbiota has not only focused on the impact it exerts on the brain and central nervous function but also on how it is intimately related to the constitutive modulation of nerve function at the peripheral central level [71].

Stress has been defined as a very complex dynamic condition in which homeostasis or the internal "resting state" is altered or threatened [85,86]. Throughout life all organisms are exposed to factors that exceed the homeostatic threshold, which results in a stress response, which may be physical, psychological or immunological. Evolution has armed most organisms with the necessary biological machinery to mount a defense response to acute stressors and restore the homeostatic balance once the stress or damage has subsided [85].

A significant number of animal studies provide abundant evidence that the medial prefrontal cortex (MPFC) plays an important role in the regulation of stress circuitry [28]. While the ventral part of the MPFC has been augmented with a stimulatory role, the more dorsal part in contrast has been described to possess an activity of HPA-axis inhibition. It has been also described that this negative feedback mechanism is mediated by the inhibition of glucocorticoid receptors (GRs) in the MPFC [28]. The amygdala is a key region in the process of stress responses in addition to being an important target for the inhibitory feedback system by the MPFC [87]. In humans, the MPFC area is involved in the modulation of amygdala activity during emotional conflicts and in the regulation of autonomic and affective responses [28,88].

Stress, particularly in the early stages of life, is one of the major predictors of the onset of major depression disorder (MDD) [89]. Early exposure to stress and MDD is associated with a significant de-regularization of the HPA-axis and the stress/cortisol response system. Exposure to stressors, HPA-axis deregulation, elevated corticosteroid levels and major depression states are related to structural alterations in the hippocampus and amygdala, key regions in the regulation of the HPA-axis [90,91].

In one study of early life maternal separation, a group of male rats were submitted to stress tests [79]. They all showed the typical pattern: poor forced swim performance while the group that was separated also showed records of high IL-6 blood levels, low NE levels in brain and higher expression of CRF gene in the amygdala [92]. By administering *L. rhamnosus R011* plus *L. helveticus R0052*, the rats downregulated their HPA axis and normalized their corticosterone levels [16,92].

Psychobiotics are now considered key elements in affective disorders. In one experiment with mice that were administered with *L. rhamnosus*, they featured lesser signs of anxiety and depression in forced swim and plus elevated maze respectively than their control counterparts, even at the same levels of corticosterone [16,93]. This suggests that the probiotic had a downregulation effect over HPA axis [93]. In the presence of *L. rhamnosus*, mice showed a lower hippocampal expression of the GABA$_{B1b}$ receptor gene and a higher expression of it in the cingulated cortex and limbic regions. Since GABA is the main inhibitory neurotransmitter of the nervous system, it would appear that psycobiotics are able to modulate the local balance of inhibition/exciting in order to control the systemic responses to stress, anxiety and depression [93].

As previously described, GF-mice exhibit an exaggerated response to stressors, with the presentation of anxious-type behaviors and cognitive deficits [94,95]. This behavior is influenced by the amygdala and the hippocampus. The signaling between the basolateral amygdala (BLA) and the ventral hippocampus modulates anxiety behaviors and social behaviors [96]. Tune changes (structural changes) in the amygdala and hippocampus are associated with anxiety disorders in humans and in rodents in early stages of development. There is evidence of hypertrophy of the dendrites of excitatory neurons in the BLA area under a state of repeated (repetitive) stress that induces atrophy of the dendrites in hippocampal neurons [94].

The "germ-free" status induces dendritic hypertrophy in inhibitory interneurons, and the excitatory pyramidal neurons of the BLA area show increased density of spines type: "thin", "stubby" and "mushroom". The absence of intestinal microbiota induces dendritic atrophy in other areas of the CNS, as is the case of hippocampal pyramidal neurons and granular cells of the dentate gyrus. In GF-animals, there is a significant loss of "stubby" and "mushroom" spines in hippocampal pyramidal neurons [94].

It has been estimated that there are 32% fewer synaptic connections in hippocampal pyramidal neurons of GF-animals when the dendrite size decreases and this is combined with a smaller size in the same dendritic spines [94].

A characteristic shared by the animal models of autism and GF-mice is an important alteration in the processes of social behavior. This type of alterations is in turn associated with alterations in the volume of the hippocampus and the amygdala. Changes in the size of these structures have been well documented in experiments with rodents, subject to severe stressors. Prenatally stressed rats experience an increase in the volume of the lateral amygdala [97,98] whereas chronic stress or treatment with corticosteroids induces hippocampal atrophy [98]. Changes in these structures of the CNS are frequently observed in human patients with anxiety disorders or with autism, clearly indicating that the volumetric alterations of the limbic structures can in turn be the result of a maladaptive response to stress [94]. In chronically stressed mice, dendrite hypertrophy is observed in inhibitory GABAergic neurons of the prefrontal cortex area [99].

The amygdala has different "target" areas that are responsible for modulating neuroendocrine responses to stress. The BLA area is activated by psychological stressors, and lesions in this area significantly reduce the HPA-axis response efficiency [94]. While, on the other hand, the area of the central nucleus of the amygdala (CeA) is not involved in the signaling of the HPA-axis induced by stressors, it is an area that also regulates autonomic responses to stress [94]. GF-mice have a lower degree of anxiety and social cognitive deficit, and it has been mentioned previously that there is an important relationship between anxiety and social behavior; the amygdala and the area of the ventral hypothalamus are directly involved in the regulation of this type of behavior [100]. In addition to having a preponderant role in the regulation of anxiety, the ventral hypothalamus is also involved in processes of sociability, and an alteration or damage in this area leads to the appearance of abnormal responses to social situations [101]. Besides, this ventral hippocampus exhibits a very important reciprocal connection with the amygdala, another area involved in anxiety and sociability [100].

The different tonsillar sub-regions have different roles in the regulation of anxiety and social behavior. The areas of the lateral amygdala (LA) and the BLA area integrate sensory information and adverse situations and then send their projections to the CeA area [100]. The stimulation of the projections from the BLA to the CeA area induces an anxiolytic phenotype in mice [102]. This is in contrast to direct stimulation of the entire BLA area, where an opposite effect is generated, suggesting that most of the BLA neurons project towards areas that regulate anxiogenic effects [102].

It has been mentioned that chronic stress in the adult stage is also capable of affecting the composition of the gut microbiota [11]. It is clear that alterations in the brain-gut axis interactions are associated with intestinal inflammatory processes, syndromes of chronic abdominal pain, and with eating disorders [11,103]. This altered modulation of the brain-gut axis is associated with alterations in the regulation of stress responses and behavioral alterations. The high co-morbidity that exists between stress and some symptoms of psychiatric illnesses such as high anxiety, gastrointestinal disorders (included in irritable bowel syndrome, IBS) is clear evidence of the importance of this axis in the pathophysiology of certain types of diseases [11].

Chronic stress on the other hand breaks the intestinal barrier, causes filtrations and alters the ability of the HPA-axis to reverse the deleterious effects of stress (Figure 5) [93,94].

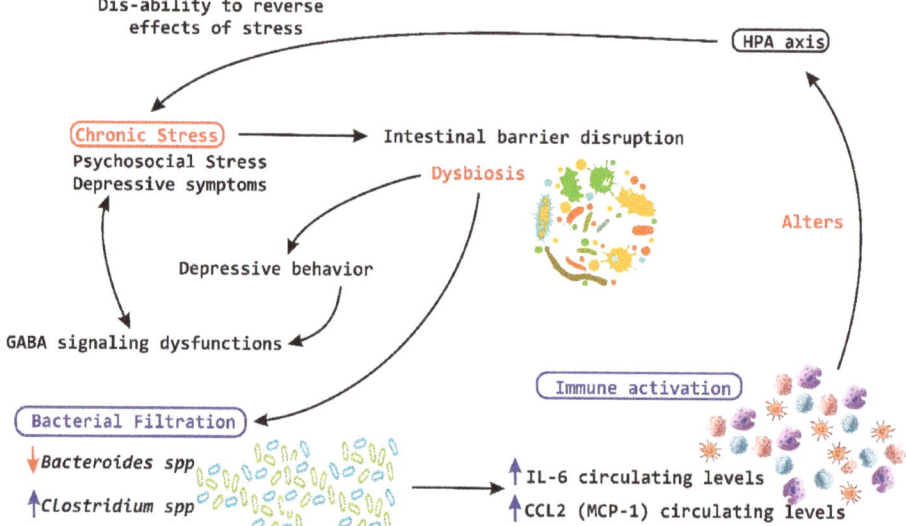

Figure 5. Chronic stress and HPA axis. A chronic stress process is capable of causing disruption at a level of the intestinal barrier and cause dysbiosis, which in turn induces the leakage of bacteria and the activation of the local immune system, leading to a significant alteration of the hypothalamic pituitary adrenal (HPA)-axis. IL, interleukin; MCP-1, monocyte chemoattractant protein; red arrow down mean decrease levels; blue arrow up mean increase levels.

GABA is the major inhibitory neurotransmitter in the CNS. Dysfunctions in GABA signaling are associated with anxiety and depression [104]. Lactobacilli and bifidobacteria are able to metabolize glutamate to produce GABA *in vitro* [62,104,105]. In an *in vivo* experiment in mice, a strain of *Lactobacillus rhamnosus* shows an effect and influence on depressive and ancestral behavior, and it can also alter the central expression of GABA receptors in key brain regions for stress management [62].

In 2006, Kamiya et al. [106] demonstrated that oral administration of *Lactobacillus* species for anesthetized rats is capable of completely suppressing colonic distension induced by pseudo-affective cardiac responses, which is reflected in the inhibition of visceral pain perception. This treatment is also effective in reducing electrical charges in fibers of the dorsal root of the ganglia [71]. The administration of these same strains of *Lactobacillus* to healthy adult rats is enough to activate calcium (Ca^{2+}) and potassium (K$^+$) channels in neurons-AH (after hyperpolarization) of the ENS in mesenteric plexus of the colon [71].

It has been shown that the oral administration of specific strains of *Lactobacillus* induces the expression of opioids-μ receptors and cannabinoids and promotes analgesic functions similar to effects of morphine. This suggests that intestinal microbiota can influence our visceral perception [107]. Altogether, these findings indicate that probiotics are able to modulate the function responsible for the visceral and somatic perception of pain [71].

Currently, there is evidence that supports the influence of intestinal microbiota on the behavior and health of SNC [1]. Patients with depressive symptoms show a significant improvement in the symptoms of depression accompanied by a reduction in plasma TRP after a fructose-restricted diet. Furthermore, fructose malabsorption provides the substrate for a rapid bacterial fermentation, which results in changes in gut motility [72]. The administration of a strain of *Bifidobacterium infantis* for 14 days increases the levels of plasma TRP, suggesting that commensal bacteria have the ability to influence the metabolism of TRP [93].

Intestinal bacteria are potent regulators of systemic and local immune responses such as that related to mucous membranes, in addition to contributing to the development of inflammatory disorders in the CNS. GF-animals or animals treated with antibiotics with an experimental autoimmune encephalomyelitis (EAE) process present reduced inflammation and a lower degree of disease compared to conventional mice, which suggest the existence of complex interactions between commensal bacteria and the inflammatory process in CNS [9,97,98]. For example, segmented filamentous bacteria (frequently associated with the intestinal epithelium) promote the development of Th17 helper T cells, which produce IL-17. They have been termed as Th17 cells in the small intestine of mice [99,108].

There is important evidence that the brain-gut axis can influence brain chemistry and is able to modulate behavior in adult mice [43]. A transient disturbance in the microbiota is able to increase the levels of BDNF in the hippocampus, as well as increase the exploratory behavior of animals. In the hippocampus, BDNF is associated with memory and learning processes and recent evidence indicates that this increase is associated with anxiolytic and antidepressant-like behavior [43]. On the other hand, the amygdala is also associated with memory and disorders in the mood and there has been an increase in the expression of BDNF in the amygdala during processes of "learning fear" [109]. Low levels of BDNF in the amygdala increase the exploratory behavior of the animals (Figure 6) [9,43].

Some other molecules with psychobiotic potential are SCFAs. These are macronutrients from non-digestible metabolites e.g., microbiome secondary degradation products of plant polysaccharides, and their production and release can be enhanced by prebiotic consumption [110,111]. These SCFAs include butyrate, acetate and propionate. It has been shown that butyrate crosses the blood-brain barrier and exhibits important neuroprotective, cognitive and anti-depressive effects [112]. Some mechanisms related to SCFAs include epigenomic histone-deacetylase gene expression regulation and HPA axis regulation [79,113,114].

Other secondary products of the psychobiotic-mediated metabolism of non-digestible fiber is DA and NE from bacilli, GABA from bifidobacteria, serotonin from enteroccocci and streptoccocci, NE and serotonin from *E. coli* and acetylcholine from lactobacilli. It is not entirely clear how much these neurotransmitters modulate the synaptic activity of the ENS [115–117].

The SCFAs regulate the metabolism of free fatty acids, glucose and cholesterol through various signaling cascades involving receptors linked to G-proteins [1,48]. It has also been found that acetylation of histones and SCFAs can improve cognitive function in animal models of neurodevelopment and neurodegenerative diseases, however, another group of researchers showed that the administration of a specific SCFAs, the propionic acid (PPA), can induce altered behavior traits in patients with ASD in addition to neurochemical changes [118]. These changes include neuroinflammation, elevation in levels of oxidative stress, and an important depletion in the efficiency of the antioxidant system; and all together can cause mitochondrial dysfunction, which is common in patients with ASD and in other neurodegenerative diseases such as AD and PD [119,120]. The PPA also exhibits neurotransmitter effects, effects on tight junctions and on immune function. SCFAs are associated with high levels of phosphorylated cAMP response element-binding (CREB), which induces a significant increase in catecholamine levels [121].

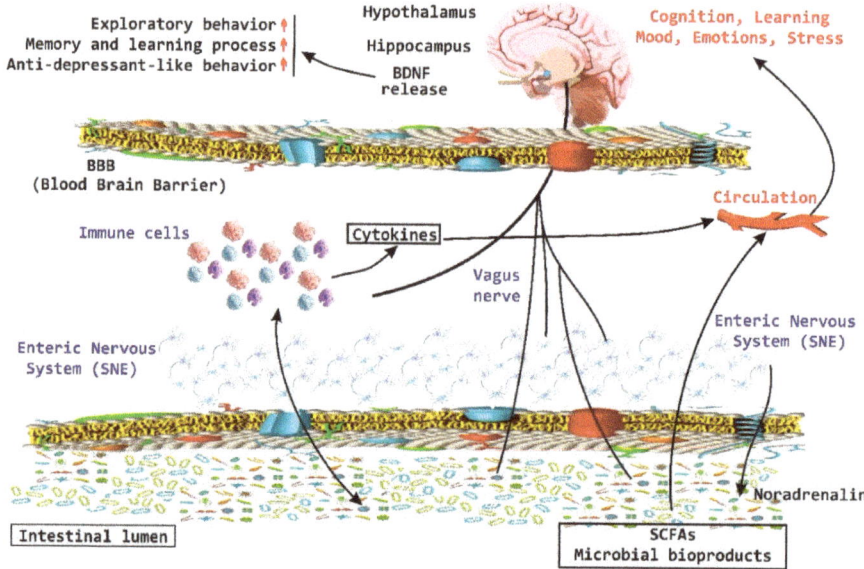

Figure 6. BDNF release system. The brain-derived neurotrophic factor (BDNF) released via the activation of the brain-gut axis has been associated with cognitive and behavioral processes, as well as with anxiolytic and antidepressive effects. SCFAs, short chain fatty acids; red arrow up mean increase levels.

A first experimental study developed in rats orally administered with FOS or GOS for 5 weeks showed that both prebiotics augmented the amount of hippocampal BDNF and NR1 subunit of glutamate N-methyl-D-aspartate receptor (NMDAR) [122]. Besides, oral administration of GOS induced an increase in NR2A subunit expression in hippocampus, NR1 subunit and D-serine expression in frontal cortex, and plasma D-alanine. Brain levels of other amino acids related with glutamate neurotransmission were not modified by either prebiotic. Authors demonstrated that both prebiotics increased the number of fecal *Bifidobacteria*, with the effect being greater with GOS intake. However, OG may be modulating brain chemistry independently of its prebiotic activity, as gut hormones such as peptide YY (PYY) were increased in plasma of GOS-fed rats in relation with BDNF increase, suggesting a direct interaction between GOS and gut mucosa that may inclusive influence the immune system. Based in these experimental results, the same research group developed a clinical study in healthy human volunteers that received FOS, Bimuno® GOS (B-GOS) or placebo daily during 3 weeks [123]. Although no effects in cortisol secretion and emotional processing were observed in relation to FOS consumption, the intake of B-GOS decreased salivary cortisol awakening response and attentional bias in participants as compared to those receiving placebo. Recently, Burokas and co-workers developed a protocol in mice supplemented with FOS, GOS or a FOS-GOS combination during 3 weeks to analyze endocrine response to stress, neurotransmitters and their receptor brain expression, gut microbiota composition, and SCFAs levels [124]. FOS-GOS treatment exhibited both antidepressant and anxiolytic effects and reduced stress-induced corticosterone release. The same decrease on corticosterone level was achieved with GOS intake, however FOS had no effect. Prebiotics also modified specific gene expression of neurotransmitters and involved-receptors in hippocampus and hypothalamus. Notably, cecal acetate and propionate concentrations were increased and that of isobutyrate was diminished by prebiotics, changes that correlated significantly with the positive effects seen on behavior. When FOS-GOS-treated mice were exposed to chronic psychosocial stress, elevations in corticosterone and proinflammatory cytokine levels, and depression- and anxiety-like behavior were reduced, as well as changes on microbiota were normalized. Thus, as previously demonstrated with probiotics, specific prebiotics may also modulate HPA axis activity and attention to emotional stimuli, suggesting a beneficial role of prebiotic treatment for stress-related behaviors.

Another path through which microbiota is able to affect functions in the CNS is by the alteration of hippocampal neurogenesis (AHN) in adults. Indeed, it has been described that the adult brain has the capacity to generate new neurons within the hippocampus and the lateral ventricles [125]. AHN is involved in memory and learning processes and can be affected by an important variety of neurological disorders such as epilepsy, major depression, AD and PD, among others [126,127]. A decrease in the number of neural stem cells and in the AHN process is observed in old age, with the concomitant cognitive decline [127]. Since metabolic and immune system pathways are involved in this process, dysbiosis of the intestinal microbiota due to diseases in the early stages of development may have long-term effects on behavior and cognitive function.

During an episode of medium stress, they observed an increase in ACTH and corticosterone release in young GF-mice, compared to young conventional specific pathogen free (SPF) mice [128]. The increases in ACTH and corticosterone levels induced by stress were completely reversed in GF mice when colonized with *B. infantis*, but only partially reversed when the mice were colonized with the microbiota of SPF mice. These findings suggest that within the microbiota of SPF mice there are bacteria that contribute to the suppression of the ACTH response.

Microbiome studies in autoimmune diseases have shown important alterations in the levels of certain bacterial groups such as *Bifidobacteria* spp. and *Lactobacillus* spp., as well as elevated levels of *Clostridia* spp., *Staphilococcus* spp. and *E. coli* [129–131], which are capable of alter the immune response, proinflammatory cytokine (TNF-α and IL-1-β) and anti-inflammatory (IL-10) levels, and generate feedback loops of dysbiosis while altering the immune responses. Celiac disease is a chronic inflammatory bowel disease caused by an autoimmune response to gluten [129]; in patients with celiac disease, the persistence of GABA has been suggested by mediating intracortical dysfunction despite dietary restriction. This hyperexcitability can be the result of a regulation in the GABAergic inhibitory interneurons mediated in the immune system or by a cortical reorganization mediated by glutamate, an excitatory neurotransmitter, which tries to compensate for the illness of the gluten disease [132]. In celiac disease, autoreactive clones of anti-tissue transglutaminase (anti-tTG)2 and anti-tTG6 antibodies have been found in intestine and areas of the nervous system (cerebellum, pons, bone marrow and blood vessels), addition to possible injury to the integrity of the BBB by infiltration of activated Th1 cell-exposing the brain parenchyma to the action of auto-antibodies [133]. This process leads to synaptic hyper-excitation and low inhibition at the cortical level [132,133], promoting the typical neurological signs of this disease.

Another important finding made by Sudo et al. [128] was a severe reduction in BDNF expression, at mRNA and protein levels, in the cortex and hippocampus of GF-mice, compared with SPF-mice. BDNF regulates important aspects of brain activity, including mood and cognitive functions [128]. Other reports have shown the influence of gut microbiota on the development of brain responses to stress and on cognitive functions in young mice [7,128].

5. Conclusions and Future Research

Nowadays, we recognize the need to study the human microbiota and probiotics as a whole ecosystem to better understand the relation between microbiota and host health or disease. One of the major limitations in using psychobiotics in humans is the lack of its possible interaction with sex hormones (estrogen and/or testosterone) and its long-term effect. Preliminary findings on how probiotic treatments, called psychobiotics, may help improve your mood, decrease your anxiety, and strengthen your memory suggest that in the near future these probiotics could be prescribed to treat depression, anxiety, and other mental health issues, by using them in the form of food or supplements to alter the gut microbiome and treat psychiatric conditions.

Author Contributions: Conceptualization, O.K.B.-Q., L.G.B.-H., J.A.M.; Compiling and curation of the state-of-the-art, O.K.B.-Q., L.G.B.-H., E.S., L.J.R.-J., G.G.O., J.A.M.; Project administration, OKB; Visualization, O.K.B.-Q., L.J.R.-J., J.A.M.; Writing—original draft, O.K.B.-Q., L.G.B.-H., E.S., L.J.R.-J., G.G.O., J.A.M.; Writing—review & editing, O.K.B.-Q., L.G.B.-H., E.S., L.J.R.-J., J.A.M.; Supervision, O.K.B.-Q., L.G.B.-H.

Funding: This research received no external funding.

Conflicts of Interest: The authors declare no conflict of interest.

References

1. Leung, K.; Thuret, S. Gut Microbiota: A Modulator of Brain Plasticity and Cognitive Function in Ageing. *Healthcare* **2015**, *3*, 898–916. [CrossRef]
2. Qin, J.; Li, R.; Raes, J.; Arumugam, M.; Burgdorf, K.S.; Manichanh, C.; Nielsen, T.; Pons, N.; Levenez, F.; Yamada, T.; et al. A human gut microbial gene catalogue established by metagenomic sequencing. *Nature* **2010**, *464*, 59–65. [CrossRef]
3. Palmer, C.; Bik, E.M.; DiGiulio, D.B.; Relman, D.A.; Brown, P.O. Development of the human infant intestinal microbiota. *PLoS Biol.* **2007**, *5*, e177. [CrossRef]
4. Jasarevic, E.; Howerton, C.L.; Howard, C.D.; Bale, T.L. Alterations in the Vaginal Microbiome by Maternal Stress Are Associated with Metabolic Reprogramming of the Offspring Gut and Brain. *Endocrinology* **2015**, *156*, 3265–3276. [CrossRef] [PubMed]
5. Bercik, P.; Collins, S.M.; Verdu, E.F. Microbes and the gut-brain axis. *Neurogastroenterol. Motil.* **2012**, *24*, 405–413. [CrossRef]
6. Kamada, N.; Seo, S.U.; Chen, G.Y.; Nunez, G. Role of the gut microbiota in immunity and inflammatory disease. *Nat. Rev. Immunol.* **2013**, *13*, 321–335. [CrossRef] [PubMed]
7. Collins, S.M.; Bercik, P. The relationship between intestinal microbiota and the central nervous system in normal gastrointestinal function and disease. *Gastroenterology* **2009**, *136*, 2003–2014. [CrossRef] [PubMed]
8. Moustafa, A.; Li, W.; Anderson, E.L.; Wong, E.H.M.; Dulai, P.S.; Sandborn, W.J.; Biggs, W.; Yooseph, S.; Jones, M.B.; Venter, J.C.; et al. Genetic risk, dysbiosis, and treatment stratification using host genome and gut microbiome in inflammatory bowel disease. *Clin. Transl. Gastroenterol.* **2018**, *9*, e132. [CrossRef] [PubMed]
9. Fung, T.C.; Olson, C.A.; Hsiao, E.Y. Interactions between the microbiota, immune and nervous systems in health and disease. *Nat. Neurosci.* **2017**, *20*, 145–155. [CrossRef]
10. Collins, S.M.; Surette, M.; Bercik, P. The interplay between the intestinal microbiota and the brain. *Nat. Rev. Microbiol.* **2012**, *10*, 735–742. [CrossRef]
11. Cryan, J.F.; Dinan, T.G. Mind-altering microorganisms: The impact of the gut microbiota on brain and behaviour. *Nat. Rev. Neurosci.* **2012**, *13*, 701–712. [CrossRef]
12. Hill, C.; Guarner, F.; Reid, G.; Gibson, G.R.; Merenstein, D.J.; Pot, B.; Morelli, L.; Canani, R.B.; Flint, H.J.; Salminen, S.; et al. Expert consensus document. The International Scientific Association for Probiotics and Prebiotics consensus statement on the scope and appropriate use of the term probiotic. *Nat. Rev. Gastroenterol. Hepatol.* **2014**, *11*, 506–514. [CrossRef]
13. Gibson, G.R.; Roberfroid, M.B. Dietary modulation of the human colonic microbiota: Introducing the concept of prebiotics. *J. Nutr.* **1995**, *125*, 1401–1412. [CrossRef] [PubMed]
14. Gibson, G.R.; Hutkins, R.; Sanders, M.E.; Prescott, S.L.; Reimer, R.A.; Salminen, S.J.; Scott, K.; Stanton, C.; Swanson, K.S.; Cani, P.D.; et al. Expert consensus document: The International Scientific Association for Probiotics and Prebiotics (ISAPP) consensus statement on the definition and scope of prebiotics. *Nat. Rev. Gastroenterol. Hepatol.* **2017**, *14*, 491–502. [CrossRef]
15. Dinan, T.G.; Stanton, C.; Cryan, J.F. Psychobiotics: A novel class of psychotropic. *Biol. Psychiatry* **2013**, *74*, 720–726. [CrossRef] [PubMed]
16. Sarkar, A.; Lehto, S.M.; Harty, S.; Dinan, T.G.; Cryan, J.F.; Burnet, P.W.J. Psychobiotics and the Manipulation of Bacteria-Gut-Brain Signals. *Trends Neurosci.* **2016**, *39*, 763–781. [CrossRef]
17. Sundman, E.; Olofsson, P.S. Neural control of the immune system. *Adv. Physiol. Educ.* **2014**, *38*, 135–139. [CrossRef]

18. Nayak, D.; Roth, T.L.; McGavern, D.B. Microglia development and function. *Annu. Rev. Immunol.* **2014**, *32*, 367–402. [CrossRef] [PubMed]
19. Nayak, D.; Zinselmeyer, B.H.; Corps, K.N.; McGavern, D.B. In vivo dynamics of innate immune sentinels in the CNS. *Intravital* **2012**, *1*, 95–106. [CrossRef] [PubMed]
20. Hu, X.; Leak, R.K.; Shi, Y.; Suenaga, J.; Gao, Y.; Zheng, P.; Chen, J. Microglial and macrophage polarization-new prospects for brain repair. *Nat. Rev. Neurol.* **2015**, *11*, 56–64. [CrossRef]
21. Matcovitch-Natan, O.; Winter, D.R.; Giladi, A.; Vargas Aguilar, S.; Spinrad, A.; Sarrazin, S.; Ben-Yehuda, H.; David, E.; Zelada González, F.; Perrin, P.; et al. Microglia development follows a stepwise program to regulate brain homeostasis. *Science* **2016**, *353*, aad8670. [CrossRef]
22. Erny, D.; Hrabe de Angelis, A.L.; Jaitin, D.; Wieghofer, P.; Staszewski, O.; David, E.; Keren-Shaul, H.; Mahlakoiv, T.; Jakobshagen, K.; Buch, T.; et al. Host microbiota constantly control maturation and function of microglia in the CNS. *Nat. Neurosci.* **2015**, *18*, 965–977. [CrossRef] [PubMed]
23. Borre, Y.E.; O'Keeffe, G.W.; Clarke, G.; Stanton, C.; Dinan, T.G.; Cryan, J.F. Microbiota and neurodevelopmental windows: Implications for brain disorders. *Trends Mol. Med.* **2014**, *20*, 509–518. [CrossRef] [PubMed]
24. Smith, S.M.; Vale, W.W. The role of the hypothalamic-pituitary-adrenal axis in neuroendocrine responses to stress. *Dialogues Clin. Neurosci.* **2006**, *8*, 383–395.
25. Dallman, M.F.; Akana, S.F.; Levin, N.; Walker, C.D.; Bradbury, M.J.; Suemaru, S.; Scribner, K.S. Corticosteroids and the control of function in the hypothalamo-pituitary-adrenal (HPA) axis. *Ann. N. Y. Acad. Sci.* **1994**, *746*, 22–31; discussion 31–32, 64–67. [CrossRef]
26. Dickmeis, T.; Weger, B.D.; Weger, M. The circadian clock and glucocorticoids—Interactions across many time scales. *Mol. Cell Endocrinol.* **2013**, *380*, 2–15. [CrossRef]
27. Mayer, E.A. The neurobiology of stress and gastrointestinal disease. *Gut* **2000**, *47*, 861–869. [CrossRef] [PubMed]
28. Ma, S.T.; Abelson, J.L.; Okada, G.; Taylor, S.F.; Liberzon, I. Neural circuitry of emotion regulation: Effects of appraisal, attention, and cortisol administration. *Cogn. Affect. Behav. Neurosci.* **2017**, *17*, 437–451. [CrossRef] [PubMed]
29. Dinan, T.G.; Cryan, J.F. Regulation of the stress response by the gut microbiota: Implications for psychoneuroendocrinology. *Psychoneuroendocrinology* **2012**, *37*, 1369–1378. [CrossRef]
30. Williams, S.; Chen, L.; Savignac, H.M.; Tzortzis, G.; Anthony, D.C.; Burnet, P.W. Neonatal prebiotic (BGOS) supplementation increases the levels of synaptophysin, GluN2A-subunits and BDNF proteins in the adult rat hippocampus. *Synapse* **2016**, *70*, 121–124. [CrossRef] [PubMed]
31. Oliveros, E.; Ramirez, M.; Vazquez, E.; Barranco, A.; Gruart, A.; Delgado-Garcia, J.M.; Buck, R.; Rueda, R.; Martin, M.J. Oral supplementation of 2'-fucosyllactose during lactation improves memory and learning in rats. *J. Nutr. Biochem.* **2016**, *31*, 20–27. [CrossRef] [PubMed]
32. Van den Berg, J.P.; Westerbeek, E.A.; Broring-Starre, T.; Garssen, J.; van Elburg, R.M. Neurodevelopment of Preterm Infants at 24 Months After Neonatal Supplementation of a Prebiotic Mix: A Randomized Trial. *J. Pediatr. Gastroenterol. Nutr.* **2016**, *63*, 270–276. [CrossRef] [PubMed]
33. LeCouffe, N.E.; Westerbeek, E.A.; van Schie, P.E.; Schaaf, V.A.; Lafeber, H.N.; van Elburg, R.M. Neurodevelopmental outcome during the first year of life in preterm infants after supplementation of a prebiotic mixture in the neonatal period: A follow-up study. *Neuropediatrics* **2014**, *45*, 22–29. [CrossRef]
34. Olofsson, P.S.; Rosas-Ballina, M.; Levine, Y.A.; Tracey, K.J. Rethinking inflammation: Neural circuits in the regulation of immunity. *Immunol. Rev.* **2012**, *248*, 188–204. [CrossRef] [PubMed]
35. Sun, J.; Singh, V.; Kajino-Sakamoto, R.; Aballay, A. Neuronal GPCR controls innate immunity by regulating noncanonical unfolded protein response genes. *Science* **2011**, *332*, 729–732. [CrossRef]
36. Nathan, C. Points of control in inflammation. *Nature* **2002**, *420*, 846–852. [CrossRef] [PubMed]
37. Chiu, I.M.; von Hehn, C.A.; Woolf, C.J. Neurogenic inflammation and the peripheral nervous system in host defense and immunopathology. *Nat. Neurosci.* **2012**, *15*, 1063–1067. [CrossRef] [PubMed]
38. Elenkov, I.J.; Wilder, R.L.; Chrousos, G.P.; Vizi, E.S. The sympathetic nerve—An integrative interface between two supersystems: The brain and the immune system. *Pharmacol. Rev.* **2000**, *52*, 595–638. [PubMed]
39. Kipnis, J.; Cardon, M.; Avidan, H.; Lewitus, G.M.; Mordechay, S.; Rolls, A.; Shani, Y.; Schwartz, M. Dopamine, through the extracellular signal-regulated kinase pathway, downregulates CD4+CD25+ regulatory T-cell activity: Implications for neurodegeneration. *J. Neurosci.* **2004**, *24*, 6133–6143. [CrossRef]

40. Prado, C.; Contreras, F.; Gonzalez, H.; Diaz, P.; Elgueta, D.; Barrientos, M.; Herrada, A.A.; Lladser, Á.; Bernales, S.; Pacheco, R. Stimulation of dopamine receptor D5 expressed on dendritic cells potentiates Th17-mediated immunity. *J. Immunol.* **2012**, *188*, 3062–3070. [CrossRef]
41. Tracey, K.J. The inflammatory reflex. *Nature* **2002**, *420*, 853–859. [CrossRef] [PubMed]
42. Rosas-Ballina, M.; Olofsson, P.S.; Ochani, M.; Valdes-Ferrer, S.I.; Levine, Y.A.; Reardon, C.; Tusche, M.W.; Pavlov, V.A.; Andersson, U.; Chavan, S.; et al. Acetylcholine-synthesizing T cells relay neural signals in a vagus nerve circuit. *Science* **2011**, *334*, 98–101. [CrossRef]
43. Bercik, P.; Denou, E.; Collins, J.; Jackson, W.; Lu, J.; Jury, J.; Deng, Y.; Blennerhassett, P.; Macri, J.; McCoy, K.D.; et al. The intestinal microbiota affect central levels of brain-derived neurotropic factor and behavior in mice. *Gastroenterology* **2011**, *141*, 599–609, 609.e1-3. [CrossRef] [PubMed]
44. Vazquez, E.; Barranco, A.; Ramirez, M.; Gruart, A.; Delgado-Garcia, J.M.; Martinez-Lara, E.; Blanco, S.; Martín, M.J.; Castanys, E.; Buck, R.; et al. Effects of a human milk oligosaccharide, 2′-fucosyllactose, on hippocampal long-term potentiation and learning capabilities in rodents. *J. Nutr. Biochem.* **2015**, *26*, 455–465. [CrossRef] [PubMed]
45. Song, L.; Gao, Y.; Zhang, X.; Le, W. Galactooligosaccharide improves the animal survival and alleviates motor neuron death in SOD1G93A mouse model of amyotrophic lateral sclerosis. *Neuroscience* **2013**, *246*, 281–290. [CrossRef] [PubMed]
46. Castro, R.; Rivera, I.; Blom, H.J.; Jakobs, C.; Tavares de Almeida, I. Homocysteine metabolism, hyperhomocysteinaemia and vascular disease: An overview. *J. Inherit. Metab Dis.* **2006**, *29*, 3–20. [CrossRef] [PubMed]
47. Savignac, H.M.; Couch, Y.; Stratford, M.; Bannerman, D.M.; Tzortzis, G.; Anthony, D.C.; Burnet, P.W.J. Prebiotic administration normalizes lipopolysaccharide (LPS)-induced anxiety and cortical 5-HT2A receptor and IL1-beta levels in male mice. *Brain Behav. Immun.* **2016**, *52*, 120–131. [CrossRef]
48. Jia, S.; Lu, Z.; Gao, Z.; An, J.; Wu, X.; Li, X.; Dai, X.; Zheng, Q.; Sun, Y. Chitosan oligosaccharides alleviate cognitive deficits in an amyloid-beta1-42-induced rat model of Alzheimer's disease. *Int. J. Biol. Macromol.* **2016**, *83*, 416–425. [CrossRef] [PubMed]
49. Chen, D.; Yang, X.; Yang, J.; Lai, G.; Yong, T.; Tang, X.; Shuai, O.; Zhou, G.; Xie, Y.; Wu, Q. Prebiotic Effect of Fructooligosaccharides from Morinda officinalis on Alzheimer's Disease in Rodent Models by Targeting the Microbiota-Gut-Brain Axis. *Front. Aging Neurosci.* **2017**, *9*, 403. [CrossRef]
50. Neufeld, K.A.; Foster, J.A. Effects of gut microbiota on the brain: Implications for psychiatry. *J. Psychiatry Neurosci.* **2009**, *34*, 230–231.
51. Carabotti, M.; Scirocco, A.; Maselli, M.A.; Severi, C. The gut-brain axis: Interactions between enteric microbiota, central and enteric nervous systems. *Ann. Gastroenterol.* **2015**, *28*, 203–209. [PubMed]
52. Ogbonnaya, E.S.; Clarke, G.; Shanahan, F.; Dinan, T.G.; Cryan, J.F.; O'Leary, O.F. Adult Hippocampal Neurogenesis Is Regulated by the Microbiome. *Biol. Psychiatry* **2015**, *78*, e7–e9. [CrossRef] [PubMed]
53. Bailey, M.T.; Dowd, S.E.; Galley, J.D.; Hufnagle, A.R.; Allen, R.G.; Lyte, M. Exposure to a social stressor alters the structure of the intestinal microbiota: Implications for stressor-induced immunomodulation. *Brain Behav. Immun.* **2011**, *25*, 397–407. [CrossRef] [PubMed]
54. Chen, C.; Brown, D.R.; Xie, Y.; Green, B.T.; Lyte, M. Catecholamines modulate Escherichia coli O157:H7 adherence to murine cecal mucosa. *Shock* **2003**, *20*, 183–188. [CrossRef] [PubMed]
55. Freestone, P.P.; Williams, P.H.; Haigh, R.D.; Maggs, A.F.; Neal, C.P.; Lyte, M. Growth stimulation of intestinal commensal Escherichia coli by catecholamines: A possible contributory factor in trauma-induced sepsis. *Shock* **2002**, *18*, 465–470. [CrossRef] [PubMed]
56. O'malley, D.; Julio-Pieper, M.; Gibney, S.M.; Gosselin, R.D.; Dinan, T.G.; Cryan, J.F. Differential stress-induced alterations of colonic corticotropin-releasing factor receptors in the Wistar Kyoto rat. *Neurogastroenterol. Motil.* **2010**, *22*, 301–311. [CrossRef] [PubMed]
57. Larauche, M.; Gourcerol, G.; Wang, L.; Pambukchian, K.; Brunnhuber, S.; Adelson, D.W.; Rivier, J.; Million, M.; Taché, Y. Cortagine, a CRF1 agonist, induces stresslike alterations of colonic function and visceral hypersensitivity in rodents primarily through peripheral pathways. *Am. J. Physiol. Gastrointest. Liver Physiol.* **2009**, *297*, G215–G227. [CrossRef]
58. Gareau, M.G.; Silva, M.A.; Perdue, M.H. Pathophysiological mechanisms of stress-induced intestinal damage. *Curr. Mol. Med.* **2008**, *8*, 274–281. [CrossRef] [PubMed]

59. Tache, Y. Corticotropin releasing factor receptor antagonists: Potential future therapy in gastroenterology? *Gut* **2004**, *53*, 919–921. [CrossRef]
60. Wu, Y.; Hu, J.; Zhang, R.; Zhou, C.; Xu, Y.; Guan, X.; Li, S. Enhanced intracellular calcium induced by urocortin is involved in degranulation of rat lung mast cells. *Cell Physiol. Biochem.* **2008**, *21*, 173–182. [CrossRef] [PubMed]
61. Teitelbaum, A.A.; Gareau, M.G.; Jury, J.; Yang, P.C.; Perdue, M.H. Chronic peripheral administration of corticotropin-releasing factor causes colonic barrier dysfunction similar to psychological stress. *Am. J. Physiol. Gastrointest. Liver Physiol.* **2008**, *295*, G452–G459. [CrossRef]
62. Foster, J.A.; McVey Neufeld, K.A. Gut-brain axis: How the microbiome influences anxiety and depression. *Trends Neurosci.* **2013**, *36*, 305–312. [CrossRef] [PubMed]
63. Leonardo, E.D.; Hen, R. Anxiety as a developmental disorder. *Neuropsychopharmacology* **2008**, *33*, 134–140. [CrossRef] [PubMed]
64. Stein, M.B.; Seedat, S.; Gelernter, J. Serotonin transporter gene promoter polymorphism predicts SSRI response in generalized social anxiety disorder. *Psychopharmacology* **2006**, *187*, 68–72. [CrossRef] [PubMed]
65. Gershon, M.D.; Tack, J. The serotonin signaling system: From basic understanding to drug development for functional GI disorders. *Gastroenterology* **2007**, *132*, 397–414. [CrossRef] [PubMed]
66. Hoffman, J.M.; Tyler, K.; MacEachern, S.J.; Balemba, O.B.; Johnson, A.C.; Brooks, E.M.; Zhao, H.; Swain, G.M.; Moses, P.L.; Galligan, J.J.; et al. Activation of colonic mucosal 5-HT(4) receptors accelerates propulsive motility and inhibits visceral hypersensitivity. *Gastroenterology* **2012**, *142*, 844-854.e4. [CrossRef]
67. Mawe, G.M.; Hoffman, J.M. Serotonin signalling in the gut–functions, dysfunctions and therapeutic targets. *Nat. Rev. Gastroenterol. Hepatol.* **2013**, *10*, 473–486. [CrossRef]
68. Baganz, N.L.; Blakely, R.D. A dialogue between the immune system and brain, spoken in the language of serotonin. *ACS Chem. Neurosci.* **2013**, *4*, 48–63. [CrossRef]
69. Yano, J.M.; Yu, K.; Donaldson, G.P.; Shastri, G.G.; Ann, P.; Ma, L.; Nagler, C.R.; Ismagilov, R.F.; Mazmanian, S.K.; Hsiao, E.Y. Indigenous bacteria from the gut microbiota regulate host serotonin biosynthesis. *Cell* **2015**, *161*, 264–276. [CrossRef] [PubMed]
70. Stasi, C.; Bellini, M.; Bassotti, G.; Blandizzi, C.; Milani, S. Serotonin receptors and their role in the pathophysiology and therapy of irritable bowel syndrome. *Tech. Coloproctol.* **2014**, *18*, 613–621. [CrossRef]
71. Forsythe, P.; Sudo, N.; Dinan, T.; Taylor, V.H.; Bienenstock, J. Mood and gut feelings. *Brain Behav. Immun.* **2010**, *24*, 9–16. [CrossRef]
72. Gibson, P.R.; Newnham, E.; Barrett, J.S.; Shepherd, S.J.; Muir, J.G. Review article: Fructose malabsorption and the bigger picture. *Aliment Pharmacol. Ther.* **2007**, *25*, 349–363. [CrossRef] [PubMed]
73. Lundin, A.; Bok, C.M.; Aronsson, L.; Bjorkholm, B.; Gustafsson, J.A.; Pott, S.; Arulampalam, V.; Hibberd, M.; Rafter, J.; Pettersson, S. Gut flora, Toll-like receptors and nuclear receptors: A tripartite communication that tunes innate immunity in large intestine. *Cell Microbiol.* **2008**, *10*, 1093–1103. [CrossRef]
74. Hosoi, J.; Murphy, G.F.; Egan, C.L.; Lerner, E.A.; Grabbe, S.; Asahina, A.; Granstein, R.D. Regulation of Langerhans cell function by nerves containing calcitonin gene-related peptide. *Nature* **1993**, *363*, 159–163. [CrossRef] [PubMed]
75. Goehler, L.E.; Gaykema, R.P.; Nguyen, K.T.; Lee, J.E.; Tilders, F.J.; Maier, S.F.; Watkins, L.R. Interleukin-1beta in immune cells of the abdominal vagus nerve: A link between the immune and nervous systems? *J. Neurosci.* **1999**, *19*, 2799–2806. [CrossRef]
76. Borovikova, L.V.; Ivanova, S.; Zhang, M.; Yang, H.; Botchkina, G.I.; Watkins, L.R.; Wang, H.; Abumrad, N.; Eaton, J.W.; Tracey, K.J. Vagus nerve stimulation attenuates the systemic inflammatory response to endotoxin. *Nature* **2000**, *405*, 458–462. [CrossRef] [PubMed]
77. Ghia, J.E.; Blennerhassett, P.; Kumar-Ondiveeran, H.; Verdu, E.F.; Collins, S.M. The vagus nerve: A tonic inhibitory influence associated with inflammatory bowel disease in a murine model. *Gastroenterology* **2006**, *131*, 1122–1130. [CrossRef]
78. Dai, C.; Zheng, C.Q.; Meng, F.J.; Zhou, Z.; Sang, L.X.; Jiang, M. VSL#3 probiotics exerts the anti-inflammatory activity via PI3k/Akt and NF-kappaB pathway in rat model of DSS-induced colitis. *Mol. Cell Biochem.* **2013**, *374*, 1–11.
79. Bambury, A.; Sandhu, K.; Cryan, J.F.; Dinan, T.G. Finding the needle in the haystack: Systematic identification of psychobiotics. *Br. J. Pharmacol.* **2018**, *175*, 4430–4438. [CrossRef]

80. Chu, H.; Mazmanian, S.K. Innate immune recognition of the microbiota promotes host-microbial symbiosis. *Nat. Immunol.* **2013**, *14*, 668–675. [CrossRef] [PubMed]
81. Takeda, K.; Akira, S. Toll-like receptors in innate immunity. *Int. Immunol.* **2005**, *17*, 1–14. [CrossRef]
82. Moussaoui, N.; Braniste, V.; Ait-Belgnaoui, A.; Gabanou, M.; Sekkal, S.; Olier, M.; Théodorou, V.; Martin, P.G.; Houdeau, E. Changes in intestinal glucocorticoid sensitivity in early life shape the risk of epithelial barrier defect in maternal-deprived rats. *PLoS ONE* **2014**, *9*, e88382. [CrossRef] [PubMed]
83. Rhee, S.H.; Pothoulakis, C.; Mayer, E.A. Principles and clinical implications of the brain-gut-enteric microbiota axis. *Nat. Rev. Gastroenterol. Hepatol.* **2009**, *6*, 306–314. [CrossRef]
84. Bercik, P.; Verdu, E.F.; Foster, J.A.; Macri, J.; Potter, M.; Huang, X.; Malinowski, P.; Jackson, W.; Blennerhassett, P.; Neufeld, K.A.; et al. Chronic gastrointestinal inflammation induces anxiety-like behavior and alters central nervous system biochemistry in mice. *Gastroenterology* **2010**, *139*, 2102-2112.e1. [CrossRef] [PubMed]
85. Rea, K.; Dinan, T.G.; Cryan, J.F. The microbiome: A key regulator of stress and neuroinflammation. *Neurobiol. Stress.* **2016**, *4*, 23–33. [CrossRef]
86. McEwen, B.S.; Gray, J.D.; Nasca, C. 60 YEARS OF NEUROENDOCRINOLOGY: Redefining neuroendocrinology: Stress, sex and cognitive and emotional regulation. *J. Endocrinol.* **2015**, *226*, T67–T83. [CrossRef]
87. Herman, J.P.; Ostrander, M.M.; Mueller, N.K.; Figueiredo, H. Limbic system mechanisms of stress regulation: Hypothalamo-pituitary-adrenocortical axis. *Prog. Neuropsychopharmacol. Biol. Psychiatry* **2005**, *29*, 1201–1213. [CrossRef]
88. De Voogd, L.D.; Klumpers, F.; Fernandez, G.; Hermans, E.J. Intrinsic functional connectivity between amygdala and hippocampus during rest predicts enhanced memory under stress. *Psychoneuroendocrinology* **2017**, *75*, 192–202. [CrossRef]
89. Pagliaccio, D.; Luby, J.L.; Bogdan, R.; Agrawal, A.; Gaffrey, M.S.; Belden, A.C.; Botteron, K.N.; Harms, M.P.; Barch, D.M. Stress-system genes and life stress predict cortisol levels and amygdala and hippocampal volumes in children. *Neuropsychopharmacology* **2014**, *39*, 1245–1253. [CrossRef]
90. Lupien, S.J.; McEwen, B.S.; Gunnar, M.R.; Heim, C. Effects of stress throughout the lifespan on the brain, behaviour and cognition. *Nat. Rev. Neurosci.* **2009**, *10*, 434–445. [CrossRef] [PubMed]
91. Montiel-Castro, A.J.; Gonzalez-Cervantes, R.M.; Bravo-Ruiseco, G.; Pacheco-Lopez, G. The microbiota-gut-brain axis: Neurobehavioral correlates, health and sociality. *Front. Integr. Neurosci.* **2013**, *7*, 70. [CrossRef] [PubMed]
92. Gareau, M.G.; Jury, J.; MacQueen, G.; Sherman, P.M.; Perdue, M.H. Probiotic treatment of rat pups normalises corticosterone release and ameliorates colonic dysfunction induced by maternal separation. *Gut* **2007**, *56*, 1522–1528. [CrossRef] [PubMed]
93. Bravo, J.A.; Forsythe, P.; Chew, M.V.; Escaravage, E.; Savignac, H.M.; Dinan, T.G.; Bienenstock, J.; Cryan, J.F. Ingestion of Lactobacillus strain regulates emotional behavior and central GABA receptor expression in a mouse via the vagus nerve. *Proc. Natl. Acad. Sci. USA* **2011**, *108*, 16050–16055. [CrossRef] [PubMed]
94. Luczynski, P.; Whelan, S.O.; O'Sullivan, C.; Clarke, G.; Shanahan, F.; Dinan, T.G.; Cryan, J.F. Adult microbiota-deficient mice have distinct dendritic morphological changes: Differential effects in the amygdala and hippocampus. *Eur. J. Neurosci.* **2016**, *44*, 2654–2666. [CrossRef]
95. Arentsen, T.; Raith, H.; Qian, Y.; Forssberg, H.; Diaz Heijtz, R. Host microbiota modulates development of social preference in mice. *Microb. Ecol. Health Dis.* **2015**, *26*, 29719. [CrossRef] [PubMed]
96. Felix-Ortiz, A.C.; Tye, K.M. Amygdala inputs to the ventral hippocampus bidirectionally modulate social behavior. *J. Neurosci.* **2014**, *34*, 586–595. [CrossRef]
97. Lee, Y.K.; Menezes, J.S.; Umesaki, Y.; Mazmanian, S.K. Proinflammatory T-cell responses to gut microbiota promote experimental autoimmune encephalomyelitis. *Proc. Natl. Acad. Sci. USA* **2011**, *108* (Suppl. 1), 4615–4622. [CrossRef] [PubMed]
98. Ochoa-Reparaz, J.; Mielcarz, D.W.; Ditrio, L.E.; Burroughs, A.R.; Foureau, D.M.; Haque-Begum, S.; Kasper, L.H. Role of gut commensal microflora in the development of experimental autoimmune encephalomyelitis. *J. Immunol.* **2009**, *183*, 6041–6050. [CrossRef]
99. Gaboriau-Routhiau, V.; Rakotobe, S.; Lecuyer, E.; Mulder, I.; Lan, A.; Bridonneau, C.; Rochet, V.; Pisi, A.; De Paepe, M.; Brandi, G.; et al. The key role of segmented filamentous bacteria in the coordinated maturation of gut helper T cell responses. *Immunity* **2009**, *31*, 677–689. [CrossRef]

100. Allsop, S.A.; Vander Weele, C.M.; Wichmann, R.; Tye, K.M. Optogenetic insights on the relationship between anxiety-related behaviors and social deficits. *Front. Behav. Neurosci.* **2014**, *8*, 241. [CrossRef]
101. Kheirbek, M.A.; Drew, L.J.; Burghardt, N.S.; Costantini, D.O.; Tannenholz, L.; Ahmari, S.E.; Zeng, H.; Fenton, A.A.; Hen, R. Differential control of learning and anxiety along the dorsoventral axis of the dentate gyrus. *Neuron* **2013**, *77*, 955–968. [CrossRef]
102. Tye, K.M.; Prakash, R.; Kim, S.Y.; Fenno, L.E.; Grosenick, L.; Zarabi, H.; Thompson, K.R.; Gradinaru, V.; Ramakrishnan, C.; Deisseroth, K. Amygdala circuitry mediating reversible and bidirectional control of anxiety. *Nature* **2011**, *471*, 358–362. [CrossRef] [PubMed]
103. Mayer, E.A. Gut feelings: The emerging biology of gut-brain communication. *Nat. Rev. Neurosci.* **2011**, *12*, 453–466. [CrossRef]
104. Cryan, J.F.; Kaupmann, K. Don't worry 'B' happy!: A role for GABA(B) receptors in anxiety and depression. *Trends Pharmacol. Sci.* **2005**, *26*, 36–43. [CrossRef]
105. Higuchi, T.; Hayashi, H.; Abe, K. Exchange of glutamate and gamma-aminobutyrate in a Lactobacillus strain. *J. Bacteriol.* **1997**, *179*, 3362–3364. [CrossRef] [PubMed]
106. Kamiya, T.; Wang, L.; Forsythe, P.; Goettsche, G.; Mao, Y.; Wang, Y.; Tougas, G.; Bienenstock, J. Inhibitory effects of Lactobacillus reuteri on visceral pain induced by colorectal distension in Sprague-Dawley rats. *Gut* **2006**, *55*, 191–196. [CrossRef] [PubMed]
107. Amaral, F.A.; Sachs, D.; Costa, V.V.; Fagundes, C.T.; Cisalpino, D.; Cunha, T.M.; Ferreira, S.H.; Cunha, F.Q.; Silva, T.A.; Nicoli, J.R.; et al. Commensal microbiota is fundamental for the development of inflammatory pain. *Proc. Natl. Acad. Sci. USA* **2008**, *105*, 2193–2197. [CrossRef] [PubMed]
108. Ivanov, I.I.; Atarashi, K.; Manel, N.; Brodie, E.L.; Shima, T.; Karaoz, U.; Wei, D.; Goldfarb, K.C.; Santee, C.A.; Lynch, S.V.; et al. Induction of intestinal Th17 cells by segmented filamentous bacteria. *Cell* **2009**, *139*, 485–498. [CrossRef]
109. Drevets, W.C. Neuroimaging studies of mood disorders. *Biol. Psychiatry* **2000**, *48*, 813–829. [CrossRef]
110. Roy, C.C.; Kien, C.L.; Bouthillier, L.; Levy, E. Short-chain fatty acids: Ready for prime time? *Nutr. Clin. Pract.* **2006**, *21*, 351–366. [CrossRef]
111. Psichas, A.; Sleeth, M.L.; Murphy, K.G.; Brooks, L.; Bewick, G.A.; Hanyaloglu, A.C.; Ghatei, M.A.; Bloom, S.R.; Frost, G. The short chain fatty acid propionate stimulates GLP-1 and PYY secretion via free fatty acid receptor 2 in rodents. *Int. J. Obes. (Lond.)* **2015**, *39*, 424–429. [CrossRef]
112. Han, A.; Sung, Y.B.; Chung, S.Y.; Kwon, M.S. Possible additional antidepressant-like mechanism of sodium butyrate: Targeting the hippocampus. *Neuropharmacology* **2014**, *81*, 292–302. [CrossRef] [PubMed]
113. Stilling, R.M.; Dinan, T.G.; Cryan, J.F. Microbial genes, brain & behavior—Epigenetic regulation of the gut-brain axis. *Genes Brain Behav.* **2014**, *13*, 69–86. [PubMed]
114. Perry, R.J.; Peng, L.; Barry, N.A.; Cline, G.W.; Zhang, D.; Cardone, R.L.; Petersen, K.F.; Kibbey, R.G.; Goodman, A.L.; Shulman, G.I. Acetate mediates a microbiome-brain-beta-cell axis to promote metabolic syndrome. *Nature* **2016**, *534*, 213–217. [CrossRef]
115. Barrett, E.; Ross, R.P.; O'Toole, P.W.; Fitzgerald, G.F.; Stanton, C. gamma-Aminobutyric acid production by culturable bacteria from the human intestine. *J. Appl. Microbiol.* **2012**, *113*, 411–417. [CrossRef]
116. Dinan, T.G.; Stilling, R.M.; Stanton, C.; Cryan, J.F. Collective unconscious: How gut microbes shape human behavior. *J. Psychiatr. Res.* **2015**, *63*, 1–9. [CrossRef] [PubMed]
117. Lyte, M. Probiotics function mechanistically as delivery vehicles for neuroactive compounds: Microbial endocrinology in the design and use of probiotics. *Bioessays* **2011**, *33*, 574–581. [CrossRef] [PubMed]
118. Macfabe, D.F. Short-chain fatty acid fermentation products of the gut microbiome: Implications in autism spectrum disorders. *Microb. Ecol. Health Dis.* **2012**, *23*. [CrossRef] [PubMed]
119. Rossignol, D.A.; Frye, R.E. Mitochondrial dysfunction in autism spectrum disorders: A systematic review and meta-analysis. *Mol. Psychiatry* **2012**, *17*, 290–314. [CrossRef]
120. Coskun, P.; Wyrembak, J.; Schriner, S.E.; Chen, H.W.; Marciniack, C.; Laferla, F.; Wallace, D.C. A mitochondrial etiology of Alzheimer and Parkinson disease. *Biochim. Biophys. Acta* **2012**, *1820*, 553–564. [CrossRef]
121. Shah, P.; Nankova, B.B.; Parab, S.; La Gamma, E.F. Short chain fatty acids induce TH gene expression via ERK-dependent phosphorylation of CREB protein. *Brain Res.* **2006**, *1107*, 13–23. [CrossRef]
122. Savignac, H.M.; Corona, G.; Mills, H.; Chen, L.; Spencer, J.P.; Tzortzis, G.; Burnet, P.W. Prebiotic feeding elevates central brain derived neurotrophic factor, N-methyl-D-aspartate receptor subunits and D-serine. *Neurochem. Int.* **2013**, *63*, 756–764. [CrossRef]

123. Schmidt, K.; Cowen, P.J.; Harmer, C.J.; Tzortzis, G.; Errington, S.; Burnet, P.W. Prebiotic intake reduces the waking cortisol response and alters emotional bias in healthy volunteers. *Psychopharmacology* **2015**, *232*, 1793–1801. [CrossRef]
124. Burokas, A.; Arboleya, S.; Moloney, R.D.; Peterson, V.L.; Murphy, K.; Clarke, G.; Stanton, C.; Dinan, T.G.; Cryan, J.F. Targeting the Microbiota-Gut-Brain Axis: Prebiotics Have Anxiolytic and Antidepressant-like Effects and Reverse the Impact of Chronic Stress in Mice. *Biol. Psychiatry* **2017**, *82*, 472–487. [CrossRef] [PubMed]
125. Gage, F.H. Mammalian neural stem cells. *Science* **2000**, *287*, 1433–1438. [CrossRef] [PubMed]
126. Zhao, C.; Deng, W.; Gage, F.H. Mechanisms and functional implications of adult neurogenesis. *Cell* **2008**, *132*, 645–660. [CrossRef] [PubMed]
127. Villeda, S.A.; Luo, J.; Mosher, K.I.; Zou, B.; Britschgi, M.; Bieri, G.; Stan, T.M.; Fainberg, N.; Ding, Z.; Eggel, A.; et al. The ageing systemic milieu negatively regulates neurogenesis and cognitive function. *Nature* **2011**, *477*, 90–94. [CrossRef]
128. Sudo, N.; Chida, Y.; Aiba, Y.; Sonoda, J.; Oyama, N.; Yu, X.N.; Kubo, C.; Koga, Y. Postnatal microbial colonization programs the hypothalamic-pituitary-adrenal system for stress response in mice. *J. Physiol.* **2004**, *558 Pt 1*, 263–275. [CrossRef]
129. Brown, K.; DeCoffe, D.; Molcan, E.; Gibson, D.L. Diet-induced dysbiosis of the intestinal microbiota and the effects on immunity and disease. *Nutrients* **2012**, *4*, 1095–1119. [CrossRef] [PubMed]
130. Cristofori, F.; Indrio, F.; Miniello, V.L.; De Angelis, M.; Francavilla, R. Probiotics in Celiac Disease. *Nutrients* **2018**, *10*, 1824. [CrossRef]
131. Ou, G.; Hedberg, M.; Horstedt, P.; Baranov, V.; Forsberg, G.; Drobni, M.; Sandström, O.; Wai, S.N.; Johansson, I.; Hammarström, M.L.; et al. Proximal small intestinal microbiota and identification of rod-shaped bacteria associated with childhood celiac disease. *Am. J. Gastroenterol.* **2009**, *104*, 3058–3067. [CrossRef] [PubMed]
132. Bella, R.; Lanza, G.; Cantone, M.; Giuffrida, S.; Puglisi, V.; Vinciguerra, L.; Pennisi, M.; Ricceri, R.; D'Agate, C.C.; Malaguarnera, G.; et al. Effect of a Gluten-Free Diet on Cortical Excitability in Adults with Celiac Disease. *PLoS ONE* **2015**, *10*, e0129218. [CrossRef] [PubMed]
133. Pennisi, M.; Bramanti, A.; Cantone, M.; Pennisi, G.; Bella, R.; Lanza, G. Neurophysiology of the "Celiac Brain": Disentangling Gut-Brain Connections. *Front. Neurosci.* **2017**, *11*, 498. [CrossRef] [PubMed]

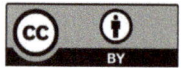

© 2019 by the authors. Licensee MDPI, Basel, Switzerland. This article is an open access article distributed under the terms and conditions of the Creative Commons Attribution (CC BY) license (http://creativecommons.org/licenses/by/4.0/).

MDPI
St. Alban-Anlage 66
4052 Basel
Switzerland
Tel. +41 61 683 77 34
Fax +41 61 302 89 18
www.mdpi.com

Nutrients Editorial Office
E-mail: nutrients@mdpi.com
www.mdpi.com/journal/nutrients

www.ingramcontent.com/pod-product-compliance
Lightning Source LLC
LaVergne TN
LVHW070653100526
838202LV00013B/949